Sleep Medicine and Physical Therapy

Cristina Frange
Fernando Morgadinho Santos Coelho
Editors

Sleep Medicine and Physical Therapy

A Comprehensive Guide for Practitioners

Springer

Editors
Cristina Frange
Neurology and Neurosurgery Department
Escola Paulista de Medicina
Federal University of São Paulo
São Paulo, Brazil

Fernando Morgadinho Santos Coelho
Neurology and Neurosurgery Department
Escola Paulista de Medicina
Federal University of São Paulo
São Paulo, Brazil

ISBN 978-3-030-85073-9 ISBN 978-3-030-85074-6 (eBook)
https://doi.org/10.1007/978-3-030-85074-6

This Springer imprint is published by the registered company Springer Nature Switzerland AG
The registered company address is: Gewerbestrasse 11, 6330 Cham, Switzerland

This book is dedicated to our families:

Matheus and Mauricio, Lucimar and Geraldo, Felício, and Ilza

Fernando, Ana Carolina, and Amanda

And to our patients

insomnia, restless legs symptom and periodic limb movement of sleep, circadian rhythm sleep disturbances, sleep bruxism, obstructive and central sleep apnea, upper airway resistance syndrome, narcolepsy, excessive daytime sleepiness, and parasomnias. Furthermore, you will improve your knowledge about sleep in specific conditions across the lifespan including gender differences, neurological disease, and pain in relation to sleep. Of course, you as a reader will get familiar in more detail with various physiotherapeutic resources, methods, and techniques to improve sleep, such as exercise, hydrotherapeutic resources, optimizing behavior strategies, and sleep ergonomics. You will also learn more about evidence-based physiotherapy in sleep medicine (especially in sleep physiotherapy and sleep and musculoskeletal system). At the end, you will learn in detail about the subjective and objective sleep assessment in physical therapy practice. Overall, the content of this book constantly reminds you that sleep problems require multidisciplinary approaches.

So, as a physiotherapist, a national health promoter, a health educator, and a senior lecturer, I would highly recommend this excellent and one-of-a-kind literature to all physiotherapists (and also other related health professionals) around the globe, who are dealing with sleep problems in their everyday clinical or education practice. This is a professional book that every physiotherapist should own, read, and use.

Andrea Backović Juričan, World Physiotherapy Network for Health Promotion in Life and Work

Ljubljana, Slovenia Andrea Backović Juričan

Preface

Many of the ideas seen in this book were germinated in a discussion section held at the World Physical Therapy Congress (WCPT) in Geneva, Switzerland, in 2019, toghether with the routine of the Excessive Daytime Sleepiness and Hypersomnia Outpatient Clinic, several supervision meetings, and physical therapy sessions (between a neurologist and a physical therapist) in São Paulo (Brazil) were fundamental for ideas, brainstorming and clinical experiences shared from both of us to become a book.

There is a set of core ideas that underlies all the chapters in this book. Some of these ideas have been roughly investigated while others are more hypotheses until this moment. Indeed, the physiotherapeutic practices and the regulation of the profession, and education policies regarding sleep health may vary between countries and cultures. In Brazil, only recently the sleep health was stated as a role for the physical therapist. This book highlights many points of sleep medicine and discusses how physical therapists can help within the interdisciplinary approach and their role in sleep medicine. The mission of physiotherapists is to promote wellness, mobility, and independence developing people's abilities to move during the course of their lives. Physiotherapists also prevent and treat several issues related to pain, illness, disability and disease, sport and work-related injuries, aging, and inactivity.

Sleep and its disturbances are related to health in general. Sleep is an example of new areas that have been constantly developed into health sciences. Continuing education ensures that they keep up to date with the latest advances in physical therapy research and practice. This book will give a basic grounding in sleep medicine to physiotherapists, healthcare providers, and related specialties, as well as to younger professionals.

The book itself has been divided into seven main parts. The first part focuses on fundamental concepts of sleep, explaining sleep and discussing disturbances and other factors that impact a good night's sleep.

Part of sleep medicine history is remembered. The knowledge of our history is fundamental to understand the present approach and drive to beyond. The second part focuses on the basic conceptions of physical therapists' understanding and working in clinical practice and research with sleep. Both sides must be seen: sleep impacting on rehabilitation/physical therapy and vice versa. The third part focuses on the most prevalent sleep disorders. There is a brief explanation of sleep diseases in each chapter, followed by evidence-based research and clinical reports by physicians, physical therapists, and other health professionals that already work with sleep issues. The fourth part focuses on specific particularities of sleep during childhood, adolescence, and old age, as well as differences between genders and women's phases during her lifespan. The clinical practice of many physiotherapists is to treat patients with pain and neurological conditions. We also debate about neurological diseases and pain, discussing the intrinsic relationship between sleep and pain/neurological diseases. In the fifth part, the chapters discuss physical therapy resources (exercise, hydrotherapy, ergonomics during sleep, and cognitive behavioral therapy) to improve sleep and to treat sleep disturbances.

There is much to grow in the interface between sleep and physical therapy field. It requires the improvement of basic sleep science knowledge, including experiment-based research (i.e., animal experiments). The sixth part explains the importance of basic research and its results from investigations on the musculoskeletal system and sleep (or lack of sleep). Finally, the seventh part focuses on subjective and objective tools to assess sleep and sleep disturbances. These tools provide useful information to practical clinics with fundamental importance in a interdisciplinary set of approaches.

The editorial process has been a pleasure due to intense work with many professionals who dedicated a lot of time and effort to this project. All these chapters have been written by experts in their respective areas, and we are extremely grateful for their contributions and willingness to donate their experience and time for this book. This book would not be possible without the authors and their wholehearted contributions and keeping up with deadlines.

We hope that this book will improve clinical practice, interdisciplinarity of healthcare professionals of many health professions and physiotherapists, and stimulate further researches in this important area. It is important always to take sleep into account on behalf of our patient's (and our) lives.

São Paulo, Brazil
November 2021

Cristina Frange
Fernando Morgadinho Santos Coelho

Acknowledgments

São Paulo Research Foundation (Fundação de Amparo à Pesquisa do Estado de São Paulo, FAPESP)

Department of Neurology and Neurosurgery from Universidade Federal de São Paulo

Post-Graduate Program of Neurology and Neurosciences, Universidade Federal de São Paulo

Department of Psychobiology from Universidade Federal de São Paulo

Post-graduate students and fellows from Excessive Daytime Sleepiness and Hypersomnia Outpatient Clinic, Universidade Federal de São Paulo

Liliane Martins Frange and Luíz Alexandre Berclaz Pinto, for the unconditional support

We are also thankful to Erika de Cassia Ferraz, Henry Rodgers, Abha Krishnan, Sasirekka Nijanthan, Arul Viveaun Sagayanathan and their staff at Springer, who were involved in the development, production and design of this volume, both online and printed ones

Part VII Sleep Assessment for Physical Therapy Clinical Practice

Contributors

Ana Carolina Aguilar, MD, MSc Department of Psychobiology, Escola Paulista de Medicina, Universidade Federal de São Paulo, São Paulo, SP, Brazil

Monica Levy Andersen, BS, PhD, Associate Professor Department of Psychobiology, Escola Paulista de Medicina, Universidade Federal de São Paulo, São Paulo, SP, Brazil

Alberto Herrero Babiloni, DDS, MS, PhD (c) Division of Experimental Medicine and Faculty of Dentistry, McGill University, Montreal, QC, Canada

Research Center of CIUSSS Nord Ile de Montréal, Sleep and Trauma Unit, Montréal, Montreal, QC, Canada

Lia Rita Azeredo Bittencourt, MD, PhD, Associate Professor Department of Psychobiology, Escola Paulista de Medicina, Universidade Federal de São Paulo, São Paulo, SP, Brazil

Evelyn Brasil, PT, MSc Department of Severe Patients, Hospital Israelita Albert Einstein, Certified in Sleep Physiotherapy by the Brazilian Sleep Society (ABS), and The Brazilian Association of Cardiorespiratory Physiotherapy and Physiotherapy in Intensive Care (ASSOBRAFIR), São Paulo, SP, Brazil

Silmara Bueno, PT Personal do Sono Sleep Consulting, São Paulo, SP, Brazil

Fernando Morgadinho Santos Coelho, MD, PhD, Full Professor Neurology and Neurosurgery Department; Department of Psychobiology, Escola Paulista de Medicina, Universidade Federal de São Paulo, São Paulo, SP, Brazil

Glaury A. Coelho, Psy, MSc, PhD (c) Department of Medicine, Escola Paulista de Medicina, Universidade Federal de São Paulo, São Paulo, SP, Brazil

Carolina Vicaria Rodrigues D'Aurea, PT, PhD Hospital Israelita Albert Einstein, São Paulo, SP, Brazil

Juliana Arcanjo Lino, PT, PhD Medical Sciences, Federal University of Ceará (UFC), Fortaleza, Ceará, Brazil

Certified in Sleep Physiotherapy by the Brazilian Sleep Society (ABS), and The Brazilian Association of Cardiorespiratory Physiotherapy and Physiotherapy in Intensive Care (ASSOBRAFIR), São Paulo, Brazil

Ozeas Lins-Filho, BPhEd, PhD Sleep and Heart Laboratory, Cardiovascular Emergency Room of Pernambuco, University of Pernambuco, Recife, PE, Brazil

Ligia Mendonça Lucchesi, MD, PhD Sleep Institute, Associação Fundo Incentivo à Pesquisa, São Paulo, SP, Brazil

Maria Julia Lyra, BPhEd, PhD (c) Associate Graduate Program in Physical Education, University of Pernambuco, Recife, PE, Brazil

Amélia Pasqual Marques, PT, PhD Department of Physical Therapy, Speech Therapy and Occupational Therapy, and Post-Graduate Program in Rehabilitation Sciences, Faculdade de Medicina da Universidade de São Paulo, São Paulo, SP, Brazil

Cinthia Santos Miotto, PT, PhD Department of Physiotherapy, Speech Therapy and Occupational Therapy, Faculty of Medicine, University of São Paulo, São Paulo, SP, Brazil

Claudia R. C. Moreno, BIOL, PhD, Associate professor Department of Health, Life Cycles and Society, School of Public Health, University of São Paulo (USP), São Paulo, SP, Brazil

Stress Research Institute, Psychology Department, Stockholm University, Stockholm, Sweden

Morgana Nicolodelli, PT Hipnos Sleep Consulting, Curitiba, Paraná, Brazil

Luciana Palombini, MD, PhD Sleep Institute, Associação Fundo Incentivo à Pesquisa, São Paulo, SP, Brazil

Giselle Soares Passos, BPhEd, PhD Health Sciences, Universidade Federal de Jataí, Jataí, Goiás, Brazil

Vivien Schmeling Piccin, PT, PhD Sleep Medicine, Pulmonary Division, Heart Institute, São Paulo, SP, Brazil

Certified in Sleep Physiotherapy by the Brazilian Sleep Society (ABS), and The Brazilian Association of Cardiorespiratory Physiotherapy and Physiotherapy in Intensive Care (ASSOBRAFIR), São Paulo, SP, Brazil

Ronaldo Delmonte Piovezan, MD, PhD Sleep Institute, Associação Fundo Incentivo à Pesquisa, São Paulo, SP, Brazil

Marcia Pradella-Hallinan, MD, PhD Treatment Center for Neuromuscular Diseases (TDN-AFIP) and Sleep Medicine Lab of Sirio Libanês Hospital, São Paulo, SP, Brazil

Maria Júlia Figueiró Reis, MD, MSc (c) Psychobiology Department, Escola Paulista de Medicina, Universidade Federal de São Paulo, São Paulo, SP, Brazil

Stavros Stathopoulos, PT, PhD Physical Therapy Department, Evaggelismos General Hospital, Athens, Greece

Postgraduate Program of the Medical School of National and Kapodistrian, University of Athens, Athens, Greece

Marconi University of Rome, Rome, Italy

Cristina Staub, PT, PhD International Organization of Physical Therapy in Mental Health, Swiss Group of Physiotherapy in Mental Health, Pro Dormo Switzerland, Zurich, Switzerland

Renato Stefanini, MD, PhD Otorhinolaryngology and Head and Neck Surgery Department, Escola Paulista de Medicina, Universidade Federal de São Paulo, São Paulo, SP, Brazil

Priscila Farias Tempaku, BS, PhD Psychobiology Department, Escola Paulista de Medicina, Universidade Federal de São Paulo, São Paulo, SP, Brazil

Sônia Maria Guimarães Pereira Togeiro, MD, PhD Department of Clínica Médica e Medicina Laboratorial, Department of Pneumology and Department of Psychobiology, Escola Paulista de Medicina, Universidade Federal de São Paulo, São Paulo, SP, Brazil

Sergio Tufik, MD, PhD, Full Professor Department of Psychobiology, Escola Paulista de Medicina, Universidade Federal de São Paulo, São Paulo, SP, Brazil

Melissa Araújo Ulhôa, PT, PhD Faculty of Medicine of Vale do Aço, School of Health and Education, Centro Universitário Católico do Leste de Minas Gerais; Centro Universitário de Caratinga, Ipatinga, Minas Gerais, Brazil

Eliana Lottenberg Vago, DMD, MSc Neurology and Neurosurgery Department, Escola Paulista de Medicina, Universidade Federal de São Paulo, São Paulo, SP, Brazil

Débora Strose Villaça, Clin Nutr, PhD Department of Pneumology, Escola Paulista de Medicina, Universidade Federal de São Paulo, São Paulo, SP, Brazil

About the Editors

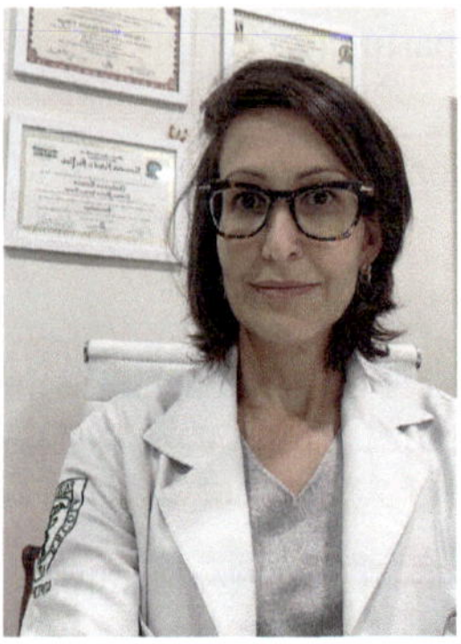

Cristina Frange Physical therapist specialized in neurorehabilitation (2010), Master of Communication (2004) from Pontificia Universidade Católica de São Paulo, and PhD in Science, Sleep Division from Universidade Federal de São Paulo, UNIFESP. Postdoctoral research fellow at Neurology and Neurosurgery Department, UNIFESP (2021). Received funding from Sao Paulo Research Foundation (FAPESP) for PhD and postdoctoral studies. Certified in Sleep Physiotherapy by the Brazilian Sleep Society (ABS), and The Brazilian Association of Cardiorespiratory Physiotherapy and Physiotherapy in Intensive Care (ASSOBRAFIR). Executive board member of the World Physiotherapy Network for Health Promotion in Life and Work. Clinical experience in neurorehabilitation, pain, and sleep medicine. Research focuses on non-pharmacological interventions to improve sleep in various population, particularly people after stroke or in chronic pain conditions. Scientific interest is the treatment of sleep disorders with physiotherapy and the improvement of rehabilitation sessions by enhancing sleep.

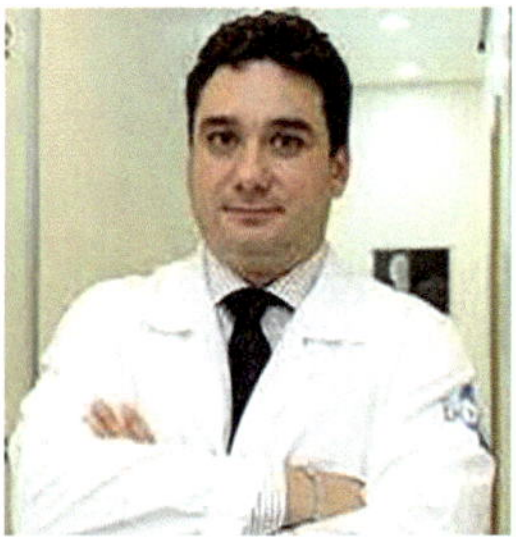

Fernando Morgadinho Santos Coelho Neurologist, Medical degree from Universidade Federal do Espírito Santo (1995), Master's degree (2005) and PhD (2009) in Science, Sleep Division from UNIFESP. Postdoctoral research fellow at the University of Toronto (2011). Full professor in the Neurology and Neurosurgery Department at UNIFESP (since 2013). Clinical experience in neurology and sleep medicine. Development of research in neurology (stroke and rehabilitation) and in sleep diseases (narcolepsy, periodic limb movements of sleep, restless legs syndrome, and obstructive sleep apnea). Author of the *Sleep and Stroke* book published in Brazilian Portuguese and of many book chapters. Highest scientific interest is the overlap between sleep and neurology focusing on an interdisciplinary approach.

Abbreviations

ACTH	adrenocorticotropic hormone
ADHD	attention deficit hyperactivity disorder
AHI	apnea hypopnea index
ARDS	ascending activator reticular system
ASD	autism spectrum disorder
ASV	adaptive servo-ventilation
BFD	biofeedback
BiPAP	bilevel ventilation
BMI	body mass index
BZD	benzodiazepines
CAI	central apnea index
CBT	cognitive-behavioral therapy
CBT-I	cognitive-behavioral therapy for insomnia
CBT-P	cognitive-behavioral therapy for pain
CBT-S	cognitive-behavioral therapy for sleep
CES	contingent electrical stimulation
CHF	congestive heart failure
CNS	central nervous system
CO_2	carbon dioxide
CRSWD	circadian rhythm sleep-wake disorders
CSB	Cheyne-Stokes breathing
CSF	cerebrospinal fluid
Ct	clinical trial
CT	computer assisted tomography
DSM-V	Diagnostic and Statistical Manual for Mental Disorders, Fifth Edition
ECG	electrocardiogram
EDS	excessive daytime sleepiness
EEG	electroencephalogram
EMG	electromyogram
EOG	electrooculogram
ESS	Epworth sleepiness scale

Part I
Basic Concepts

Sleep: Definition, Concept, New Area for Physical Therapy

Cristina Frange, Ana Carolina Aguilar, and Fernando Morgadinho Santos Coelho

Sleep is often characterized by a reversible reduction in consciousness, an increase in arousal threshold, behavioral quiescence, closed eyes, and a recumbent body posture. Sleep is an essential physiological phenomenon for the maintenance of homeostasis of our organism, being a state of intense brain activity. Yes, you read it right: intense activity! Sleep was considered a passive state until the discovery of rapid eye movements (REM) sleep in 1951, today called R stage [1]. At that time, and prior to that time, no distinction was seen between sleep and other states of quiescence such as comma, stupor, intoxication, hypnosis, anesthesia, and hibernation. Sleep represents an essential element for health and well-being, including cognitive performance, physiological processes, emotion regulation, physical development, and quality of life [2].

Sleep (and why we sleep) remains a scientific enigma and we do not know sleep functions precisely. We do know that we cannot survive without it. Many scientific investigations on the function of sleep have proposed a variety of theories: sleep serves an immune function, reduces caloric usage, restores brain energy stores, has a glymphatic function (house cleaning duties such as removal of extracellular amyloid-β from the brain), restores waking-induced performance degradation, and

C. Frange (✉)
Department of Neurology and Neurosurgery, Escola Paulista de Medicina, Universidade Federal de São Paulo, São Paulo, SP, Brazil

Certified in Sleep Physiotherapy by the Brazilian Sleep Society (ABS), and The Brazilian Association of Cardiorespiratory Physiotherapy and Physiotherapy in Intensive Care (ASSOBRAFIR), São Paulo, SP, Brazil

World Physiotherapy Network for Health Promotion in Life and Work, São Paulo, SP, Brazil

A. C. Aguilar
Department of Psychobiology, Escola Paulista de Medicina, Universidade Federal de São Paulo, São Paulo, SP, Brazil

F. M. S. Coelho
Neurology and Neurosurgery Department; Department of Psychobiology, Escola Paulista de Medicina, Universidade Federal de São Paulo, São Paulo, SP, Brazil

C. Frange, F. M. S. Coelho (eds.), *Sleep Medicine and Physical Therapy*,
https://doi.org/10.1007/978-3-030-85074-6_1

The identification and classification of sleep stages are made by polysomnography examination (PSG, see Chap. 36 for more information). In PSG, the characteristics of each of the stages are well defined and measured through the electroencephalography (EEG) waves, according to their frequency and amplitude. Sleep has two separate stages, defined based on an assemblage of physiologic parameters: the R stage (REM sleep) and the non-REM stage (NREM). The NREM stage is further subdivided into stage 1 (N1), stage 2 (N2), and stage 3 (N3) sleep. A sleep cycle is composed of consecutive alternations between the NREM and R stage and lasts about 70–110 minutes each. Humans experience about 4 to 6 sleep cycles per night, with different proportions of each stage throughout the night (Fig. 2) [27] and vary according to age, sex, exposition to daylight, diseases, etc. In normal individuals, NREM sleep predominates in the first half of the night, while REM sleep is more frequent in the second half of the night. The schematic representation of sleep architecture (sleep structure, sleep pattern) can be seen in polysomnographic examination in the hypnogram, a graph that characterizes the sleep stages as a function of time (Fig. 3). There exists a protocol defined by the AASM for sleep scoring.

Normal sleep pattern begins at the N1 stage of NREM sleep, which constitutes the transition from wakefulness to sleep and is predominantly characterized by the transition from alpha rhythm to theta rhythm, from 4 to 7.5 Hz. From the time an individual goes to bed to sleep and the time he/she effectively starts to sleep is called sleep latency. During stage N1 sleep, the heart rate decreases and the eyes exhibit lenient movement. N1 sleep stage presents typical graphic elements in the EEG, such as the vertex waves (i.e., focal sharp transients' waves with duration <0.5 seconds, with greater amplitude (Fig. 4). The vertex waves progress through deeper NREM stages N2 and N3, before the first episode of REM sleep, which occurs about 80 to 100 minutes after N1. Here the time from the begining of sleep to the first REM sleep stage in a cycle is called REM sleep latency. Back to sleep pattern,

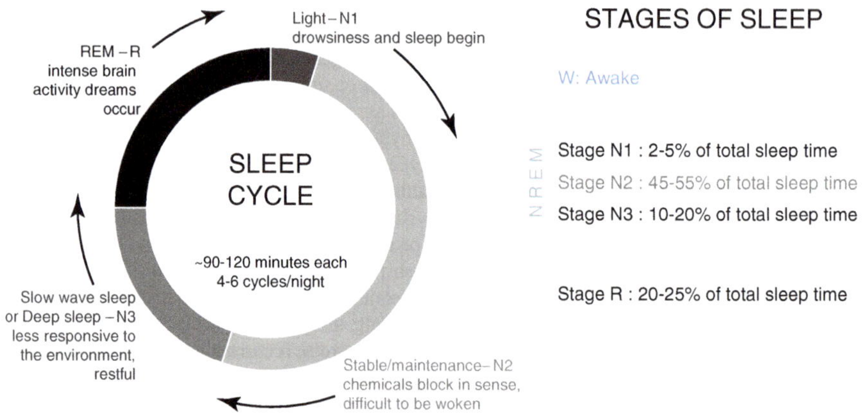

Fig. 2 Sleep "architecture," sleep pattern, sleep structure: distribution of sleep stages during the total sleep time/sleep duration, which is composed of 4–6 sleep cycles each night. A sleep cycle is composed of stages NREM: N1, N2, N3, and R

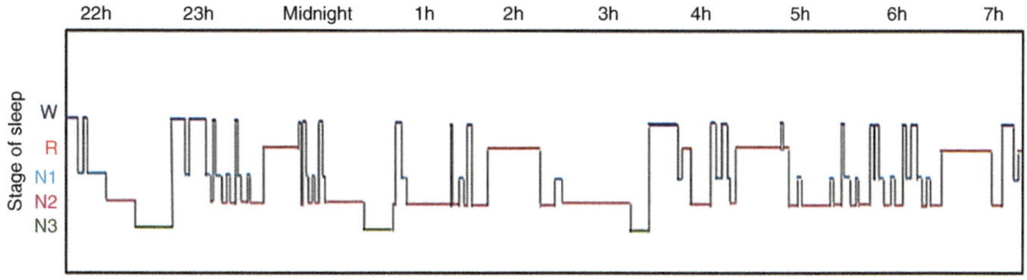

Fig. 3 Hypnogram representing the sleep pattern, extracted from the polysomnography exam. Note that the sleep stages repeat, although with different durations throughout the night. In addition, generally, the N3 stage is predominant in the first half of the night and the R stage in the second half of the night. (Image courtesy from Dr. Cristina Frange)

most of the night's sleep occurs in stage N2, characterized by slow waves (i.e., theta waves, with decreased frequency, low amplitude, and graphic elements such as sleep spindles and K-complexes) (Fig. 4), related to sleep maintenance [28]. Sleep spindles are bursts of neural oscillatory activity that are generated by the interplay of the thalamic reticular nucleus and other thalamic nuclei in a frequency range of 11–16 Hz (usually 12–14 Hz) with a duration of 0.5–1.5 seconds [29]. Sleep spindles are an EEG hallmark of NREM sleep and are believed to mediate many sleep-related functions, from memory consolidation to cortical development. K-complexes have the functions of suppressing cortical arousal in response to stimuli that the sleeping brain evaluates not to signal danger and supporting sleep-based memory consolidation [30]. At the N2 sleep stage, there are slow or absent eye movement and moderate muscle tone. The N3 stage of NREM sleep is composed of high amplitude waves, $\geq$75 μV – with low frequency <3.5 Hz (delta wave activity, that is why it is also called slow-wave sleep, deep sleep, or delta sleep (Fig. 4) – called delta waves, which makes it the "deepest" sleep, with a higher threshold for awakening and more intense brain synchronization seen in the EEG. Night terrors and sleepwalking can occur during N3 sleep. In NREM sleep, there is a regular decrease in ventilation, effectiveness of proprioceptive reflexes and chemoreceptors is maintained, and intercostal muscles are active. There is also maintenance of muscle tone of the upper airways, eurythmic decrease in heart rate, and regular decrease in blood pressure and cardiac output. Therefore, the EEG pattern in NREM sleep is commonly described as synchronous, with such characteristic waveforms as sleep spindles, K-complexes, and high-voltage slow waves. Finally, REM sleep is characterized by EEG activation, muscle atonia, and episodic bursts of rapid eye movements, presenting with a mixed frequency of fast brain waves, with theta and alpha waves, desynchronized, indicating (very) intense brain activity, with or without the presence of sawtooth waves (triangular, 2–6 Hz, with greater amplitude in central regions (Fig. 4)). In the REM sleep stage, there is muscle hypotonia (also called by some researchers as muscle atonia), as the brain blocks motor neurons; consequently, the body does not "act" the dreamed orders or waxes them. Brain activity is intense, similar (or even higher!) to the state of awakeness [25, 31]. REM sleep stage was once known (not anymore) as paradoxical sleep, exactly by the paradox

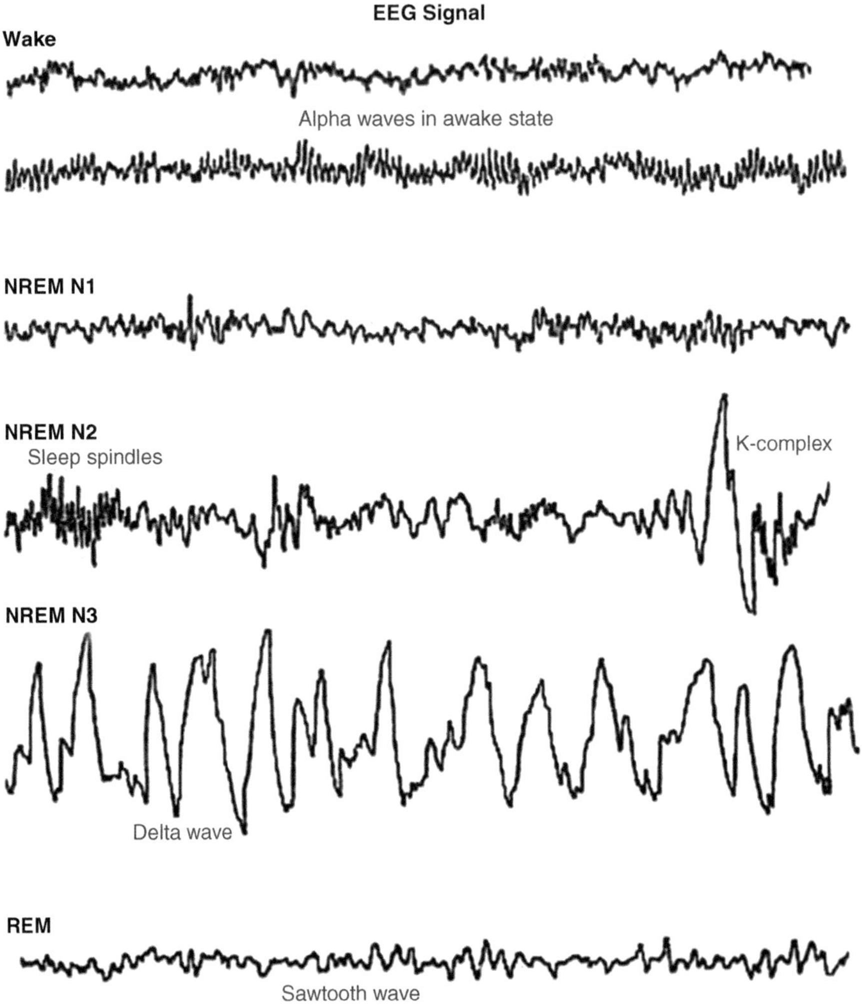

Fig. 4 Sleep stages and their brain waves acquired by electroencephalography in the polysomnography exam and its typical graphic elements

of being in a very intense activity of the mind and extreme relaxation of muscles. In REM sleep, ventilation is variable and quick, proprioceptive reflexes and chemoreceptors are abolished, intercostal muscles are inactive, hypotonia of the upper airway muscles is observed, heart rate becomes faster, and irregular oscillations of blood pressure and cardiac output occurs. Therefore, a quick definition of REM sleep is "an activated brain in a paralyzed body."

For the first sleep cycle, sleep does not always start in N1 and goes through N2, N3, and REM sleep stages. Individuals who are deprived of sleep, for example, may initiate sleep in the REM sleep stage, a condition called sleep rebound, a strategy of our organism to compensate for some functions of the body going directly to the needed sleep stage. Sleep deprivation and issues regarding sleep may, in a long time, lead to sleep disorders comorbid with other diseases, with a negative impact on health and functioning.

In this sense, physiotherapists (PTs) are in an ideal position to promote health and wellness, prescribing physical activity and exercises, educating patients and clients to adopt a regular physical activity regimen, performing hands-on interventions consistent with the biopsychosocial paradigm, and educating patients and clients about sleep. PTs are in ideal position due to the nature of PT's scope of practice, having constant and persistent access to their patients and clients. As the profession changes and improve over time, based on scientific developments PTs practice in contemporary times include sleep health.

The World Health Organization (WHO) has an international classification of occupational professions, essentially reflecting the distinction of subgroups of the health workforce according to assumed differences in skill level and skill specialization required to fulfill the tasks and duties of jobs. PTs are under the classification of health professionals focused on the study, advise on, or provide preventive, curative, rehabilitative, and promotional health services based on an extensive body of theoretical and factual knowledge in diagnosis and treatment of disease, health difficulties and conditions:

> Physiotherapists assess, plan and implement rehabilitative programs that improve or restore human motor functions, maximize movement ability, relieve pain syndromes, and treat or prevent physical challenges associated with injuries, diseases, and other impairments. They apply a broad range of physical therapies and techniques such as movement, ultrasound, heating, laser, and other techniques. They may develop and implement programs for screening and prevention of common physical ailments and disorders.

On the one hand, for the patient, many diseases or conditions may ameliorate if sleep is properly assessed and treated (e.g., knowledge of sleep basics and the importance of sleep for health), as sleep has an imperative function in most of our body's systems, such as modulating pain and mood disorders (e.g., anxiety and depression), memory and learning (and include motor learning), cognitive function, immune function, cardiovascular health, and many more. So, adequate sleep with regard to amount and quality can aid within rehabilitation and physical therapy. On the other hand, PTs can perceive sleep issues in their patients, access and refer to physician and other health professionals, and treat the disturbance along with the physician and other health care providers in an interdisciplinary manner. Therefore, PTs can treat sleep disturbances by a variety of techniques, methods, and resources, addressed in the course of this book.

References

1. Kryger MHRT, Dement WC. Principles and practices of sleep medicine. 6th ed. Philadelphia: Elsevier; 2017.
2. Hirshkowitz M, Whiton K, Albert SM, Alessi C, Bruni O, DonCarlos L, et al. National Sleep Foundation's updated sleep duration recommendations: final report. Sleep Health. 2015;1(4):233–43.

Normal Sleep: Interindividual Differences and Sleep Variability

Maria Júlia Figueiró Reis

Normal sleep is characterized by multiple cycles of defined stages that comprise cerebral and behavioral features. Central nervous system (CNS) maturation and aging processes are intimately linked to changes in normal sleep patterns. Additionally, there are variations related to gender and individual night-by-night oscillations. These normal variants will be the matter of this chapter.

1 Circadian Rhythm and Homeostasis

Sleep-wake machinery is composed of two independent forces – circadian (C) and homeostatic (S) processes – that can be modulated by internal and external cues, leading to a nearly 24-hour cycle [1], as explained in Chap. 1. These cues include body temperature, light, physical exercise, among others [2]. Sleep onset normally occurs in association with body temperature decrease, while sleep offset occurs when temperature rises [3].

The homeostatic process is mediated mainly by adenosine, which is a direct product of the cleavage of adenosine triphosphate (ATP) in the synaptic cleft. ATP is coreleased with neurotransmitters and leads to the accumulation of adenosine in the extracellular space as neuronal activity is stimulated, leading to an increase in the drive to sleep by the end of the day [4]. On the other hand, it is believed that the circadian process promotes maximum wakefulness by that same time, to

The original version of this chapter was revised. The correction to this chapter can be found at https://doi.org/10.1007/978-3-030-85074-6_38

M. J. F. Reis (✉)
Psychobiology Department, Escola Paulista de Medicina, Universidade Federal de São Paulo, São Paulo, SP, Brazil

C. Frange, F. M. S. Coelho (eds.), *Sleep Medicine and Physical Therapy*, https://doi.org/10.1007/978-3-030-85074-6_2

counterbalance homeostatic drive [1]. This system is mediated by the retinohypothalamic pathway, by which light stimuli are transduced to promote rhythm adjustment of the suprachiasmatic nucleus – also known as a master clock – by means of transcription of clock genes [5]. Also, there is a light mediated continuous inhibition of melatonin release by the pineal gland. By twilight, as it becomes dimmer, there is a disinhibition of this pathway, leading to an increase in melatonin levels, which occurs about 2 hours before usual sleep onset [6]. Finally, at the end of the night, wake is promoted by a suprachiasmatic nucleus-mediated increase in cortisol levels around 2–3 hours before usual wake time, by the same time when the lowest core body temperatures are registered, and the peak of melatonin levels occurs [7].

Usually, some circadian preferences within healthy individuals are described, referred to as morningness-eveningness. On the other hand, chronotypes are defined as an activity/behavior measure: late types are more active and productive by night, whereas early types have increased activity in the morning hours [8]. Human populations, in the majority, show a slight tendency for late chronotypes.

Circadian rhythms have progressive expression in the course of development and the aging process is related to changes mainly in the entrainment of the master clock and gene expression. It has been demonstrated that human fetuses show circadian rhythms for cardiovascular function, behavior, and hormonal regulation. Cycles of heart rate and body temperature within the 24-hour period were demonstrated in both preterm and full-term infants. Cortisol rhythms appear approximately 2–4 months after birth, while melatonin secretion starts to cycle around 48 to 52 weeks post-conception [9].

2 Sleep Duration

Normal sleep duration in young adults varies from 7.5 to 8.5 hours, considering weekday and weekend nights, respectively. It is known that duration depends not only on volitional but also on genetic features. Circadian and homeostatic factors also contribute to bout length [3]. A recent meta-analysis suggests that this difference in sleep duration for weekend nights occurs only in age groups that have a school or work schedule during weekdays [10].

In childhood, most recommendations on normal sleep duration are based on expert consensus opinions. American National Sleep Foundation opinion is the most cited of them [11]. Sleep requirements normally decrease over the lifespan in healthy populations, and it is assumed that lower needs occur in older subjects (Fig. 1).

There are also defined criteria for sleep durations that are out of the recommended range, although without clear daytime dysfunction or sleep/wake complaints, putting these special cases as part of the normal range. Short sleepers are the ones who report to sleep six or fewer hours a day and long sleepers are the ones who need nine or more hours of sleep per day. The clinical significance of these patterns remains unclear [12]. Although some studies suggest an increase in morbidity in the extremes of sleep hours per day [13], they might be unable to distinguish genuine

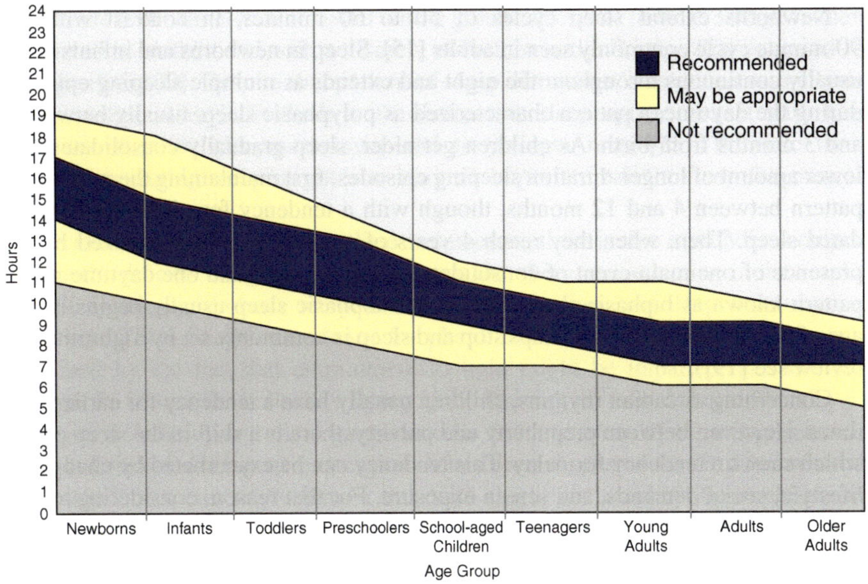

Fig. 1 Sleep duration recommendations across the lifespan. Note that there is a progressive decrease of average sleep needs over the lifespan, as assumed for this consensus. (Reprinted with permission from Hirshkowitz et al. [11])

short and long sleepers from individuals who present with a sleep pathology that leads to secondarily short or long periods of sleep [12].

3 Sleep Particularities in Childhood

Clear wakefulness and sleep states can already be defined around 27–28 weeks post-conception. By this time, active sleep (REM, R stage) corresponds to approximately 80% of total sleep time. By 40 weeks post-conception, active sleep is reduced to approximately 50% of total sleep time, counterbalanced by quiet (NREM) sleep. R stage is progressively reduced until ages 3–4 years, by which it corresponds to 20–25% of total sleep time, similar to adults [14].

In neonates, sleep usually begins with an active sleep (R stage), differently from older infants [15]. Along the first year, quiet (NREM) sleep sequences become progressively more prominent, with N3 predominance over other sleep stages in the first part of the night during early childhood. This can lead to one or more episodes of suppression of the R stage in the first sleep cycles [16, 17]. N3 amount gradually decreases to reach the adult pattern by the second decade of life [18].

Considering electroencephalogram (EEG) components linked to brain development, K-complexes and sleep spindles can first be seen in full-term infants around 2–3 months of age and are linked to thalamocortical maturation. Around 4–6 months of age, sleep stages N1 to N3 become more defined. N3 is important for growth hormone release and memory consolidation [14].

Table 1 Sleep in childhood and aging. Note the main differential elements in the macro and microstructure of sleep across the aging process

Children	Older ones
Increased percentage of R stage (up to 3–4 years of age)	Progressive reduction of R stage
Increased percentage of N3 (up to the second decade of life)	Progressive reduction of N3 stage leading to probable cognitive implications
Progressive consolidation into a monophasic sleep	Progressive return to a polyphasic pattern
A tendency for phase delay in adolescence	A tendency for phase advance
An increased amount of spindles and K-complexes	Reduction in spindles and K-complexes
Difficulty in waking up in the N3 stage of the first sleep cycle	Sleep fragmentation + increase in WASO

R Stage rapid eye movement stage, *WASO* wake after sleep onset

5 Final Considerations

There is a wide range of individual variations within the concept of normality. Ontogeny also adds a component of difficulty in analyzing the patient sleep complaints – or the absence of them. Knowing to interpret such subtlety can help clinicians and researchers to adequately predict outcomes and plan clinical interventions.

Although a lot has been made to elucidate the causes and consequences of changes in sleep architecture, sleep duration, and circadian patterns, there are still unanswered questions. Defining subgroup analyses that comprise the different normal variants will help to better understand this challenging field and to build an adequate epidemiological database for clinical support.

References

1. Borbély AA. A two process model of sleep regulation. Hum Neurobiol. 1982;1(3):195–204.
2. Yamanaka Y. Basic concepts and unique features of human circadian rhythms: implications for human health. Nutr Rev. 2020;78(S3):91–6. https://doi.org/10.1093/nutrit/nuaa072.
3. Carskadon MA, Dement WC. Normal human sleep: an overview. In: Kryger M, Roth T, Dement WC, editors. Principles and practice of sleep medicine. 6th ed. Philadelphia: Elsevier; 2017. p. 15–24.
4. Schneider LD. Anatomy and physiology of normal sleep. In: Miglis MG, editor. Sleep neurological disease. 1st ed. London: Elsevier Science; 2017. p. 1–28.
5. Welsh DK, Takahashi JS, Kay SA. Suprachiasmatic nucleus: cell autonomy and network properties. Annu Rev Physiol. 2010;72:551–77. https://doi.org/10.1146/annurev-physiol-021909-135919.
6. Ma MA, Morrison EH. Neuroanatomy, Nucleus Suprachiasmatic. In: StatPearls [Internet]. Treasure Island (FL): StatPearls, 2020. Available in: https://www.ncbi.nlm.nih.gov/books/NBK546664/. Accessed on: December 30, 2020.

7. Schneider L. Neurobiology and neuroprotective benefits of sleep. Continuum (minneap minn). 2020; 26(4, sleep neurology): 848–870. doi: https://doi.org/10.1212/CON.0000000000000878.
8. Bauducco S, Richardson C, Gradisar M. Chronotype, circadian rhythms and mood. Curr Opin Psychol. 2020;34:77–83. https://doi.org/10.1016/j.copsyc.2019.09.002.
9. Finger AM, Kramer A. Mammalian circadian systems: organization and modern life challenges. Acta Physiol. 2020; https://doi.org/10.1111/apha.13548.
10. Kocevska D, Lysen TS, Dotinga A, Koopman-Verhoeff ME, Luijk MPCM, Antypa N, et al. Sleep characteristics across the lifespan in 1.1 million people from the Netherlands, United Kingdom and United States: a systematic review and meta-analysis. Nat Hum Behav. 2020; https://doi.org/10.1038/s41562-020-00965-x.
11. Hirshkowitz M, Whiton K, Albert SM, Alessi C, Bruni O, DonCarlos L, et al. National Sleep Foundation's updated sleep duration recommendations: final report. Sleep Health. 2015;1(4):233–43. https://doi.org/10.1016/j.sleh.2015.10.004.
12. American Academy of Sleep Medicine. International classification of sleep disorders. 3rd ed. Darien: American Academy of Sleep Medicine; 2014.
13. He M, Deng X, Zhu Y, Huan L, Niu W. The relationship between sleep duration and all-cause mortality in the older people: an updated and dose-response meta-analysis. BMC Public Health. 2020;20(1):1179. https://doi.org/10.1186/s12889-020-09275-3.
14. Kotagal S. Sleep-wake disorders of childhood. Continuum (Minneap Minn). 2017;23(4, Sleep Neurology):1132–50. https://doi.org/10.1212/CON.0000000000000504.
15. Dereymaeker A, Pillay K, Vervisch J, De Vos M, Van Huffel S, Jansen K, et al. Review of sleep-EEG in preterm and term neonates. Early Hum Dev. 2017;113:87–103. https://doi.org/10.1016/j.earlhumdev.2017.07.003.
16. Bes F, Schulz H, Navelet Y, Salzarulo P. The distribution of slow-wave sleep across the night: a comparison for infants, children, and adults. Sleep. 1991;14(1):5–12. https://doi.org/10.1093/sleep/14.1.5.
17. Fattinger S, Jenni OG, Schmitt B, Achermann P, Huber R. Overnight changes in the slope of sleep slow waves during infancy. Sleep. 2014;37(2):245–53. https://doi.org/10.5665/sleep.3390.
18. Baker FC, Willoughby AR, de Zambotti M, Franzen PL, Prouty D, Javitz H, et al. Age-related differences in sleep architecture and electroencephalogram in adolescents in the National Consortium on alcohol and neurodevelopment in adolescence sample. Sleep. 2016;39(7):1429–39. https://doi.org/10.5665/sleep.5978.
19. Chaput JP, Dutil C, Sampasa-Kanyinga H. Sleeping hours: what is the ideal number and how does age impact this? Nat Sci Sleep. 2018;10:421–30. https://doi.org/10.2147/NSS.S163071.
20. Danner F, Phillips B. Adolescent sleep, school start times, and teen motor vehicle crashes. J Clin Sleep Med. 2008;4(6):533–5.
21. Ohayon MM, Carskadon MA, Guilleminault C, Vitiello MV. Meta-analysis of quantitative sleep parameters from childhood to old age in healthy individuals: developing normative sleep values across the human lifespan. Sleep. 2004;27(7):1255–73. https://doi.org/10.1093/sleep/27.7.1255.
22. Redline S, Kirchner HL, Quan SF, Gottlieb DJ, Kapur V, Newman A. The effects of age, sex, ethnicity, and sleep-disordered breathing on sleep architecture. Arch Intern Med. 2004;164(4):406–18. https://doi.org/10.1001/archinte.164.4.406.
23. Schwarz JFA, Åkerstedt T, Lindberg E, Gruber G, Fischer H, Theorell-Haglöw J. Age affects sleep microstructure more than sleep macrostructure. J Sleep Res. 2017;26(3):277–87. https://doi.org/10.1111/jsr.12478.
24. Klerman EB, Davis JB, Duffy JF, Dijk DJ, Kronauer RE. Older people awaken more frequently but fall back asleep at the same rate as younger people. Sleep. 2004;27(4):793–8. https://doi.org/10.1093/sleep/27.4.793.
25. Iannella G, Vicini C, Colizza A, Meccariello G, Polimeni A, Greco A, et al. Aging effect on sleepiness and apneas severity in patients with obstructive sleep apnea syndrome:

a meta-analysis study. Eur Arch Otorhinolaryngol. 2019;276(12):3549–56. https://doi.org/10.1007/s00405-019-05616-0.
26. Miner B, Kryger MH. Sleep in the aging population. Sleep Med Clin. 2017;12(1):31–8. https://doi.org/10.1016/j.jsmc.2016.10.008.
27. Bliwise DL, Scullin MK. Normal aging. In: Kryger M, Roth T, Dement WC, editors. Principles and practice of sleep medicine. 6th ed. Philadelphia: Elsevier; 2017. p. 25–38.
28. Kessel L, Siganos G, Jørgensen T, Larsen M. Sleep disturbances are related to decreased transmission of blue light to the retina caused by lens yellowing. Sleep. 2011;34(9):1215–9. https://doi.org/10.5665/SLEEP.1242.
29. La Morgia C, Ross-Cisneros FN, Koronyo Y, Hannibal J, Gallassi R, Cantalupo G, et al. Melanopsin retinal ganglion cell loss in Alzheimer disease. Ann Neurol. 2016;79(1):90–109. https://doi.org/10.1002/ana.24548.
30. Musiek ES, Holtzman DM. Mechanisms linking circadian clocks, sleep, and neurodegeneration. Science. 2016;354(6315):1004–8. https://doi.org/10.1126/science.aah4968.
31. Ostrin LA. Ocular and systemic melatonin and the influence of light exposure. Clin Exp Optom. 2019;102(2):99–108. https://doi.org/10.1111/cxo.12824.
32. Daneault V, Dumont M, Massé É, Vandewalle G, Carrier J. Light-sensitive brain pathways and aging. J Physiol Anthropol. 2016;35:9. https://doi.org/10.1186/s40101-016-0091-9.
33. Puentes-Mestril C, Roach J, Niethard N, Zochowski M, Aton SJ. How rhythms of the sleeping brain tune memory and synaptic plasticity. Sleep. 2019;42(7):zsz095. https://doi.org/10.1093/sleep/zsz095.
34. Cai S, Li T, Zhang L, Shi L, Liao J, Li W, et al. Characteristics of sleep structure assessed by objective measurements in patients with amnestic mild cognitive impairment: a Meta-analysis. Front Neurol. 2020;11:577126. https://doi.org/10.3389/fneur.2020.577126.
35. Reeves BC, Karimy JK, Kundishora AJ, Mestre H, Cerci HM, Matouk C. Glymphatic system impairment in Alzheimer's disease and idiopathic Normal pressure hydrocephalus. Trends Mol Med. 2020;26(3):285–95. https://doi.org/10.1016/j.molmed.2019.11.008.
36. La AL, Walsh CM, Neylan TC, Vossel KA, Yaffe K, Krystal AD, et al. Long-term trazodone use and cognition: a potential therapeutic role for slow-wave sleep enhancers. J Alzheimers Dis. 2019;67(3):911–21. https://doi.org/10.3233/JAD-181145.
37. Akbari V, Ghobadi S, Mohammadi S, Khodarahmi R. The antidepressant drug; trazodone inhibits tau amyloidogenesis: prospects for prophylaxis and treatment of AD. Arch Biochem Biophys. 2020;679:108218. https://doi.org/10.1016/j.abb.2019.108218.

Brief History of Sleep Medicine and Its Importance for Overall Health

Monica Levy Andersen and Sergio Tufik

Sleep has been a target of human imagination since ancient times, a period when inexplicable happenings, such as dreams and sleepwalking, were surrounded by mysticism. With the development of science, our knowledge became more refined and new investigation methods were conceived, resulting in the current level of understanding. This knowledge, however, is not yet complete, seen that some elementary problems, such as the evolutive origins of sleep, its biological causes, and the main question of why we sleep, remain unsolved.

Proper tools to study sleep were not available for a long time, making it a particularly elusive physiological process when compared to more tangible ones, such as blood flow and pulmonary respiration. It was only by the middle of the nineteenth century that the development of adequate techniques happened. Initially, auditory and tactile stimuli were employed to measure the depth of sleep (see [1]), but the true revolution in sleep neurology was reached with the discovery of electrooculography by Hans Berger in 1929 (see [2]). This technique, which measures neuroelectric activity, later established the basis for modern electroencephalograms (EEG).

With this new tool, it was possible, for the first time, to measure neuroencephalic activity during sleep, which led to numerous discoveries about its mechanisms and disorders. An important finding was that encephalic neurons trigger at different levels of synchrony, forming patterns or waves with distinct frequencies and amplitudes. These patterns are measured in Hertz (Hz) and are classified, by convention, as delta (slowest waves), theta, alpha, beta, and gamma (fastest waves).

Another elementary discovery was that human sleep occurs in phases, characterized according to different patterns detected by EEG, as described in the previous chapters.

M. L. Andersen (✉) · S. Tufik
Department of Psychobiology, Escola Paulista de Medicina, Universidade Federal de São Paulo, São Paulo, SP, Brazil

C. Frange, F. M. S. Coelho (eds.), *Sleep Medicine and Physical Therapy*,
https://doi.org/10.1007/978-3-030-85074-6_3

Sono is responsible for the research Sleep Epidemiology in the City of São Paulo, designated EPISONO Project. Epidemiological studies permit the assessment of the prevalence of pathologies in the general population through a representative sample of individuals. In the case of sleep science, they also allow other measurements, including the average duration of sleep, the quality of sleep, its impact during the vigil, and the prevalence of sleep disorders. EPISONO's first edition, concentrated in the city of São Paulo, was done in 1986, followed by three more editions in 1995, 2007 [15, 16] and 2018/2019, which allowed the longitudinal assessment of sleep patterns in the city.

In the 2007 edition, the largest and most complete so far, EPISONO recruited 1042 subjects for polysomnography, actigraphy, blood tests, genetic exams, and questionnaires [16]. The results indicated that 42% of São Paulo's population suffered from snoring, 24% registered frequent nightmares, and 9% and 3% had bruxism and sleepwalking, respectively [17]. The most common sleep disorder was sleep obstructive apnea, with a prevalence of 32.8% [18].

The 2007 EPISONO was one of the largest epidemiological sleep investigations in the world to utilize a modern and complete methodology, which provided invaluable data referring to populational habits and sleep disorders prevalence, thus allowing the realization of conscientization campaigns and the implementation of public policies specifically aimed at these patients. In the case of sleep obstructive apnea, for example, it was detected that its prevalence was 5–10 times higher than previously described [19], demonstrating the importance of employing adequate methodology in this type of research.

1 Sleep Medicine

Human beings consume one-third of their lives sleeping, an activity that leaves them inert for about 8 hours every day and drastically decreases their reaction capacity, making them vulnerable to predators and to other environmental factors, which lead us to question the evolutive importance of sleep in terms of its physiological utility. Today, it is known that this state is fundamental for the maintenance of organic systems, besides being responsible for numerous cognitive and homeostatic processes, such as metabolic clearance of the brain and the recovery of the musculoskeletal, nervous, and immune systems.

Another function of sleep is to conserve energy by reducing physical activity, besides the maintenance of encephalic energetic homeostasis. This happens through metabolic dynamics specific to REM sleep and depends upon regulatory mechanisms of energetic molecules such as adenosine triphosphate, glucose, and glycogen [19].

Several studies pointed out that the occurrence of infections or exposure to microbiotic antigens alters sleep patterns [19]. It is also known that the incidence of sleep results in improved immune response, while the lack of sleep impairs the response to infections [20]; for example, patients that slept better after a round of hepatitis A vaccine obtained superior results in the establishment of immune memory against the viral antigen [21]. These data show the importance of sleep in the response against infections and in the patient's recovery after disease.

Another proposed function for sleep is the clearance of metabolites originated from cell activity, removing them from the cerebrospinal fluid and leading them to the bloodstream [22], in a process denominated "glymphatic function" (in reference to the analogous function of the lymphatic system). The glymphatic activity of sleep is responsible for cleaning products originated from the vigil period which, besides protecting the brain against neurotoxic compounds, results in the decrease of osmotic pressure in the extracellular medium due to the presence of these metabolites [23]. It has been proposed that the correct function of the glymphatic process may prevent against Alzheimer's disease, as one of its causes is the accumulation of beta-amyloid peptides in the cerebrospinal fluid [24].

Sleep is intimately related to cognitive and behavioral functions. Sleep deprivation impairs decision-making, reduces speed and precision when performing tasks, causes fatigue, and negatively affects the mood [25]. On the other hand, the incidence of sleep recovers these impaired functions in a way directly proportional to the time spent sleeping [26]. At the cellular level, it has been proposed that the quality of sleep maintains neuronal plasticity in a way that improves memory consolidation and learning [27]. These effects are not static and depend upon factors such as the patient's age and type of experience before sleeping, but they demonstrate the general importance of sleep upon cognition and in the maintenance of mental health.

Bearing in mind sleep's physiological functions and the negative consequences of its deprivation, it is fundamental to point out the importance of sleep hygiene to our health. This concept involves the habits practiced by each individual in order to preserve the quality and efficiency of sleep, including the regular practice of exercises, good nutrition, noise reduction at the time of sleep, and avoidance of caffeine, nicotine, and alcohol consumption, among others (see Chap. 31 for more info). Sleep hygiene is becoming more and more important within the clinical context due to the fact that it has a very low financial cost, is promptly available, and has the potential to significantly improve the quality of life. Laboral impositions and the prevalence of electronic media affect the circadian rhythm of a great portion of the population, leading to deregulation of sleep and of the biological clock, which may become public health issues. Information campaigns about sleep are relatively easy to realize and have an extensive reach when compared to medical consultations and individualized pharmacological treatments, which makes them an important tool in sleep medicine and public health [28]. It is important to point out that there are numerous disorders for which sleep hygiene may not be enough. These have several biological origins (including physiological, psychological, and genetic), and, therefore, need proper therapies. In these cases, sleep hygiene may be indicated as ancillary treatment.

2 Final words

Reference to healthy habits usually implies good nutrition or the practice of physical exercises, but one should bear in mind that care with his or her sleep is equally important. Fortunately, we have observed an increase in the population's awareness about sleep practices, partly due to the growth of science in this area and partly due to the promotion of this knowledge to the population. In this context, the education of health professionals about the importance of sleep is critical, as they act at the front line of the clinical practice and establish direct contact with the patients.

We must point out that the knowledge of sleep disorders by professionals is essential, as their prevalence among the general population is greater than previously thought. Because they occur during the night, away from the clinic, they may easily go unnoticed by the patient and by the health professional. A critical look is necessary for their identification, as well as the patient's forwarding to a specialized professional for exams and proper treatment. This book aims to educate health practictioners about sleep and its disorders, and we expect to help them become better and more conscientious professionals on this so-important factor to human health.

References

1. Tufik S. Medicina e Biologia do Sono. 1st ed. São Paulo: Manole; 2008.
2. Karakas S, Barry RJ. A brief historical perspective on the advent of brain oscillations in the biological and psychological disciplines. Neurosci Biobehav Rev. 2017;75:335–47.
3. Stone JL, Hughes JR. Early history of electroencephalography and establishment of the American Clinical Neurophysiology Society. J Clin Neurophysiol. 2013;30(1):28–44.
4. Aserinsky E, Kleitman N. Regularly occurring periods of eye motility, and concomitant phenomena, during sleep. Science. 1953;118(3062):273–4.
5. Dement W, Kleitman N. Cyclic variations in EEG during sleep and their relation to eye movements, body motility, and dreaming. Electroencephalogr Clin Neurophysiol. 1957;9(4):673–90.
6. Jouvet M, Michel F. On the neural tract responsible for the rapid cortical activity during the course of physiological sleep in the cat (paradoxal phase). C R Seances Soc Biol Fil. 1960;154:995–8.
7. Guilleminault C, Eldridge F, Dement WC. Insomnia, narcolepsy, and sleep apneas. Bull Physiopathol Respir (Nancy). 1972;8(5):1127–38.
8. Guilleminault C, Dement WC, Monod N. [Sudden (infant) death syndrome: apnea during sleep. New hypothesis]. Nouv Press Med, 1973;2(20):1355–8.
9. Diagnostic classification of sleep and arousal disorders. 1979 first edition. Association of sleep disorders centers and the association for the psychophysiological study of Sleep. Sleep. 1979;2(1):1–154.
10. Sullivan CE, et al. Reversal of obstructive sleep apnoea by continuous positive airway pressure applied through the nares. Lancet. 1981;1(8225):862–5.
11. Meir H, Kryger TR, Dement WC. Principles and practice of sleep medicine. 6th ed. Elsevier; 2017.
12. PubMed. 2020. [cited 2020 November, 11]; Available from: https://pubmed.ncbi.nlm.nih.gov/?term=sleep+rat&sort=date.

13. Timo-Iaria C, et al. Phases and states of sleep in the rat. Physiol Behav. 1970;5(9):1057–62.
14. Pedemonte M, et al. Past, present, and future of sleep medicine research in Latin America. J Clin Sleep Med. 2021;17(5):1133–9.
15. Pires ML, et al. Sleep habits and complaints of adults in the city of Sao Paulo, Brazil, in 1987 and 1995. Braz J Med Biol Res. 2007;40(11):1505–15.
16. Santos-Silva R, et al. Sao Paulo Epidemiologic Sleep Study: rationale, design, sampling, and procedures. Sleep Med. 2009;10(6):679–85.
17. Santos-Silva R, et al. Increasing trends of sleep complaints in the city of Sao Paulo, Brazil. Sleep Med. 2010;11(6):520–4.
18. Tufik S, et al. Obstructive sleep apnea syndrome in the Sao Paulo Epidemiologic Sleep Study. Sleep Med. 2010;11(5):441–6.
19. Punjabi NM. The epidemiology of adult obstructive sleep apnea. Proc Am Thorac Soc. 2008;5(2):136–43.
20. Besedovsky L, Lange T, Born J. Sleep and immune function. Pflugers Arch. 2012;463(1):121–37.
21. Lange T, et al. Sleep after vaccination boosts immunological memory. J Immunol. 2011;187(1):283–90.
22. Xie L, et al. Sleep drives metabolite clearance from the adult brain. Science. 2013;342(6156):373–7.
23. Krueger JM, et al. Sleep function: toward elucidating an enigma. Sleep Med Rev. 2016;28:46–54.
24. Kang JE, et al. Amyloid-beta dynamics are regulated by orexin and the sleep-wake cycle. Science. 2009;326(5955):1005–7.
25. Troynikov O, Watson CG, Nawaz N. Sleep environments and sleep physiology: a review. J Therm Biol. 2018;78:192–203.
26. Rosa RR, Bonnet MH, Warm JS. Recovery of performance during sleep following sleep deprivation. Psychophysiology. 1983;20(2):152–9.
27. Frank MG, Cantera R. Sleep, clocks, and synaptic plasticity. Trends Neurosci. 2014;37(9):491–501.
28. Irish LA, et al. The role of sleep hygiene in promoting public health: a review of empirical evidence. Sleep Med Rev. 2015;22:23–36.

Basic Principles of Sleep Physiotherapy Practice

Cristina Frange, Cristina Staub, and Stavros Stathopoulos

According to the World Physiotherapy, the global body for national physiotherapy associations, physiotherapists (PTs) provide services that develop, maintain, and restore people's maximum movement and functional ability. They can help people at any stage of life when movement and function are threatened by aging, injury, diseases, disorders, conditions, or environmental factors.

PTs help people maximize their quality of life, looking at physical, psychological, emotional, and social well-being. They work in the health spheres of promotion, prevention, treatment, and rehabilitation. PTs are qualified and professionally required to:

1. Undertake a comprehensive examination/assessment of the patient/client or needs of a client group
2. Evaluate the findings from the examination/assessment to make clinical judgments regarding patients/clients

---

C. Frange (✉)
Department of Neurology and Neurosurgery, Escola Paulista de Medicina, Universidade Federal de São Paulo, São Paulo, SP, Brazil

Certified in Sleep Physiotherapy by the Brazilian Sleep Society (ABS), and The Brazilian Association of Cardiorespiratory Physiotherapy and Physiotherapy in Intensive Care (ASSOBRAFIR), São Paulo, SP, Brazil

World Physiotherapy Network for Health Promotion in Life and Work, São Paulo, SP, Brazil

C. Staub
International Organization of Physical Therapy in Mental Health, Swiss Group of Physiotherapy in Mental Health, Pro Dormo Switzerland, Zurich, Switzerland

S. Stathopoulos
Physical Therapy Department, Evaggelismos General Hospital, Athens, Greece

Postgraduate Program of the Medical School of National and Kapodistrian, University of Athens, Athens, Greece

Marconi University of Rome, Rome, Italy

C. Frange, F. M. S. Coelho (eds.), *Sleep Medicine and Physical Therapy*,
https://doi.org/10.1007/978-3-030-85074-6_4

3. Formulate a diagnosis, prognosis, and plan
4. Provide consultation within their expertise and determine when patients/clients need to be referred to another healthcare professional
5. Implement a physiotherapist intervention/treatment program
6. Determine the outcomes of any interventions/treatments
7. Make recommendations for self-management

According to the American Physical Therapy Association (APTA) of the position of house delegates updated in 2020:

> Physical therapists are part of an interdisciplinary team of licensed health services providers in prevention and management of sleep impairments and promotion of healthy sleep behaviors. The PTs role includes using the best available evidence and standards of practice to screen for sleep dysfunction; identify impairments related to sleep dysfunction; implement and progress therapeutic interventions to address impairments that interfere with sleep; educate society, patients and clients, caregivers and providers on healthy sleep behaviors and the relationship between sleep, pain, physical activity, function, health, and well-being; monitor and, if indicated, manage sleep quality and quantity in patients and clients to enhance physical therapy outcomes, and refer to sleep medicine professionals as indicated.

Contemporary PTs, who are function specialists and movement experts, need to understand the impact of the sleep deprivation and disorders singularity on the health and well-being of the patients they attend. In this sense, knowledge about sleep (function, physiology, duration, etc.) and skills to screen sleep disorders and to promote quality sleep are important components for PTs to promote (and treat) health and wellness. Sleep must be listed within our priorities and be part of the anamnesis and of clinical practice. PTs must guise at the topic sleep more precisely – in research, in education, and in everyday practice [1, 2]. Therefore, the regulations/practice of physical therapy in each country is different and depends on the governmental system and health care system. PTs must respect local, regional and cultural differences and act within our scope of practice, in an interdisciplinary manner, and focused on patient-centered care.

1 Why PTs May Treat Sleep Disturbances

A network for Health Promotion in Life and Work (HPLW) has been established into World Physiotherapy. It encourages the members to forward with their health promotion strategies and share views and ideas which can be implemented for sustainable development of various problems such as sleep problems.

Sleep has a vital role in life. In fact, sleep is a behavior that occupies plenty of time in our lives. To be more specific, one-third of our life is spent asleep. In this sense, it must have an imperative function – or many functions, that we don't know yet for sure. However, we know that we cannot survive without sleep. Sleep is an important protagonist of the proper functioning of most, if not all, body systems. We know it because of much scientific evidence on lack of sleep, or disturbed sleep stages from experimental, epidemiological, longitudinal, and trial investigations that showed that we cannot survive without sleep. In fact, since the 1960s, a variety of investigations using animal models have been conducted in order to study the effects of sleep deprivation on the system or organs and to see which would fail first [3–5]. The researchers found for example that after 2 weeks of sleep deprivation, the rodents died from massive multi-organ failure. The cause of death was not clear: the deterioration in appearance, skin lesions, and changes in brain activity resisted simple explication. Several organs failed, and not just one, as they expected to see. These experiments led a group of researchers to investigate the role of immune function in different organs and systems, and they started to investigate in humans the purpose of sleep. Until now we know that sleep is a biological necessity and that extended sleep loss reliably produces a syndrome of specific substantial physiological changes. Sleep functions are still a mystery. Impaired sleep affects our overall health.

Lack of sleep (both in appropriate quantity and quality) and circadian misalignment have been implicated in numerous adverse health outcomes and can lead to several physiological, neuropsychological, and mental health changes.

2 How PTs May Treat Sleep Disturbances

The physical therapy session, beyond being an external cue for the alignment of the peripheral oscillators, is also capable of adding to the sleep pressure, by many biochemicals endogenously induced during exercise and diverse PTs techniques. PTs' diagnoses are often based on single time point assessments during the day, ignoring circadian influences on physiology. Even when time is considered, using (external) clock time, it ignores the large interindividual differences in internal timing (chronotypes: morning, evening, and intermediate types; amount of sleep needed: short, intermediate, and long sleepers). These themes must be addressed by PTs in order to optimize not only sleep but also rehabilitation in physical therapy practice.

PTs as experts in movement and exercise and with a thorough knowledge of risk factors and pathology and their effects on all systems are the ideal professionals to promote, guide, and manage physical and exercise activities and efforts [6].

PTs are protagonists in promoting wellness, mobility, and independence, in a broad range of diseases. Why not sleep? As we have seen, all of our systems depend on the sleep-wake cycle, either in health or in disease. PTs can help with health promotion and with the prevention of disease conditions by enhancing sleep quantity and improving sleep quality.

In this context, to incorporate sleep health in PTs practice, we must address prevention, health promotion, and wellness interventions: evaluate general sleep health and screen for risk of sleep disorders; refer to a physician when a suspected disorder requires diagnosis and further investigation; arrange for sleep hygiene education; prescribe an appropriate and individualized exercise program to increase homeostatic sleep pressure and also breathing exercises for some

Given the context, there are many opportunities for PTs to provide sleep health education and to treat sleep disorders and conditions in their patients/clients that will be discussed in this book.

References

1. Staub C et al. Integrate sleep into physiotherapy. Oral presentation. In Fifth European Congress of the European Region WCPT on Physiotherapy – Education. 2020; World Confederation of Physiocal Therapy.
2. Staub C. Concept of diverse sleep treatments in physiotherapy. Eur J Phys. 2019; 21(3):177–84. https://doi.org/10.1080/21679169.2018.1505948.
3. Levitt RA. Sleep deprivation in the rat. Science. 1966;153(3731):85–7.
4. Rechtschaffen A, et al. Sleep deprivation in the rat: I. Conceptual issues. Sleep. 1989;12(1):1–4.
5. Rechtschaffen A, et al. Sleep deprivation in the rat: X. Integration and discussion of the findings. Sleep. 1989;12(1):68–87.
6. WCPT Policy statement: Physical therapists as exercise and physical activity experts across the life span. Revised and re-approved at the 19th General Meeting of WCPT. May 2019. https://world.physio/policy/ps-exercise-experts.
7. Biswas A, et al. Sedentary time and its association with risk for disease incidence, mortality, and hospitalization in adults: a systematic review and meta-analysis. Ann Intern Med. 2015;162(2):123–32.
8. Healy GN, et al. Sedentary time and cardio-metabolic biomarkers in US adults: NHANES 2003-06. Eur Heart J. 2011;32(5):590–7.
9. Benatti FB, Ried-Larsen M. The effects of breaking up prolonged sitting time: a review of experimental studies. Med Sci Sports Exerc. 2015;47(10):2053–61.
10. Chastin SF, et al. Meta-analysis of the relationship between breaks in sedentary behavior and cardiometabolic health. Obesity (Silver Spring). 2015;23(9):1800–10.
11. Bassetti CLA. Sleep and stroke: a bidirectional relationship with clinical implications. Sleep Med Rev. 2019;45:127–8.
12. Silveira SL, et al. Symptom clusters and quality of life in persons with multiple sclerosis across the lifespan. Qual Life Res. 2021;30(4):1061–71.
13. MacKintosh EW, Chen ML, Benditt JO. Lifetime care of Duchenne muscular dystrophy. Sleep Med Clin. 2020;15(4):485–95.
14. Aydin T, et al. Sleep quality in individuals with short-duration chronic spinal cord injury. Int J Rehabil Res. 2020;43(4):369–75.
15. Bugalho P, et al. Polysomnographic predictors of sleep, motor and cognitive dysfunction progression in Parkinson's disease: a longitudinal study. Sleep Med. 2021;77:205–8.
16. Shi L, et al. Sleep disturbances increase the risk of dementia: a systematic review and meta-analysis. Sleep Med Rev. 2018;40:4–16.
17. Bubu OM, et al. Sleep, cognitive impairment, and Alzheimer's disease: a systematic review and meta-analysis. Sleep. 2017;40(1):1-18.
18. Andersen ML, et al. Sleep disturbance and pain: a tale of two common problems. Chest. 2018;154(5):1249–59.
19. Herrero Babiloni A, et al. Sleep and pain: recent insights, mechanisms, and future directions in the investigation of this relationship. J Neural Transm (Vienna). 2020;127(4):647–60.
20. Amiri S, Behnezhad S. Sleep disturbances and back pain: systematic review and meta-analysis. Neuropsychiatrie. 2020;34(2):74–84.

21. Moldofsky H. The significance of dysfunctions of the sleeping/waking brain to the pathogenesis and treatment of fibromyalgia syndrome. Rheum Dis Clin N Am. 2009;35(2):275–83.
22. Lavigne GJ, Sessle BJ. The neurobiology of orofacial pain and sleep and their interactions. J Dent Res. 2016;95(10):1109–16.
23. Chouchou F, et al. Postoperative sleep disruptions: a potential catalyst of acute pain? Sleep Med Rev. 2014;18(3):273–82.
24. Lavigne GJ, et al. Does sleep differ among patients with common musculoskeletal pain disorders? Curr Rheumatol Rep. 2011;13(6):535–42.
25. Smith MT, et al. Mechanisms by which sleep disturbance contributes to osteoarthritis pain: a conceptual model. Curr Pain Headache Rep. 2009;13(6):447–54.
26. Hu F, et al. Improvement of sleep quality in patients with ankylosing spondylitis kyphosis after corrective surgery. Spine (Phila Pa 1976). 2020;45(23):E1596–603.
27. Longo UG, et al. Sleep disturbance and rotator cuff tears: a systematic review. Medicina (Kaunas). 2019;55(8):453-63.
28. Swann MC, et al. Sleep disturbance in orthopaedic trauma patients. J Orthop Trauma. 2018;32(10):500–4.

Sleep Physiology and Neuroendocrinology for Physiotherapists

Priscila Farias Tempaku

Far from being a simple absence of wakefulness, sleep is characterized by an active, regulated, consciousness, and metabolically distinct state, essential for the health and well-being of several species. Sleep has an important modulatory effect on neuroendocrine, metabolic, and immunological functions that will be discussed in this chapter and are summarized in Table 1.

The three main states of the sleep-wakefulness cycle (i.e., wakefulness, NREM, and R stages) are usually identified based on electroencephalogram (EEG) rhythms, muscle tone level, and in the presence of eye movements [1]. However, the physiological definition and the understanding of these states cannot disregard the evaluation of respiratory, cardiovascular, and metabolic parameters, which are under the integrated control of the autonomic and endocrine systems [2].

This definition goes beyond the standard, largely based on the level of cortical and somatomotor activity of the brain. The hypothalamus plays a fundamental role in this complex integrative activity [3], in arousal, and in regulating transitions between sleep and waking states, which are critical for the maintenance of body homeostasis and for both the survival of the body (fight or flight response) and reproduction. This activity leads to the formation of bodily functions, largely based on external and internal sensory information, according to the physiological meaning and objectives of the different behavioral states [2, 3].

The neural fundamentals of the sleep-wake cycle involve interactions between sleep-promoting areas, such as the anterior hypothalamus, and waking systems [4]. During sleep, gabaergic and glycinergic neurons located in the ventrolateral preoptic area of the anterior hypothalamus are activated and the alternation between REM and NREM sleep is controlled by the multiple cell populations located in the hypothalamus, basal forebrain, and brainstem [5]. Transitions for wakefulness

P. F. Tempaku (✉)
Psychobiology Department, Escola Paulista de Medicina, Universidade Federal de São Paulo, São Paulo, SP, Brazil

C. Frange, F. M. S. Coelho (eds.), *Sleep Medicine and Physical Therapy*,
https://doi.org/10.1007/978-3-030-85074-6_5

and energy expenditure, and the probability of active interaction with the external environment is quite reduced. Although in the human adult, the decrease in energy expenditure during sleep is apparently moderate compared to silent waking, sleep may play a relevant role in energy conservation in animals with a less favorable surface-to-volume ratio (babies or small mammals), in which energy conservation is more persistent [8]. In general, the expenditure of body energy decreases during sleep.

The brain energy metabolism decreases widely during NREM sleep and increases during REM sleep to similar levels, or even slightly higher than those of waking [9]. Thermoregulatory responses can be experimentally induced by the delivery of external or internal thermal loads. These responses are present both in silent vigil and in NREM sleep but are depressed during REM sleep [7]. While the thermoregulatory differences between waking and NREM sleep depend only on the different levels of energy metabolism in the two states, a profound functional change occurs during REM sleep. This change alters the normal homeostatic regulatory modality from closed to open net [7]. In particular, during episodes of REM sleep that occur under a positive (hot) thermal charge, sweating is limited at the beginning of the sleep episode and subsequently depressed. On the other hand, under a negative thermal charge (cold), the tremor is suppressed and the vasoconstriction of the heat exchanger is reduced [10].

2 Respiratory System

The respiratory system is the result of a complex interaction between the central nervous system, motor neurons, and respiratory muscles, providing continuous homeostasis of arterial oxygen pressures, carbon dioxide, and pH levels during distinct physiological conditions and responding promptly to subtle metabolic variations. The ventilation control is mediated by two mechanisms: one is voluntary and related to cortical activity and the other is involuntary, being responsive to factors such as hypercapnia and hypoxemia [11].

The regulation of breathing differs significantly between wakefulness and sleep. With sleep onset, important changes occur in the various processes that regulate respiratory control, such as the cessation of voluntary breath control during the sleep onset. In addition, breathing is a function closely related to the sleep phase, in which great differences are observed between NREM and REM sleep [12].

2.1 NREM Sleep

When compared with waking, the frequency and amplitude of breathing are lower during NREM sleep, generating hypoventilation. These sleep-related changes are the result of a decreased tonic impulse of the respiratory network and increased resistance of the upper airways. A quantitative analysis of neural activity during sleep showed that neurons with a higher proportion of tonic activity are predominantly affected by sleep [13].

2.2 *REM Sleep*

During the R sleep stage, the amplitude and respiratory frequency are marked by oscillations, so that ventilation acquires an irregular dynamic nature, accompanied by the occasional presence of central apnea [14]. Thus, ventilation during this sleep stage may be unchanged, increased, or decreased. During periods of hypoventilation, rapid eye movements are observed. As for the periods of hypoventilation, they are due primarily to the reduction of the activity of the thoracic muscles [15].

3 Cardiovascular System

Normal human sleep is accompanied by changes in blood pressure and heart rate [16]. These hemodynamic changes are mediated mainly by changes in the autonomic nervous system. During NREM sleep, sympathetic inhibition is associated with a decrease in blood pressure and heart rate. Already during REM sleep, there is an intermittent sympathetic activation with rapid fluctuations in blood pressure and heart rate [17]. Thus, in general, baseline cardiovascular activity is higher in wakefulness than during sleep and tends to decrease gradually from stage N1 to N3 of NREM sleep. Considering that NREM sleep is characterized by autonomic stability with parasympathetic predominance and sympathetic inhibition, there is a gradual decrease in sympathetic nerve activity, blood pressure, and heart rate progressing from stage N1 to N3 of NREM sleep. Blood pressure decreases as much as 30% [17, 18]. These changes are consistent with decreased metabolic demand during sleep. The drop in blood pressure is mediated by a reduction in cardiac output and a decrease in peripheral vascular resistance. During sleep, the arterial baroreflex has a reduced adjustment point that allows the reduction of blood pressure levels without activation of the sympathetic nervous system [19]. Transient excitation stimuli may give rise to high-amplitude K-complexes in the electroencephalogram during stage N2 of NREM sleep, which may be accompanied by transient explosions in sympathetic activity with brief increases in blood pressure [20].

REM sleep is associated with sympathetic activation. Although REM is a predominantly parasympathetic state, marked fluctuations in autonomic nervous system activity are typically seen. REM sleep can be divided into two distinct patterns: tonic and phasic. The tonic pattern is persistent throughout the sleep stage. On the other hand, the phase component is intermittent, superimposed,

and characterized by explosions of sympathetic activity, fast eye movements, and brief irregular muscle contractions superimposed on muscular atony [17]. Blood pressure is high during REM compared to NREM sleep, particularly during phasic episodes. The increase of sympathetic activation during phasic REM leads to abrupt peaks in blood pressure [17, 18]. Heart rate variability increases during REM [21]. Heart rate during phase REM is faster compared to tonic REM sleep, consistent with sympathetic activation.

4 Endocrine System

The physiology of endocrine and sleep systems interacts in a complex and bidirectional way. In general, sleep and the circadian system modulate endocrine functions following two different patterns: (1) one is the influence of sleep or certain stages of sleep on hormone release; this is an ultradian process, as the frequency of change is greater than once every 24 hours; (2) another is the influence of circadian rhythm. More commonly, a combination of both types is found [22].

Most endocrine functions follow a more or less pronounced circadian rhythm. As sleep usually occurs at night, it becomes difficult to distinguish sleep influences from circadian influences. To elucidate the basis of the mechanisms, experimental protocols with night sleep restriction and daytime sleep periods were evaluated. A classic example of a predominantly circadian system is the hypothalamus-pituitary-adrenal axis (HPA) that determines cortisol release. A classic example of hormone release triggered by sleep is found in the case of growth hormone.

4.1 Hypothalamus-Pituitary-Adrenal Axis

Plasma levels of adrenocorticotropic hormone (ACTH) and cortisol are associated with circadian rhythm. Predisposing to the onset and maintenance of sleep, a decrease in cortisol is found in the late afternoon and evening hours with a minimum around 2–3 h, called cortisol nadir. In the short term, cortisol inhibition is reported to be derived from the onset of sleep. Around dawn, cortisol levels increase in order to prepare the body for the waking state with the peak around awakening. The increase in cortisol levels is linked to the predicted awakening time, as shown by plasma levels of ACTH. The real awakening is followed by an extra pulse of ACTH secretion. In the case of early awakening, time is preceded by real awakening, and the following ACTH pulse is most pronounced as a means of compensation [23]. Inhibition of HPA feedback is attenuated in the sleep state but becomes sensitive again in light sleep and wakefulness. Cortisol pulses occur as an unspecific reaction to excitation stimuli during sleep. However, the total release of cortisol is not reported to differ between sleep deprivation and fragmented and undisturbed sleep [24].

4.2 Growth Hormone

The observation that the growth hormone (GH) secretion is stimulated during sleep in normal adults was made more than 30 years ago [25]. The 24-hour plasma GH profile presents stable low levels interrupted abruptly by secretion outbreaks and the most reproducible pulse occurs soon after the onset of sleep [26]. In normal men, the GH pulse in early sleep is often the only daily episode of active secretion detectable in middle age and adulthood. In women with normal cycling, the daytime pulses of GH are more frequent, and the pulse associated with the onset of sleep, although present in most cases, usually does not take into account most of the release of 24 hours of GH [27].

The onset of sleep causes a pulse in the GH secretion, whether the sleep is advanced, delayed or interrupted, and restarted. There is a consistent relationship between the appearance of delta waves in the EEG and the high concentrations of GH, and its maximum release occurs minutes after the beginning of the slow-wave sleep [28].

4.3 Progesterone

Progesterone is an endogenous steroid hormone commonly produced by the adrenal cortex, as well as the gonads, which consists of the ovaries and testicles. Progesterone is also secreted by the ovarian corpus luteum during the first 10 weeks of pregnancy, followed by the placenta in the later stage of pregnancy. Progesterone is primarily known as the pregnancy hormone in women, and most of its function is related to maintaining pregnancy. It also plays a role in the menstrual cycle, causing hair growth and development as a result of increased vascularity and blood flow.

Evidence indicates that when progesterone is added to the hormone therapy regimen, there is no improvement in sleep [29]. However, there is a possibility that several types of progesterone may affect sleep differently. Montplaisir and collaborators [30] tested the sedative effects of progesterone by comparing hormone therapy with two different progestogens. They found that women treated with micronized progesterone had improved sleep efficiency. On the other hand, a study investigating the effects of estrogen-progestin treatment on pre-menopausal and post-menopausal women's sleep revealed that both groups receiving treatment had a significantly higher number of awakenings than the corresponding placebo group [31]. Also, progesterone is an important respiratory stimulant. Both progesterone [32] and estrogen [33] increase the contractility of the genioglossus, neutralizing the collapsibility of the upper airways during sleep. Progesterone prevents sleep disorders [34] and can therefore stabilize night breathing.

7. Parmeggiani P, Bartsch R, Ivanov P. Physiologic regulation in sleep. In: Kryger M, editor. Physiologic regulation in sleep. Philadelphia: Elsevier Inc.; 2005.
8. Krauchi K, Deboer T. The interrelationship between sleep regulation and thermoregulation. Front Biosci (Landmark Ed). 2010;15:604–25. https://doi.org/10.2741/3636.
9. Harding EC, Franks NP, Wisden W. Sleep and thermoregulation. Curr Opin Physiol. 2020;15:7–13. https://doi.org/10.1016/j.cophys.2019.11.008.
10. Sagot JC, Amoros C, Candas V, Libert JP. Sweating responses and body temperatures during nocturnal sleep in humans. Am J Phys. 1987;252(3 Pt 2):R462–70. https://doi.org/10.1152/ajpregu.1987.252.3.R462.
11. Chowdhuri S, Badr MS. Control of ventilation in health and disease. Chest. 2017;151(4):917–29. https://doi.org/10.1016/j.chest.2016.12.002.
12. Newton K, Malik V, Lee-Chiong T. Sleep and breathing. Clin Chest Med. 2014;35(3):451–6. https://doi.org/10.1016/j.ccm.2014.06.001.
13. Long X, Foussier J, Fonseca P, Haakma R, Aarts RM. Respiration amplitude analysis for REM and NREM sleep classification. Annu Int Conf IEEE Eng Med Biol Soc. 2013;2013:5017–20. https://doi.org/10.1109/EMBC.2013.6610675.
14. Gould GA, Gugger M, Molloy J, Tsara V, Shapiro CM, Douglas NJ. Breathing pattern and eye movement density during REM sleep in humans. Am Rev Respir Dis. 1988;138(4):874–7. https://doi.org/10.1164/ajrccm/138.4.874.
15. McNicholas WT. Impact of sleep on respiratory muscle function. Monaldi Arch Chest Dis. 2002;57(5–6):277–80.
16. Snyder F, Hobson JA, Morrison DF, Goldfrank F. Changes in respiration, heart rate, and systolic blood pressure in human sleep. J Appl Physiol. 1964;19:417–22. https://doi.org/10.1152/jappl.1964.19.3.417.
17. Somers VK, Dyken ME, Mark AL, Abboud FM. Sympathetic-nerve activity during sleep in normal subjects. N Engl J Med. 1993;328(5):303–7. https://doi.org/10.1056/NEJM199302043280502.
18. Mancia G. Autonomic modulation of the cardiovascular system during sleep. N Engl J Med. 1993;328(5):347–9. https://doi.org/10.1056/NEJM199302043280511.
19. Conway J, Boon N, Jones JV, Sleight P. Involvement of the baroreceptor reflexes in the changes in blood pressure with sleep and mental arousal. Hypertension. 1983;5(5):746–8. https://doi.org/10.1161/01.hyp.5.5.746.
20. Hornyak M, Cejnar M, Elam M, Matousek M, Wallin BG. Sympathetic muscle nerve activity during sleep in man. Brain. 1991;114(Pt 3):1281–95. https://doi.org/10.1093/brain/114.3.1281.
21. Boudreau P, Yeh WH, Dumont GA, Boivin DB. Circadian variation of heart rate variability across sleep stages. Sleep. 2013;36(12):1919–28. https://doi.org/10.5665/sleep.3230.
22. Morgan D, Tsai SC. Sleep and the endocrine system. Sleep Med Clin. 2016;11(1):115–26. https://doi.org/10.1016/j.jsmc.2015.10.002.
23. Born J, Hansen K, Marshall L, Mölle M, Fehm HL. Timing the end of nocturnal sleep. Nature. 1999;397(6714):29–30. https://doi.org/10.1038/16166.
24. Späth-Schwalbe E, Gofferje M, Kern W, Born J, Fehm HL. Sleep disruption alters nocturnal ACTH and cortisol secretory patterns. Biol Psychiatry. 1991;29(6):575–84. https://doi.org/10.1016/0006-3223(91)90093-2.
25. Van Cauter E, Plat L. Physiology of growth hormone secretion during sleep. J Pediatr. 1996;128(5 Pt 2):S32–7. https://doi.org/10.1016/s0022-3476(96)70008-2.
26. Steiger A. Neurochemical regulation of sleep. J Psychiatr Res. 2007;41(7):537–52. https://doi.org/10.1016/j.jpsychires.2006.04.007.
27. Latta F, Leproult R, Tasali E, Hofmann E, L'Hermite-Balériaux M, Copinschi G, et al. Sex differences in nocturnal growth hormone and prolactin secretion in healthy older adults: relationships with sleep EEG variables. Sleep. 2005;28(12):1519–24. https://doi.org/10.1093/sleep/28.12.1519.
28. Obal F, Krueger JM. GHRH and sleep. Sleep Med Rev. 2004;8(5):367–77. https://doi.org/10.1016/j.smrv.2004.03.005.

29. Natale V, Albertazzi P, Zini M, Di Micco R. Exploration of cyclical changes in memory and mood in postmenopausal women taking sequential combined oestrogen and progestogen preparations. BJOG. 2001;108(3):286–90. https://doi.org/10.1111/j.1471-0528.2001.00070.x.
30. Montplaisir J, Lorrain J, Denesle R, Petit D. Sleep in menopause: differential effects of two forms of hormone replacement therapy. Menopause. 2001;8(1):10–6. https://doi.org/10.1097/00042192-200101000-00004.
31. Kalleinen N, Polo O, Himanen SL, Joutsen A, Polo-Kantola P. The effect of estrogen plus progestin treatment on sleep: a randomized, placebo-controlled, double-blind trial in premenopausal and late postmenopausal women. Climacteric. 2008;11(3):233–43. https://doi.org/10.1080/13697130802112033.
32. Popovic RM, White DP. Upper airway muscle activity in normal women: influence of hormonal status. J Appl Physiol (1985). 1998;84(3):1055–62. https://doi.org/10.1152/jappl.1998.84.3.1055.
33. Hou YX, Jia SS, Liu YH. 17beta-estradiol accentuates contractility of rat genioglossal muscle via regulation of estrogen receptor alpha. Arch Oral Biol. 2010;55(4):309–17. https://doi.org/10.1016/j.archoralbio.2010.02.002.
34. Caufriez A, Leproult R, L'Hermite-Balériaux M, Kerkhofs M, Copinschi G. Progesterone prevents sleep disturbances and modulates GH, TSH, and melatonin secretion in postmenopausal women. J Clin Endocrinol Metab. 2011;96(4):E614–23. https://doi.org/10.1210/jc.2010-2558.
35. Marrama P, Carani C, Baraghini GF, Volpe A, Zini D, Celani MF, et al. Circadian rhythm of testosterone and prolactin in the ageing. Maturitas. 1982;4(2):131–8. https://doi.org/10.1016/0378-5122(82)90039-1.
36. Schiavi RC, White D, Mandeli J. Pituitary-gonadal function during sleep in healthy aging men. Psychoneuroendocrinology. 1992;17(6):599–609. https://doi.org/10.1016/0306-4530(92)90018-3.
37. Luboshitzky R, Herer P, Levi M, Shen-Orr Z, Lavie P. Relationship between rapid eye movement sleep and testosterone secretion in normal men. J Androl. 1999;20(6):731–7.
38. Grandner MA, Kripke DF, Naidoo N, Langer RD. Relationships among dietary nutrients and subjective sleep, objective sleep, and napping in women. Sleep Med. 2010;11(2):180–4. https://doi.org/10.1016/j.sleep.2009.07.014.
39. Brondel L, Romer MA, Nougues PM, Touyarou P, Davenne D. Acute partial sleep deprivation increases food intake in healthy men. Am J Clin Nutr. 2010;91(6):1550–9. https://doi.org/10.3945/ajcn.2009.28523.
40. Izadi V, Saraf-Bank S, Azadbakht L. Dietary intakes and leptin concentrations. ARYA Atheroscler. 2014;10(5):266–72.
41. Mullington JM, Chan JL, Van Dongen HP, Szuba MP, Samaras J, Price NJ, et al. Sleep loss reduces diurnal rhythm amplitude of leptin in healthy men. J Neuroendocrinol. 2003;15(9):851–4. https://doi.org/10.1046/j.1365-2826.2003.01069.x.
42. Schmid SM, Hallschmid M, Jauch-Chara K, Born J, Schultes B. A single night of sleep deprivation increases ghrelin levels and feelings of hunger in normal-weight healthy men. J Sleep Res. 2008;17(3):331–4. https://doi.org/10.1111/j.1365-2869.2008.00662.x.
43. Eckerbom P, Hansell P, Cox E, Buchanan C, Weis J, Palm F, et al. Circadian variation in renal blood flow and kidney function in healthy volunteers monitored with noninvasive magnetic resonance imaging. Am J Physiol Renal Physiol. 2020;319(6):F966–F78. https://doi.org/10.1152/ajprenal.00311.2020.
44. Maung SC, El Sara A, Chapman C, Cohen D, Cukor D. Sleep disorders and chronic kidney disease. World J Nephrol. 2016;5(3):224–32. https://doi.org/10.5527/wjn.v5.i3.224.
45. Adeseun GA, Rosas SE. The impact of obstructive sleep apnea on chronic kidney disease. Curr Hypertens Rep. 2010;12(5):378–83. https://doi.org/10.1007/s11906-010-0135-1.
46. Moore JG, Englert E. Circadian rhythm of gastric acid secretion in man. Nature. 1970;226(5252):1261–2. https://doi.org/10.1038/2261261a0.
47. Feldman M, Richardson CT. Total 24-hour gastric acid secretion in patients with duodenal ulcer. Comparison with normal subjects and effects of cimetidine and parietal cell vagotomy. Gastroenterology. 1986;90(3):540–4. https://doi.org/10.1016/0016-5085(86)91106-6.

Part III
Physiotherapeutic Management of Sleep Disturbances

Table 1 Diagnostic criteria for chronic insomnia disorder according to ICSD-3

A. The patient reports, or the patient's parent or caregiver observes, one or more of the following: Difficulty initiating sleep Difficulty maintaining sleep Waking up earlier than the desired schedule Difficulty sleeping without parent or caregiver intervention
B. The patient reports, or the patient's parent or caregiver observes, one or more of the following related to the nighttime sleep difficulty: Fatigue Attention, concentration, or memory impairment Impaired social, family, occupational, or academic performance Mood disturbance/irritability Daytime sleepiness Behavioral problems (e.g., hyperactivity, impulsivity, aggression) Reduced motivation/energy/initiative Proneness for errors/accidents Concerns about or dissatisfaction with sleep
C. The reported sleep/wake complaints cannot be explained purely by an inadequate opportunity (i.e., enough time is allotted for sleep) or inadequate circumstances (i.e., the environment is safe, dark, quiet, and comfortable) for sleep
D. The sleep disturbance and associated daytime symptoms occur at least 3 times per week
E. The sleep disturbance and associated daytime symptoms have been present for at least 3 months
F. The sleep/wake difficulty is not better explained by another sleep disorder

The prevalence of insomnia varies between 10% and 30%, sometimes reaching 60% in some countries [2, 3]. Insomnia complaints were found in 45% of the population, while insomnia diagnosis was found in 32% of the Brazilian population [4]. It is important to emphasize that the complaint of dissatisfaction with sleep is not characterized as a diagnosis of insomnia. Insomnia can be a symptom, an isolated one, a secondary one due to a medication, an event (e.g., marriage), or a stressor factor (e.g., death). Therefore, insomnia complaints may not characterize a diagnosis of insomnia (Fig. 1).

Diagnosis of insomnia disorder is clinical, made by a physician, and requires clinical examination. The recommended procedure for the diagnostic management of insomnia disorder and its co-morbidities by the European Guideline for the Diagnosis and Treatment *of Insomnia* [5] incorporates medical history and examination (anamnesis, present somatic disorders, medication, alcohol, caffeine, nicotine, illegal drugs); physical examination; laboratory testing (e.g., blood count, thyroid, hepatic and renal parameters, c-reactive protein test, hemoglobin, ferritin, and vitamin B12); ECG, EEG, CT/MRT and circadian markers if necessary (melatonin, core body temperature); psychiatric/psychological history; former and present mental disorders; personality factors; work and partnership situation; interpersonal conflicts; and sleep history, including triggering factors; information from bed partner (periodic limb movements during sleep, pauses in breathing); work time/circadian factors (shift- and night-work, phase advance, delay); sleep-wake pattern, including daytime sleep (sleep diary for 10–14 days is strongly

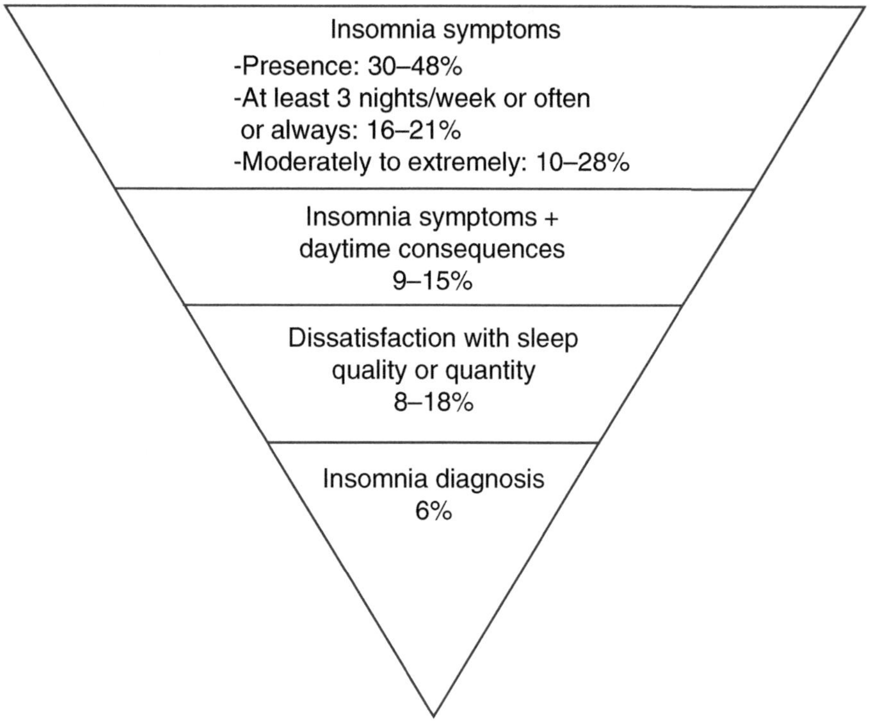

Fig. 1 Prevalence (average in the general population) of symptoms and diagnosis of insomnia. (Reprinted with permission from Ohayon [1])

recommended, which is a simple tool and very efficient that helps in the diagnosis of insomnia as it demonstrates the sleep routine of the patient); and actigraphy (if there is clinical suspicion of irregular sleep-wake schedules or circadian rhythm disorders, as it may also help with the follow-up of patients with insomnia, being useful to rule out circadian rhythm disorders, which may sometimes be confused with insomnia). Polysomnography is not usually indicated, except for ruling out other sleep disorders.

Despite polysomnography (PSG) not being indicated for insomnia diagnosis, many investigations focused on the macrostructure (the cycling between NREM and REM periods) and microstructure (power spectral analysis of the sleep EEG, a method that can be used to quantify the amount of frequency power in a specific frequency band, including arousals and specific elements) of sleep to better understand insomnia. PSG findings in insomnia patients demonstrate reduced sleep duration, long-lasting sleep-onset latencies, increased number of nocturnal awakenings and amount of time awake during the night, and reduced N3 NREM and R stages [6]. Other findings were characterized by an increased frequency of brief events, for instance, shifts in sleep stages between NREM and REM sleep, and among NREM stages (i.e., N1, N2, N3), brief periods of awakening, and microarousals (brief and transient changes in EEG frequency suggestive of an awake state), and not by enormously long periods of wakefulness [7]. Other investigations failed to deliver objective changes in insomnia disorder or no clinically significant changes in PSG macrostructure. But, when analyzing the microstructure of sleep in, within both NREM and REM periods, a disorder of the switch between sleep and wakefulness can be found, as patients with insomnia havc the most pronounced differences in the EEG fast frequency range (β power), compared with healthy sleepers [8] (Fig. 2).

Insomnia has been suggested to be a transitional state between "normal" sleep and "objectively verifiable" insomnia, leading to the use of terms such as "sleep misperception," "pseudoinsomnia," or "paradoxical insomnia." Polysomnographic investigations have shown that insomniacs often underestimate their total sleep time

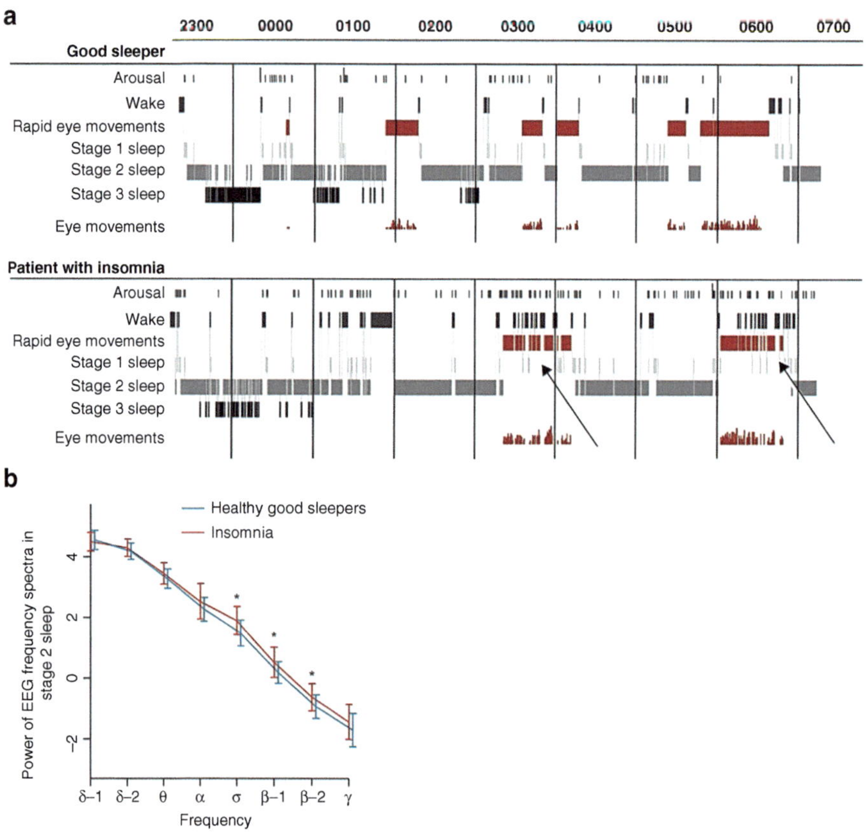

Fig. 2 Polysomnographic and power density differences between good and poor sleepers. (**a**) Comparison of the polysomnogram of a good sleeper and a patient with insomnia. With respect to the macrostructure of sleep, the sleep pattern of this patient with insomnia is mostly intact – the disturbance is mainly expressed through an increased frequency of stage shifts and increased brief waking periods and microarousals (arrows); (**b**) Asterisks show significant ($p < 0.05$) alterations in the sleep electroencephalogram of patients with insomnia as compared with healthy good sleepers, as shown by enhanced power in fast frequencies (derived from spectral analysis). (Reprinted with permission from Riemann et al. [9])

and sleep efficiency while overestimating the time it takes them to fall asleep [10]. Therefore, we may have a lack of correlation between objective findings of a PSG examination and subjective complaints of the patient, leading to a mismatch – a discrepancy between PSG outcomes and the patient's complaints and perception of sleep.

Insomnia is a risk factor for several diseases, such as arterial hypertension, myocardial infarction and chronic heart failure [11, 12], cardiovascular diseases [8, 13], type 2 diabetes [14], neurodegenerative disease, especially dementia [8], and also brain disorders [15]. Psychiatric disorders are among the most common comorbidities in insomnia, as it is present in most people; among them, the most common include substance use disorders and mood disorders. Clinical diseases and sleep disorders can also trigger or aggravate insomnia episodes, such as hyperthyroidism, fibromyalgia, sleep apnea, restless legs syndrome, mood disturbances such as anxiety and depression, and chronic pain [8, 16]. Furthermore, insomnia associated with short sleep duration (sleep <6 h) is associated with hypervigilance, increased physiological stimulation, and cardiometabolic and neurocognitive morbidities [8].

1 Pathophysiology

The pathophysiology of insomnia is not entirely clear; there seems little doubt that a self-sustaining cycle of misperception, apprehension about sleeplessness and its consequences, an exaggerated focus on sleep, and the concomitant physiological and cognitive processes accompanying these conditions are key components in the evolution and maintenance of many forms of chronic insomnia and, therefore, must be addressed.

The etiology and pathophysiology of insomnia involve genetic, environmental, behavioral, and physiological factors that culminate in cerebral hyperexcitation, causing this *"on"* and system to be unbalanced, leaving the patient in a state of hypervigilance. Evidence of hyperexcitation in insomnia includes high metabolic rate during sleep and wakefulness, elevation of cortisol and adrenocorticotropic hormone during the initial sleep period, heart rate variability, and high frequency of EEG activity during sleep. Functional imaging studies demonstrate minor differences between wakefulness and sleep in regional brain metabolism in individuals with insomnia disorder compared to people without insomnia [17].

From the perspective of behavioral science, the multidimensional model of chronic insomnia "3P" helps explain how acute insomnia becomes chronic, establishes the basis for evaluating insomnia in individual patients, and focuses on predisposing, precipitating (triggering), and perpetuating factors in the long-term evolution of insomnia [18]. Predisposing factors, which are generally not modifiable, include genetic and personality characteristics (for example, being worrisome, family history of unsatisfactory sleep), leading to physiological and cognitive hyperexcitation. Precipitating factors that trigger insomnia are typically stressful events, such as problems related to health, family, work or school, and anxiety [8].

Insomnia: Physiotherapeutic Approach

Carolina Vicaria Rodrigues D'Aurea, Giselle Soares Passos, and Cristina Frange

1 The Role of Physical Therapy in Insomnia Disorder

Physiotherapy can act on chronic insomnia as adjuvant treatment or, in some cases, being the treatment per se, depending on the type of insomnia, duration, clinical condition of the patient, and various contextual issues. A priori, the physiotherapist should consider how insomnia negatively affects the physical condition and overall health of the patient, but certainly how the physical condition interferes with insomnia, which can help to direct physiotherapy intervention. For example, a patient complaining of knee pain and telling the physiotherapist that he will need a surgical approach may not be able to sleep well from the moment of injury (or surgical indication). This may direct the physiotherapist to focus on pre-surgical interventions that can control pain, prepare local condition (knee), and improve the patient's sleep pattern *before* surgery.

Insomnia may result from an acute or chronic condition, and it will negatively impact the rehabilitation process. Insomnia may be a symptom of a disease, and depending on the diagnosis, the physiotherapeutic approach will be different. In the above example, insomnia in conjunction with the knee injury may generate kinesiophobia, pain, and fear from the surgery and the whole process, which could disrupt

C. V. R. D'Aurea (✉)
Hospital Israelita Albert Einstein, São Paulo, SP, Brazil

G. S. Passos
Health Sciences, Universidade Federal de Jataí, Jataí, Goiás, Brazil

C. Frange
Department of Neurology and Neurosurgery, Escola Paulista de Medicina, Universidade Federal de São Paulo, São Paulo, SP, Brazil

Certified in Sleep Physiotherapy by the Brazilian Sleep Society (ABS), and The Brazilian Association of Cardiorespiratory Physiotherapy and Physiotherapy in Intensive Care (ASSOBRAFIR), São Paulo, SP, Brazil

World Physiotherapy Network for Health Promotion in Life and Work, São Paulo, SP, Brazil

C. Frange, F. M. S. Coelho (eds.), *Sleep Medicine and Physical Therapy*,
https://doi.org/10.1007/978-3-030-85074-6_7

sleep and generate many thoughts as the patient goes to sleep. The patient may refer that he began with this knee pain a long time ago, and since then sleep was unrefreshing and fragmented and has worsened a lot after the surgery suggestion. He also may report concerns about the surgery, the rehabilitation process, functional difficulties such as walking and getting up/sitting, and getting back to work and social life. So, every night he stays in bed, thinking about the possibilities that may happen and fearing them. The next day, he feels more pain, tired, exhausted, anxious, and sleepy. Along the time, he starts to feel depressed. This clinical picture is often frequent and demands a need for investigation of the insomnia etiology (and in this case, refer the patient to a sleep specialist physician). The purpose here for physiotherapy is to indicate a therapeutic program to achieve the treatment objectives, not only for the pain and the knee itself (strength, flexibility, range of motion, etc.) but also for insomnia. These approaches will prepare the knee and the body as a whole for surgery and for the rehabilitation process and to dissociate the sleep-pain relationship that has been established in this patient (see Chap. 28 for more on sleep and pain relationship). Thus, the physiotherapist can treat insomnia, whether being a symptom or a disease, as an adjuvant or complementary treatment, by using many non-pharmacological resources.

The treatment of insomnia disorder is mainly cognitive and should include sleep hygiene, physical activities such as exercise, increasing the activities at work and at home (climbing stairs instead of the elevator, walking instead of driving, etc.), light therapy mindfulness, and manual therapies, such as acupuncture and soft tissue massage.

2 Cognitive Behavioral Therapy for Insomnia (CBT-I)

Current guidelines have indicated cognitive behavioral therapy for insomnia (CBT-I) as a first-line choice for the treatment of insomnia [1]. CBT-I is a structured program that aids patients to recognize and change thoughts and behaviors that cause or worsen sleep issues with habits that promote sleep, affecting the ability to sleep. CBT-I works with the precipitating, predisposing, and perpetuating factors of insomnia, intending to break the cycle of negative emotions, thoughts, and behaviors related to sleep (or the lack of). Pharmacological intervention should be adopted by a physician in case of failure or impossibility of CBT-I treatment [1, 2]. A detailed sleep diary for 10–14 days may help the patient to understand his/her sleep issue. CBT-I works with some techniques that will be defined by the physiotherapist according to the patient's need and can be seen in detail in Chap. 31.

To be considered effective, non-pharmacological therapies should reduce sleep onset latency and fragmented sleep, and the daytime repercussions such as sleepiness, unrefreshing feeling, and lack of concentration increase total sleep time [3]. However, very often, therapies may not demonstrate altered objective outcomes. The therapies can have positive impacts on patients' functional complaints, reducing symptoms of anxiety and depression and improving quality of life.

3 Sleep Hygiene

Sleep hygiene is the most widely used behavioral intervention in the treatment of insomnia [4, 5]. This method was developed to guide patients about healthy habits to promote sleep and prevent and treat insomnia (and many other sleep disturbances). Nevertheless, it has become a behavioral treatment for chronic insomnia. This technique can be combined with other resources, and the patient must understand why changes in his/her habits are needed (please refer to Chap. 31).

4 Physical Exercise

Epidemiological studies have described the influence of physical activity [6] and physical inactivity [7] in the natural history of insomnia. Some conditions such as low physical health, depressed mood, and low levels of physical activity were risk factors for the incidence of insomnia; physical activity was highlighted as a protective factor for the evolution of insomnia [6].

In recent decades, the regular practice of physical exercises has been studied as a treatment for insomnia [8]. The exercise characteristics such as type, intensity, duration, and time of the day practiced, as well as the mechanisms responsible for improvements in sleep, have been investigated in clinical studies. Studies investigating the acute effect of physical exercise on insomnia disorder have identified that acute moderate-intensity aerobic exercise is effective in improving sleep and reducing pre-sleep anxiety when performed in the late afternoon [9], and acute morning exercise can improve nocturnal sleep quality in individuals with difficulty initiating sleep, especially during the latter part of the night [10] (Table 1). For the chronic effect of exercise on insomnia disorder, aerobic exercises performed at moderate intensity [11–13], resistance exercise (i.e., muscle strength) performed at moderate intensity, and stretching [14] have been considered effective (Table 2).

Some mechanisms that can explain the effects of exercise on sleep are as follows:

- Thermogenic effect [15–18]: according to this theory, the increase in central temperature caused by exercise would facilitate the onset of sleep due to heat activation by hypothalamus-controlled dissipation mechanisms. Patients with insomnia presented a reduction of nocturnal temperature [19].
- Anxiety reduction: anxiety is one of the markers of insomnia; reducing it via exercise could improve sleep quality [20], and this effect has been observed in patients with insomnia [9].
- *Serotonin increase* (*5-hydroxytryptamine, 5-HT*): chronic insomnia may be the result of a serotonergic deficit [21]. Acute exercise (running) increased the synthesis of 5-HT [22].
- *Antidepressant effect*: there exists evidence on the chronic effects of physical exercise on depression in insomnia [11–13, 23], which correlated with improvement in sleep quality [11, 12].

Table 2 (continued)

Study	Number of sessions	Population	Intervention	Outcomes	Results
Hartescu et al. [13]	6 months (a monitored program of ≥150 min of moderate- to vigorous-intensity physical activity per week)	Average age and women/men: Intervention: 60.10–15/6; Control: 59.50–15/5.	150 minutes of physical activity, moderate to vigorous, per week vs. no exercise (control)	ISI Epworth Sleepiness Scale EuroQoL5D-5 L	The physical activity group showed significantly reduced insomnia symptom severity, with an average reduction of four points on the Insomnia Severity Index and significantly reduced depression and anxiety scores
Reid et al. [12]	Chronic insomnia patients 16 weeks (4 times/week)	Average age and women/men: Intervention: 62–10/0; Control: 63.5–6/1.	Aerobic physical activity plus sleep hygiene vs. sleep hygiene only	PSQI Epworth Sleepiness Scale SF-36	The physical activity group improved in sleep quality on the global PSQI, SOL, sleep duration, daytime dysfunction, and SE (PSQI sub-scores compared to the control group). The physical activity group also had reductions in depressive symptoms, daytime sleepiness, and improvements in vitality compared to baseline scores
Passos et al. [23]	Chronic insomnia patients 4 months (3 times/week)	Homens/women Age 30–55 years	MAE, baseline vs. post-exercise	PSG PSQI BDI Cortisol Immune system	PSG: reduction on SOL, WASO, and REM latency and increase on TST, SE, and in the percentage of REM sleep. Latency of stages 2, 3, and 4 decreased significantly. Decrease in PSQI score, depression, cortisol, CD4, and CD8 and increased in apoA

(continued)

Table 2 (continued)

Study	Number of sessions	Population	Intervention	Outcomes	Results
Passos et al. [11]	Chronic insomnia patients 6 months (3 times/week)	Homens/ women Age 30–55 years	MAE, baseline vs. post-exercise	PSG Sleep diary POMS SF-36	Polysomnographic data shows a significant decrease in SOL and WASO and a significant increase in SE. Data from sleep diaries revealed significant improvement in SOL, sleep quality, and feeling rested in the morning. Some quality-of-life measures improved significantly and a significant decrease in the POMS measures of tension-anxiety, depression, and total mood disturbance

ACT actigraphy, *HAE* high-intensity aerobic exercise, *MAE* moderate-intensity aerobic exercise, *MRE* moderate-intensity resistance exercise, *DIS* difficulty in initiating sleep, *EMA* early morning awakening, *apoA* plasma apolipoprotein A, *RCT* randomized controlled trial, *SE* sleep efficiency, *ISI* Insomnia Severity Index, *BDI* Beck Depression Inventory, *POMS* profile of mood states, *PSG* polysomnography, *PSQI* Pittsburgh Sleep Quality Index, *REM* rapid eye movement, *SF-36* Short Form Health Survey-36, *SWS* slow-wave sleep, *WASO* wake time after sleep onset, *TST* total sleep time, *SOL* sleep onset latency, *TWT* total wake time

(PSG), such as total sleep time, sleep efficiency, sleep latency, and WASO. Unfortunately, this data obtained was considered exceptionally low quality of evidence, due to the heterogeneity of the investigations that composed the meta-analysis.

In general, the studies cited have low reliability, and there are several potential limitations, such as methodological limitations, small sample sizes, more women at old age, and a predominance of moderate-intensity aerobic exercise, among others. Moreover, the absence of data (and protocols) on the characteristics of physical exercises such as a place of practice, time of the day practiced, frequency, duration, type of supervision, and individual or group makes it impossible to infer whether these variables influenced the results of the meta-analysis [29–31].

5 Light Therapy

Several studies have identified the effectiveness of light therapy for patients with insomnia, mainly in those with difficulty starting sleep (initial insomnia) [32]. The treatment consists of luminous stimulation shortly after awakening, from a light box with blue wavelength, positioned at eye level, at an approximate distance of 75 cm [32]. For the treatment of insomnia, the power of light is 10,000 lux [32], applied between 30 minutes and 2 hours [33]. Exposure to light in the early morning will facilitate sleep at the beginning of the evening [34]. Additionally, in patients with Parkinson's disease and insomnia disorder, a recent study showed that 1 hour of exposure to light, just before retiring/leaving the job market, significantly improved insomnia. Still, light therapy reduced symptoms of other sleep disorders such as REM sleep behavioral disorder by 1 month after the start of light therapy. Furthermore, improvements were maintained while light therapy was continued, for a period of 4–6 years, showing the importance of treating insomnia adjunct to Parkinson's disease [35], for example.

There is little evidence about phototherapeutic treatment in physiotherapy. According to the *European Guideline for the Diagnosis and Treatment of Insomnia*, published in 2017, the level of and evidence of the use of light therapy for insomnia is of low quality, and its recommendation is weak to be used as a single treatment. However, even in the face of these cautions, light therapy is a promising treatment for insomnia, used concomitantly with other treatments [1], still needing more studies in specific populations for a better understanding of its mechanisms and the possible creation of a consensus.

6 Massage

The search for manual therapies has been growing considerably, including massage. From constant skin stimuli on the body surface, touch, pressure, heat, vibration, and pain receptors are activated and transported to the somatic, autonomous, and central systems, triggering important neurochemical reactions [36]. The effects of massage on the circulatory, lymphatic, and muscular systems are already well established [37, 38]. Massage improves visceral functioning and restores body homeostasis.

Massage is pointed out as a pleasant intervention, as it promotes relaxation and sleep [39], as well by patients with insomnia to treat sleep complaints [40]. For instance, when investigating the severity of insomnia related to the postmenopausal period, the authors identified an improvement in the quality of sleep after the massage, as all participants fell asleep more quickly and reported better well-being upon awakening – probably due to the activation of the autonomous nervous system. Polysomnographic findings showed a decrease in REM sleep latency and an increase in the NREM stage N3 (slow-wave sleep) [37, 38].

In a multicenter investigation, massage was applied for the treatment of insomnia, and after subjective evaluations of symptoms, 96% of participants reported significant improvement of insomnia [41]. Despite some findings, massage alone is not recommended for the treatment of chronic insomnia due to an exceptionally low level of evidence [1]. However, due to few side effects and its high power of relaxation, massage can be used adjunctly to the treatment of insomnia.

7 Acupuncture

Acupuncture is an ancient technique of traditional Chinese medicine. Its effectiveness in the treatment of chronic insomnia has been described in several systematic reviews [42, 43]. For specific acupuncture points for insomnia, please see [42].

Some mechanisms have been suggested to explain the effects of acupuncture on sleep: acupuncture affects the central nervous system through structures in the spinal cord and the brain that regulate some neurotransmitters such as dopamine, norepinephrine, and acetylcholine [44]. Acupuncture can increase nocturnal melatonin secretion [45]. However, acupuncture alone is not recommended for the treatment of chronic insomnia due to the level of evidence [1].

8 Mindfulness

Many individuals with insomnia have sought alternative medicine and complement different approaches to try to expand the result of the various treatments already proposed. Data from the 2007 *National Health Interview Survey* (NHIS) indicate that 45% of adults with insomnia symptoms use some type of alternative medicine annually [46]. The physiotherapist can also act with the practice of mindfulness.

During mindfulness, the person intentionally seeks to "be attentive with his inner, thoughts and emotions," as well as the external perceptions that occur at present, without applying any form of judgment to them [47, 48]. The practitioner begins to observe the events that occur in his/her mind and let them go, without judgments, reflections, or desire to change the things that are happening around him/her.

The practice of mindfulness began in Eastern traditions, and the practice of meditation is considered a key point for its realization. This technique has been used in several clinical protocols, and its applicability in insomnia has been increasingly frequent, with encouraging results. Most sleep research has applied two types of interventions: mindfulness-based cognitive therapy (MBCT) and mindfulness-based stress reduction (MBSR) [47].

Some studies suggest that the practice of mindfulness can improve the quality and the amount of sleep in individuals with insomnia. The results are promising and point out that this method can significantly reduce the severity of insomnia, sleep latency, and pre-sleep hyperstimulation (presented in most patients with insomnia). Other benefits such as increased total sleep time, sleep efficiency, and sleep quality have already been reported by individuals with chronic insomnia after practicing mindfulness [48–51].

In addition, mindfulness is effective in secondary insomnia and in individuals who present other comorbidities such as cancer, depression, anxiety, and obesity [52–54]. The interesting fact is that mindfulness is a process of learning self-regularization of the body itself, of its emotions and needs, and, after learning, can be practiced whenever needed. For example, women in the postmenopausal period with insomnia demonstrated, after the practice of mindfulness, excellent results in

12. Reid KJ, et al. Aerobic exercise improves self-reported sleep and quality of life in older adults with insomnia. Sleep Med. 2010;11(9):934–40.
13. Hartescu I, Morgan K, Stevinson CD. Increased physical activity improves sleep and mood outcomes in inactive people with insomnia: a randomized controlled trial. J Sleep Res. 2015;24(5):526–34.
14. D'Aurea CVR, et al. Effects of resistance exercise training and stretching on chronic insomnia. Braz J Psychiat. 2019;41(1):51–7.
15. Horne JA, L.H. Staff. Exercise and sleep: body-heating effects. Sleep. 1983;6(1):36–46.
16. Horne JA, Moore VJ. Sleep EEG effects of exercise with and without additional body cooling. Electroencephalogr Clin Neurophysiol. 1985;60(1):33–8.
17. Murphy PJ, Campbell SS. Nighttime drop in body temperature: a physiological trigger for sleep onset? Sleep. 1997;20(7):505–11.
18. Krauchi K, et al. Warm feet promote the rapid onset of sleep. Nature. 1999;401(6748):36–7.
19. Glotzbach SF, Heller HC. Temperature regulation. In: Roth T, Kryger MH, Dement WC, editors. Principles and practice of sleep medicine. Philadelphia: W.B. Saunders Co; 1994. p. 260–75.
20. Herring MP, O'Connor PJ, Dishman RK. The effect of exercise training on anxiety symptoms among patients: a systematic review. Arch Intern Med. 2010;170(4):321–31.
21. Petitjean F, et al. Insomnia caused by administration of para-chlorophenylalanine: reversibility by peripheral or central injection of 5-hydroxytryptophan and serotonin. Sleep. 1985;8(1):56–67.
22. Chaouloff F. Effects of acute physical exercise on central serotonergic systems. Med Sci Sports Exerc. 1997;29(1):58–62.
23. Passos GS, et al. Exercise improves immune function, antidepressive response, and sleep quality in patients with chronic primary insomnia. Biomed Res Int. 2014;2014:1–7.
24. Nehlsen-Cannarella SL, et al. The effects of moderate exercise training on immune response. Med Sci Sports Exerc. 1991;23(1):64–70.
25. Motivala SJ, et al. Inflammatory markers and sleep disturbance in major depression. Psychosom Med. 2005;67(2):187–94.
26. Hall M, et al. Sleep as a mediator of the stress-immune relationship. Psychosom Med. 1998;60(1):48–51.
27. Cover H, Irwin M. Immunity and depression: insomnia, retardation, and reduction of natural killer cell activity. J Behav Med. 1994;17(2):217–23.
28. Savard J, et al. Chronic insomnia and immune functioning. Psychosom Med. 2003;65(2):211–21.
29. Rubio-Arias JA, et al. Effect of exercise on sleep quality and insomnia in middle-aged women: a systematic review and meta-analysis of randomized controlled trials. Maturitas. 2017;100:49–56.
30. Banno M, et al. Exercise can improve sleep quality: a systematic review and meta-analysis. PeerJ. 2018;6:e5172.
31. Lowe H, et al. Does exercise improve sleep for adults with insomnia? A systematic review with quality appraisal. Clin Psychol Rev. 2019;68:1–12.
32. Kirisoglu C, Guilleminault C. Twenty minutes versus forty-five minutes morning bright light treatment on sleep onset insomnia in elderly subjects. J Psychosom Res. 2004;56(5):537–42.
33. Passos GS, et al. Nonpharmacologic treatment of chronic insomnia. Rev Bras Psiquiatr. 2007;29(3):279–82.
34. Rosenthal NE, et al. Phase-shifting effects of bright morning light as treatment for delayed sleep phase syndrome. Sleep. 1990;13(4):354–61.
35. Martino JK, Freelance CB, Willis GL. The effect of light exposure on insomnia and nocturnal movement in Parkinson's disease: an open label, retrospective, longitudinal study. Sleep Med. 2018;44:24–31.
36. Goats GC. Massage--the scientific basis of an ancient art: Part 2. Physiological and therapeutic effects. Br J Sports Med. 1994;28(3):153–6.

37. Oliveira D, et al. Effect of massage in postmenopausal women with insomnia: a pilot study. Clinics (Sao Paulo). 2011;66(2):343–6.
38. Oliveira DS, et al. Effect of therapeutic massage on insomnia and climacteric symptoms in postmenopausal women. Climacteric. 2012;15(1):21–9.
39. Song RH, Kim DH. The effects of foot reflexion massage on sleep disturbance, depression disorder and the physiological index of the elderly. Taehan Kanho Hakhoe Chi. 2006;36:10.
40. Newton KM, et al. Use of alternative therapies for menopause symptoms: results of a population-based survey. Obstet Gynecol. 2002;100(1):18–25.
41. Zhou YF, et al. Multi-central controlled study on three-part massage therapy for treatment of insomnia of deficiency of both the heart and spleen. Zhongguo Zhen Jiu. 2006;26(6):385–8.
42. Yeung WF, et al. Acupressure, reflexology, and auricular acupressure for insomnia: a systematic review of randomized controlled trials. Sleep Med. 2012;13(8):971–84.
43. Shergis J, et al. A systematic review of acupuncture for sleep quality in people with insomnia. Complement Ther Med. 2016;26:11–20.
44. Lin Y. Acupuncture treatment for insomnia and acupuncture analgesia. Psychiatry Clin Neurosci. 1995;49(2):119–20.
45. Spence DW, et al. Acupuncture increases nocturnal melatonin secretion and reduces insomnia and anxiety: a preliminary report. J Neuropsychiatry Clin Neurosci. 2004;16(1):19–28.
46. Bertisch SM, et al. Use of relaxation techniques and complementary and alternative medicine by American adults with insomnia symptoms: results from a national survey. J Clin Sleep Med. 2012;8(6):681–91.
47. Garcia MC, et al. The effects of mindfulness and relaxation training for insomnia (MRTI) on postmenopausal women: a pilot study. Menopause. 2018;25(9):992–1003.
48. Ong JC, et al. A randomized controlled trial of mindfulness meditation for chronic insomnia. Sleep. 2014;37(9):1553–63.
49. Hubbling A, et al. How mindfulness changed my sleep: focus groups with chronic insomnia patients. BMC Complement Altern Med. 2014;14:50.
50. Gross CR, et al. Mindfulness-based stress reduction versus pharmacotherapy for chronic primary insomnia: a randomized controlled clinical trial. Explore (NY). 2011;7(2):76–87.
51. Zhang JX, et al. Mindfulness-based stress reduction for chronic insomnia in adults older than 75 years: a randomized, controlled, single-blind clinical trial. Explore (NY). 2015;11(3):180–5.
52. Adler E, et al. Impact of a mindfulness-based weight-loss intervention on sleep quality among adults with obesity: data from the SHINE randomized controlled trial. J Altern Complement Med. 2017;23(3):188–95.
53. Britton WB, et al. Mindfulness-based cognitive therapy improves polysomnographic and subjective sleep profiles in antidepressant users with sleep complaints. Psychother Psychosom. 2012;81(5):296–304.
54. Yook K, et al. Usefulness of mindfulness-based cognitive therapy for treating insomnia in patients with anxiety disorders: a pilot study. J Nerv Ment Dis. 2008;196(6):501–3.
55. Yang M, et al. Interpreting score differences in the Insomnia Severity Index: using health-related outcomes to define the minimally important difference. Curr Med Res Opin. 2009;25(10):2487–94.
56. Buman MP, et al. Does nighttime exercise really disturb sleep? Results from the 2013 national sleep foundation sleep in America poll. Sleep Med. 2014;15(7):755–61.
57. Flausino NH, et al. Physical exercise performed before bedtime improves the sleep pattern of healthy young good sleepers. Psychophysiology. 2012;49(2):186–92.
58. Hill EE, et al. Exercise and circulating cortisol levels: the intensity threshold effect. J Endocrinol Investig. 2008;31(7):587–91.
59. Youngstedt SD, et al. Testing the sleep hygiene recommendation against nighttime exercise. Sleep Breath. 2021;

Restless Legs Syndrome (Willis-Ekbom Disease) and Periodic Limb Movements of Sleep: An Overview

Ana Carolina Dias Gomes and Fernando Morgadinho Santos Coelho

1 Restless Legs Syndrome/Willis-Ekbom Disease

Restless legs syndrome (RLS) or Willis-Ekbom disease (WED) is a common neurological disease characterized by unpleasant sensations that are relieved with movement and aggravated at night and by rest. The diagnostic criteria are based on the main clinical characteristics of the disease. Polysomnography (PSG) is not usually useful, but complementary exams are needed, especially in the assessment of differential diagnoses [1].

Thomas Willis first described RLS in 1685; however, only in 1945, Karl-Axel Ekbom described the main clinical features and coined the term RLS. For this reason, RLS is also recognized as WED. WED is currently the preferred name because although the lower limbs are most commonly affected, there is an involvement of other regions of the body. In this chapter and the next one, WED will be passed over to RLS for its easy recognition in the literature and current use [2].

The prevalence of RLS ranges from 5% to 10% worldwide. In a study in a Brazilian city, the prevalence of RLS was estimated at 6.4% [2, 3]. The prevalence of clinically significant RLS is 2–3% in Europe and North America. Pediatric prevalence rates are 2–4% in studies in the UK/USA and Turkey [1, 3].

The prevalence rates of RLS increase with age until the end of adulthood, stabilizing or decreasing slightly in the elderly. The prevalence of RLS is higher in older people and in women, but there is no difference between genders until the end of adolescence. Possible justifications for the higher prevalence in adult women

A. C. D. Gomes (✉)
Psychobiology Department, Escola Paulista de Medicina, Universidade Federal de São Paulo, São Paulo, SP, Brazil

F. M. S. Coelho
Neurology and Neurosurgery Department; Department of Psychobiology, Escola Paulista de Medicina, Universidade Federal de São Paulo, São Paulo, SP, Brazil

C. Frange, F. M. S. Coelho (eds.), *Sleep Medicine and Physical Therapy*,
https://doi.org/10.1007/978-3-030-85074-6_8

include women's reports and perceptions differ from men; a hormonal difference; the reduction of iron stores in women; and effect of pregnancy [4].

The strong associations with anxiety, mood disorders, and reduced quality of life indices remain in people of older ages. The diagnostic criteria for restless legs syndrome in elderly people with cognitive impairment have been suggested, but not validated [5].

The diagnostic criteria and the clinical picture of RLS were grouped, characterizing a medical condition, whose diagnostic criteria cover these main clinical features. The diagnosis of RLS is clinical, and all of the items below must be present (Table 1).

RLS, according to the criteria of the *International Classification of Sleep Disorders* (ICSD-3) of 2014, is one of the diagnoses grouped in the chapter "Sleep Movement Disorders," where they are also located periodic limb movements (PLMS), sleep-related leg cramps, sleep-related bruxism, sleep-related rhythmic movement disorder, benign sleep myoclonus, propriospinal myoclonus in early sleep, sleep-related movement disorder due to a disorder medication or substance, and unspecified sleep-related movement disorder.

The diagnosis of RLS is not always obvious; patients often seek medical attention complaining of insomnia and do not report RLS symptoms spontaneously. A significant number of patients, 60% to 90%, have worsened sleep quality and complaints such as difficulty in initiating and maintaining sleep [1].

Another complaint that needs attention is those seen in disturbances of the sleep-wake cycle. Studies that evaluated symptoms based on circadian rhythm show that it is worse at night, regardless of the level of activity. Interestingly, patients who work at night and sleep during the day have their symptoms more tolerable.

Although the legs are the most affected, "restless legs" is an inappropriate name, since 21% to 57% of individuals describe some sensations in the upper limbs [1].

There are many ways to describe these sensations in different languages. References used may vary from one country to another, and, within the same country, regionalisms can influence the way the patient refers to them. It is important to note that the symptoms usually involve both legs, but they generally alternate between the legs and are rarely unilateral [6].

When symptoms are very severe, relief with activity may not be noticeable, as well as worsening at night. In cases of doubt, it is important to ask about symptoms

Table 1 Criteria for diagnosis of restless legs syndrome (*International Classification of Sleep Disorders* (ICSD-3))

A. Need to move the legs almost always accompanied by uncomfortable sensations, most commonly in the legs, that:
A1. Worsens at rest
A2. Improves with movement
A3. Worsens at the end of the day or early evening
B. The symptoms cause worry, distress, worsening sleep quality, or impairment in mental, physical, social, occupational, educational, behavioral, or other important areas
C. The symptoms cannot be explained by another medical or behavioral condition

in the past, as these characteristics have probably been present before. In the most challenging cases, the presence of a family history of RLS and response to dopaminergic drug therapy can help in the diagnosis [1].

PSG is not necessary for diagnosis and should not be ordered routinely; however, it can also help in a few cases. About 80% of patients with RLS have PLMS, whose diagnosis is essentially by PSG (PLMS can be seen in more than 90% of the exams of RLS patients if PSG is repeated). Other objective changes that may be present in PSG are the greater sleep latency and the higher rate of awakenings [7].

The outcome of RLS is different depending on the age of onset of symptoms. Two-thirds of patients who manifest symptoms before the age of 45 (early onset) have a slower progression of symptoms. Familial RLS has an onset of symptoms in the third and fourth decades on average. Adolescents tend to have more severe symptoms than younger children. When symptoms start at an older age, progression tends to be faster, and RLS tends to have many aggravating factors [1].

The most prevalent aggravating factors are iron deficiency, medications, pregnancy, chronic kidney failure, and prolonged immobility. Some drugs that can precipitate or worsen RLS and/or PLMS include sedative antihistamines, centrally active dopamine receptor antagonists, and antidepressants (Table 2). An exception is antidepressant bupropion, with its dopamine-promoting activity.

Complimentary exams are very important and should include at least complete blood count, complete iron profile, biochemistry, renal function, and thyroid function, in addition to the dosage of vitamins B12 and folate.

Pregnancy predisposes to the onset or worsening of RLS symptoms. The third trimester represents the worst period for pregnant women, and the resolution of symptoms, for most women, occurs after delivery. When faced with a pregnant woman with complaints of RLS, one should assess whether there is a family history of RLS or a diagnosis in the past, symptoms during pregnancy, and hemoglobin ≤11 g/dL [1].

In patients with chronic renal failure, the prevalence of RLS is two to five times higher than in the general population. Compared to patients with chronic renal failure without RLS, those with RLS have greater sleep disturbance and report worse quality of life, and many of them interrupt dialysis prematurely. Typically, the symptoms of RLS improve dramatically within a month after kidney transplantation, but they become severe again following the failure of the transplant [1].

OSA patients can increase symptoms of RLS due to sleep fragmentation, generating awakenings, and a higher probability of perception of the symptoms [6].

Table 2 Medications that precipitate or worsen restless legs syndrome

The action of medications that precipitate or worsen RLS	Medications that precipitate or worsen RLS
CNS-acting antihistamines	Dexchlorpheniramine
Dopamine receptor antagonists	Metoclopramide, haloperidol, etc.
Antidepressants (except bupropion)	Citalopram, amitriptyline, venlafaxine

RLS can begin in childhood, and it is essential that the peculiarities of evaluating younger patients are understood. Children can express their discomfort in their limbs very differently from adults: they say, for example, that their legs "need to move" or refer to the presence of insects, tremors, strange or even funny sensations, and tingling, among others. From the age of 6, the descriptors for the symptoms of RLS are more similar to those of adults [1].

It is important to exemplify situations of stillness that can worsen symptoms: sitting in the classroom, reading a book, doing homework, or riding a car, which are everyday situations. The same reasoning extends to the easing of discomfort in the limbs, which is usually achieved when moving, walking, rubbing, or kicking; it is important to try to pay attention to children's vocabulary. A child's drawing of RLS symptoms can be a good clue for diagnosis (Fig. 1). For younger children or those with developmental delay, a diagnosis of PLMS may be the initial diagnosis, with complete symptomatology of RLS evident over time [8].

The A3 diagnostic criterion, as seen in Table 1 (worse in the afternoon/evening), can also be clear only when comparing the same situation during the day and at night, for example, doing homework during the day or at night. However, even with these comparisons, many children do not report worsening at night, but meet all other diagnostic criteria and have supportive features for RLS, including positive family history [8].

As pediatric RLS is highly familiar, the presence of RLS in a first-degree relative helps to increase diagnostic certainty in childhood RLS. Likewise, the presence of PLMS can be very useful in supporting the diagnosis of RLS in children. Approximately 70% of children with RLS demonstrate PLMS ≥5/hour in a single night and almost 90%, when sampling multiple nights recordings. Pediatric RLS is comorbid to attention-deficit/hyperactivity disorder (ADHD) in about a quarter of cases, and, as in adults, higher rates of anxiety and depressive symptoms are found [8].

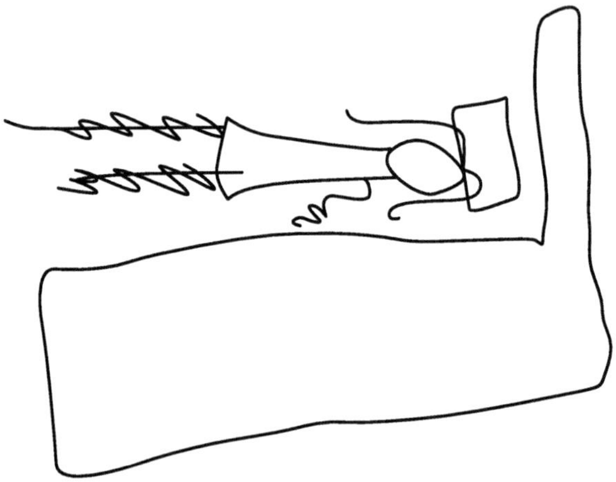

Fig. 1 Child's drawing of restless legs syndrome symptoms. (Image courtesy from Dr. Fernando Morgadinho Santos Coelho)

Table 3 Immobility testing procedure

1. At a time when the patient has more symptoms, usually in the afternoon or the first hour of the night, the patient remains in bed elevated at 45 degrees
2. The lower limbs must be resting on the bed and the eyes open; it is allowed to move the lower limbs without restriction to relieve the symptoms; the duration of the test is 1 hour
3. EMG activity is measured in the same way as in sleep, except for a maximum duration of 10 seconds
4. Every 5 minutes, the patient must report if he has discomfort
5. Discomfort on the 12 occasions has a sensitivity of 82% and specificity of 84%
6. The number of periodic limb movements is measured during the test (high specificity, but low sensitivity); values above 50/h are highly suggestive of RLS

EMG, electromyography; *RLS*, restless legs syndrome

The questionnaire of RLS severity is a very important tool and should be used routinely in these patients. Another instrument is the Restless Legs Syndrome-6 Scale (RLS-6), a smaller scale, involving six items classified on a scale from 0 to 10 (no symptoms at 0 to very severe at 10). The questions address the severity of RLS in the past week in four different circumstances: while falling asleep, at night, during the day sitting or lying down, and during the day on the move. The "RLS-6" appears to be a reliable and accurate instrument for assessing the severity of RLS in a specific and pragmatic way [9].

Immobility testing is not a routine test, but it can provide a standardized test condition for measuring symptoms of RLS, and it can be useful for confirming the diagnosis in difficult cases [10] (Table 3).

2 Periodic Limb Movements of Sleep

Periodic limb movements of sleep (PLMS) are characterized by limb movements that occur during NREM sleep, often without the patient's perception. The movements are characterized by involuntary dorsiflexion of the toes and ankles associated or not with flexion of the hip and knee. There is a difficulty in consolidating sleep and fragmentation by multiple awakenings. The diagnosis is confirmed by PSG, and the PLMS index is used to determine severity (Table 4, Fig. 2). Severity of PLMS is classified as PLM index (PLMi) in adults as normal, PLMi $\leq$5 n°/hour; mild, >5 n°/hour PLMi <25 n°/hour; moderate, >25 n°/hour PLMi <50 n°/hour; and severe, PLMi $\geq$50 n°/hour [1].

PLMS can be related to peripheral and central neurological diseases, just as it is prevalent in 50 to 90% of patients with RLS. The use of some medications may predispose to the appearance of PLMS such as lithium, antidepressants, and antipsychotics.

Activity monitors with high-frequency sampling and body position monitoring can be attached to the ankle or foot to provide an alternative measure of PLMS (see Chap. 37). Recordings assess the frequency and variability of PLMS overnight, usually three to five nights.

Table 4 Polysomnographic criteria for periodic limb movements of sleep

Frequency: minimum of four movements lasting between 0.5 and 10 seconds per movement
Interval: start of the first movement to the beginning of the second
Minimum of 4 seconds
Maximum of 90 seconds

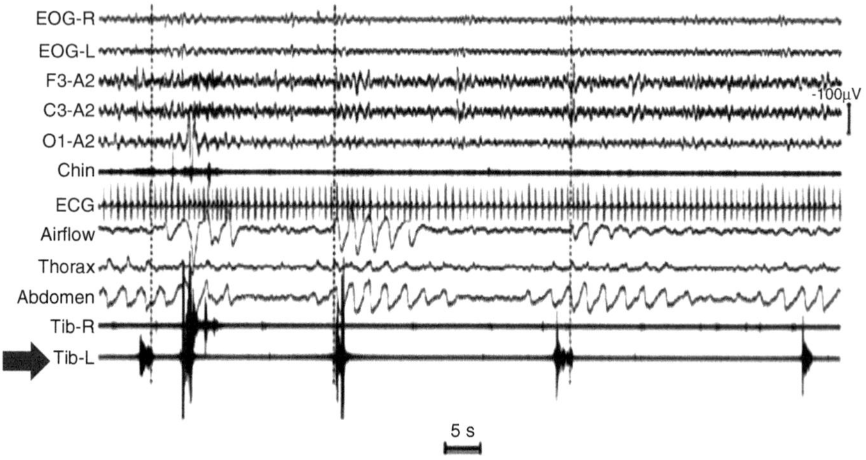

Fig. 2 A 30-second epoch of polysomnography elucidating a periodic limb movement (gray arrow indicates left tibialis anterior periodic movement). (Image courtesy from Dr. Fernando Morgadinho Santos Coelho)

When the PLMS disrupts sleep and is responsible for daytime symptoms without RLS, we name it periodic limb movements disorder (PLMD). Pharmacological treatment of PLMS is still controversial, except when associated with RLS or in patients with PLMD [1].

3 Differential Diagnosis

The differential diagnosis of RLS is not easy. About 40% of the general population who have RLS report some desire to move their lower limbs at rest. If the patient has the diagnostic criteria A2 (better with movement) and A3 (worse in the afternoon/night) as seen previously in Table 1, the specificity of diagnosis of RLS is about 70%. When we exclude leg cramps and positional discomfort, the specificity reaches 94%. Other confounders that should be part of the initial approach of a patient with suspected RLS are arthralgia/arthritis, myalgia, edema in the lower limbs, peripheral neuropathy, radiculopathy, and people who have the habit of moving their feet.

The main clues to exclude RLS are vigorous muscle contractions in the case of cramps, relief with a single postural dislocation when it comes to positional discomfort, limitation of the joints in arthralgia/arthritis, pain on muscle palpation for myalgia, and radiated neuropathic pain for radiculopathy [1].

Other conditions that may confuse the examiner are akathisia induced by neuroleptics (a possible medication exposition must be detailed and, in the akathisia, need for movement involving the whole body), myelopathy, venous insufficiency, peripheral arterial disease, eczema, orthopedic problems, and anxiety-induced restlessness.

A patient with pain due to various causes may have a nocturnal presentation and may worsen at rest, but relief with movement may not be present, or a single movement could already bring some relief, and the person makes the movement in a planned way to obtain relief. However, be very careful when excluding the diagnosis of RLS when the complaint is pain; about 50% of RLS patients refer to the symptoms as painful. In addition, it is important to keep in mind that patients with RLS are not exempt from having cramps and arthritis, among others.

When the diagnosis of RLS is not yet certain, there are still supporting characteristics such as the presence of a family history of RLS, PLMS in PSG, disproportional drowsiness in relation to what is expected due to poor sleep quality, and assessing response to low-dose dopaminergic drug therapy. The exclusion of these differential diagnoses greatly increases the chance of a correct diagnosis of RLS, with sensitivity and specificity greater than 90% [11].

4 Pathophysiology of RLS and PLMS

RLS can be considered a continuous spectrum with two temporal extremes: one with a greater contribution of genetic factors and another with a bigger contribution of environmental factors or comorbidities. The pathophysiology of RLS includes genetic factors, neurotransmitter dysfunction, and iron deficiency [1].

Many studies have attempted to identify the genes involved with increased susceptibility to RLS. No monogenic causes have been found. Thirteen genes, represented by nucleotide polymorphisms, were identified on chromosomes 6p21.2 (BTBD9), 2p14 (MEIS1), 9p24.1-p23 (PTPRD), 15q23 (MAP2K5/SKOR1), and 16q12.1 (TOX3/BC034767). Of these, four were replicated: BTBD9, MEIS1, MAP2K5/LBXCOR, and PTPRD. It is estimated that BTBD9 confers a risk attributable to the population (PAR) of 50% for the RLS. Together, BTBD9, MEIS1, and MAP2K5/LBXCOR represent 70% of PAR for RLS in individuals of European descent. The association of these genes with familial RLS still requires further studies [12].

In addition, more recent studies have identified seven additional susceptibility loci, related to neurological development in the embryonic limbs, for RLS (12q12-q21, RLS2 in 14q13-q21, RLS3 in 9p24-p22, RLS4 in 2q33, RLS5 in 20p13, RLS6 in 19p13, and RLS7 in 16p12.1). However, these variants in the genomic loci represent only a small proportion of genetic susceptibility whose pathophysiological functions have not yet been specified [12].

Iron deficiency has been associated with RLS since its initial description by Ekbom. Iron is needed for dopamine generation, synaptic density, and myelin synthesis. There are autopsy data, MRI, brain sonography, and cerebrospinal fluid analysis supporting the link between RLS and low brain iron.

Low levels of iron have been found in brain tissue samples and in the evaluation of cerebrospinal fluid of patients with RLS. The areas of the brain where this can be seen mainly are the substance nigra, the putamen, and the caudate nucleus. Indeed, there is a correlation between the severity of RLS symptoms and brain iron. The disruption of iron transport across the blood-brain barrier could explain the low levels of iron in the brain.

Unfortunately, serum iron parameters are not good predictors of central iron levels. The current guidelines established by the International RLS Study Group recommend the prescription of oral iron replacement if serum ferritin levels are less than 75 mg/L. However, it is not possible to say that patients with serum ferritin greater than this value do not have a reduction in iron in the CNS [13].

The evidence for the involvement of the dopaminergic system is supported by the almost immediate improvement in the symptoms of the disease after the administration of dopaminergic agents. However, there is evidence suggesting hyperactivity of the dopaminergic system. The D1 receptor seems to have a leading role, which is in line with the increase in the symptoms of RLS over the years. A pre-synaptic hyperdopaminergic state also appears to have implications for PLMS and changes in glutamatergic neurotransmission, which in turn would be involved in hypervigilance and PLMS [14].

Studies about adenosine may help explain the link between these neurotransmitters and the overlap of RLS and PLMS. The deficiency of cerebral iron reduces the adenosine A1 receptors in the striatum and cortex. The lower stimulation of adenosine incites the dopaminergic and glutamatergic corticostriatal pathways. Directly, low adenosine would make hypersensitive receptors, generating PLMS. The depletion of A1 receptor in the cortex, basal forebrain, and hypothalamus could generate hypervigilance. Tests with dipyridamole, which increases extracellular adenosine, corroborate this hypothesis [12, 15].

5 Prognosis

A condition that reduces the quality or quantity of sleep is expected to generate excessive daytime sleepiness, but the assessment of sleepiness (e.g., Epworth Sleepiness Scale) in RLS generally shows results in the normal range. Sleep is affected in several ways in this disease; first, the sensory symptoms of RLS impair the return to sleep and, therefore, result in a prolonged awakening.

In addition, PLMS contributes to the primary morbidity of sleep disorder by RLS. About a third of PLMS are associated with cortical excitations, and most are associated with autonomic excitations. PLMS are associated with increases of 10–20% in heart rate and large increases in blood pressure (10–15 mmHg diastolic and 25–30 mmHg systolic), contributing to the development of daytime hypertension in patients who had a periodic member movement index above 30. In the Sleep Heart Health Study, patients with a higher frequency or severity of RLS symptoms had a higher risk of coronary artery disease and cerebrovascular disease compared to control subjects [16].

Several studies have shown an increased prevalence of mood and anxiety disorders in individuals with RLS, such as depressive symptoms (OR 1.95 and 3.67), major depression (OR 2.6), major depressive disorder (OR 2.57 and 4.7), generalized anxiety disorder (OR 3.5), panic (OR 4.7, 12.9 and 18.9), and post-traumatic stress (OR 3.76). In addition, a positive correlation was found between the severity of RLS and the symptoms of depression/anxiety. Indeed, the treatment of RLS improves depressive symptoms [17].

Other conditions have increased rates in patients with RLS, such as attention-deficit/hyperactivity disorder (ADHD), narcolepsy, migraine, chronic obstructive pulmonary disease, Parkinson's disease, multiple sclerosis, peripheral neuropathy, obstructive sleep apnea, diabetes mellitus, fibromyalgia in both children and adults, rheumatoid arthritis, food night, obesity, thyroid disease, and heart disease. About a quarter of individuals with RLS have symptoms of ADHD, and 12% to 35% of those with ADHD meet the criteria for RLS [18].

Physical and mental health scores were consistently lower for individuals with RLS, using standard quality of life (QoL) assessment tools. Deficiencies in QoL are strongly associated with the severity of RLS and remain after controlling for age, sex, and comorbidity of the disease. In addition, patients with other comorbidities and RLS associated had a worse QoL than those who did not have RLS [19].]

6 Treatment

The treatment of RLS starts with an accurate diagnosis, the identification of reversible contributing factors, and the use of non-pharmacological and pharmacological therapies when indicated. Non-pharmacological treatment with increased physical activity; regular sleep times; withdrawal of precipitating factors such as medication, coffee, and alcohol; as well as iron and vitamin replacement solve the problem in many patients.

Daily treatment with any kind of medication should start only when symptoms have a significant impact on quality of life in terms of frequency and severity. An intermittent treatment can be considered in cases with short periods of worsening [18].

Many pharmacological agents can be effective in managing symptoms. Until recently, first-line treatment consisted of low doses of dopaminergic agonists; however, the use of dopaminergic agonists for a long period of time can worsen the symptoms. Therefore, international guidelines recommend that, whenever possible, the initial treatment should be done with $\alpha 2\delta$ ligands. If prescribed, dopaminergic agonists should be prescribed in the lowest effective dose and for the shortest possible time. Iron therapy can be considered in patients with refractory RLS (Tables 5 and 6). New treatments based on pathophysiology may become reality; drugs with a focus on glutamatergic and adenosine pathways (dipyridamole) are examples and are being studied [18].

Table 5 Pharmacological treatment of restless legs syndrome

	Dose range (mg)	Initial dose <65 years (mg)	Initial dose >65 years (mg)
Dopaminergic agonists			
Levodopa	100–200		
Pramipexole	0.125–0.75	0.125	0.125
Rotigotine	1–3	1	1
Anticonvulsants			
Gabapentin	900–2400	300	100
Gabapentin enacarbil	600–1200	600	300
Pregabalin	150–450	75	50
Opioids			
Codeine	15–120		
Tramadol	50–150		
Oxycodone	10–40	5–10	5–10
Methadone	5–30	5–10	2.5

Table 6 A rational approach for pharmacological options for the treatment of restless legs syndrome

Characteristics of the patient	Rational choice
Daytime symptoms	Medication with a long half-life or two takes of a shorter half-life one
Sleep changes disproportionately to the symptoms of RLS	α2δ ligand
Comorbid insomnia	α2δ ligand
Risk of pregnancy	Consider iron supplementation
Renal dysfunction	Choose medications not excreted by the kidney or adjust the doses
Increased risk of falls	Dopamine agonist
RLS with painful symptoms	α2δ ligand
Chronic pain comorbid	α2δ ligand
History of compulsions	α2δ ligand
Past abuse of licit or illicit substances	Avoid opioids
Very severe symptoms of RLS	Dopamine agonist
Overweight/metabolic syndrome	Dopamine agonist
Availability/cost of medication	Dopamine agonist
Comorbid depression	Dopamine agonist
Comorbid anxiety	α2δ ligand
Risk of drug interactions	The select drug that does not have hepatic metabolism
Symptomatic PLMS	Dopamine agonist

7 Augmentation

The prescription of levodopa for the treatment of RLS was initially considered very promising, but it soon became clear that its effectiveness decreased over time. Subsequently, its use was still associated with a worsening of patients' symptoms after chronic use. It was named augmentation [1]. The main criteria for augmentation are symptom onset earlier (2–4 hours), shorter latency of symptoms at rest, dissemination of symptoms to other parts of the body, greater intensity of symptoms, and paradoxical response to treatment.

With the role of dopamine in the pathophysiology of RLS in mind, dopaminergic agonists could be interesting therapeutic options. Ropinirole and pramipexole, whose half-lives are longer than that of levodopa, were approved for the treatment of RLS about 15 years ago. In the randomized clinical trials, it was clear that they were effective in the short term. However, the worsening of symptoms observed with levodopa has also occurred, although the treatment time required for this to happen has been longer. One study estimated that 76% of all patients treated with dopaminergic agents showed evidence of partial increase with an annual incidence rate of approximately 8%. There is insufficient evidence that longer-acting drugs (cabergoline, rotigotine) have a lower rate of increase in incidence [18].

As well as the beginning of the treatment of RLS, whenever possible, it should start with the elimination of factors that can exacerbate the symptoms (iron level, antidepressants, and antihistamines). Iron replacement should be considered if serum ferritin levels are <50–75 μg/mL or if transferrin saturation is less than 20%, and treatment can be done with oral or intravenous iron depending on the clinical picture, as already mentioned. This can be done in combination with any of the other options [18].

In milder cases of augmentation, therapy with dopaminergic agonists can be continued by dividing or advancing the dose of the agonist, or rotigotine may be tried. Alternatively, treatment can be switched to an a2δ ligand, especially in more severe cases. These drugs are effective and have little risk of augmentation. However, in cases where dopaminergic drugs are prescribed, the daily dose should be as low as possible and should not exceed that recommended for the treatment of RLS [20].

For patients with almost 24 hours of symptoms, an opioid may be considered. According to the latest consensus, it is suggested that prolonged-release oxycodone or methadone should be considered if the other approaches fail. There are, however, precautions inherent in the prescription of opioids and the physician must be aware: family or personal history of alcohol or drug abuse and psychiatric comorbidities, severe constipation, and prolonged QT interval, in addition to the risk of recreational use. When patients are chosen appropriately, low-dose opioid therapy is effective and safe, even when used for long-term therapy [20].

8 Final Words

RLS is a prevalent disease with several differential diagnoses, whose consequences for the individual's QoL is well documented. Therefore, it is imperative the knowledge about this condition and regular screen for all patients with sleep complaints. Once diagnosed, an assessment of confounders and associated conditions should be detailed. The iron depletion should be promptly corrected. The $\alpha 2\delta$ ligands should be prioritized as an initial treatment in most patients. If the physician does not feel able to manage the treatment for any reason, the patient should be referred to a sleep medicine specialist.

References

1. International classification of sleep disorders – third edition (ICSD-3). 3rd ed. American Academy of Sleep Medicine; 2014.
2. Ekbom KA. Restless legs; a report of 70 new cases. Acta Med Scand Suppl. 1950;246:64–8.
3. Eckeli AL, Gitai LL, Dach F, Ceretta H, Sander HH, Passos AD, et al. Prevalence of restless legs syndrome in the rural town of Cassia dos Coqueiros in Brazil. Sleep Med. 2011;12(8):762–7.
4. Chen SJ, Shi L, Bao YP, Sun YK, Lin X, Que JY, et al. Prevalence of restless legs syndrome during pregnancy: a systematic review and meta-analysis. Sleep Med Rev. 2018;40:43–54.
5. Stevens MS. Restless legs syndrome/Willis-Ekbom disease morbidity: burden, quality of life, cardiovascular aspects, and sleep. Sleep Med Clin. 2015;10(3):369–73, xv–xvi.
6. Romero-Peralta S, Cano-Pumarega I, Garcia-Malo C, Agudelo Ramos L, García-Borreguero D. Treating restless legs syndrome in the context of sleep disordered breathing comorbidity. Eur Respir Rev. 2019;28(153):190061. Published 2019 Oct 1. https://doi.org/10.1183/16000617.0061-2019.
7. Montplaisir J, Boucher S, Poirier G, Lavigne G, Lapierre O, Lesperance P. Clinical, polysomnographic, and genetic characteristics of restless legs syndrome: a study of 133 patients diagnosed with new standard criteria. Mov Disord. 1997;12(1):61–5.
8. Picchietti D, Allen RP, Walters AS, Davidson JE, Myers A, Ferini-Strambi L. Restless legs syndrome: prevalence and impact in children and adolescents--the Peds REST study. Pediatrics. 2007;120(2):253–66.
9. Walters AS, LeBrocq C, Dhar A, Hening W, Rosen R, Allen RP, et al. Validation of the International Restless Legs Syndrome Study Group rating scale for restless legs syndrome. Sleep Med. 2003;4(2):121–32.
10. Michaud M, Lavigne G, Desautels A, Poirier G, Montplaisir J. Effects of immobility on sensory and motor symptoms of restless legs syndrome. Mov Disord. 2002;17(1):112–5.
11. Cho YW, Song ML, Earley CJ, Allen RP. Prevalence and clinical characteristics of patients with restless legs syndrome with painful symptoms. Sleep Med. 2015;16(6):775–8.
12. Romero-Peralta S, Cano-Pumarega I, Garcia-Borreguero D. Emerging concepts of the pathophysiology and adverse outcomes of restless legs syndrome. Chest. 2020;158(3):1218–29.
13. Allen RP, Picchietti DL, Garcia-Borreguero D, Ondo WG, Walters AS, Winkelman JW, et al. Restless legs syndrome/Willis-Ekbom disease diagnostic criteria: updated International Restless Legs Syndrome Study Group (IRLSSG) consensus criteria–history, rationale, description, and significance. Sleep Med. 2014;15(8):860–73.

14. Trotti LM, Becker LA. Iron for the treatment of restless legs syndrome. Cochrane Database Syst Rev. 2019;1:CD007834.
15. Ferre S, Quiroz C, Guitart X, Rea W, Seyedian A, Moreno E, et al. Pivotal role of adenosine neurotransmission in restless legs syndrome. Front Neurosci. 2017;11:722.
16. Javaheri S, Zhao YY, Punjabi NM, Quan SF, Gottlieb DJ, Redline S. Slow-wave sleep is associated with incident hypertension: the sleep heart health study. Sleep. 2018;41(1):zsx179. https://doi.org/10.1093/sleep/zsx179.
17. Winkelmann J, Prager M, Lieb R, Pfister H, Spiegel B, Wittchen HU, et al. "Anxietas tibiarum". Depression and anxiety disorders in patients with restless legs syndrome. J Neurol. 2005;252(1):67–71.
18. Trenkwalder C, Allen R, Hogl B, Paulus W, Winkelmann J. Restless legs syndrome associated with major diseases: a systematic review and new concept. Neurology. 2016;86(14):1336–43.
19. Walters AS, Frauscher B, Allen R, Benes H, Chaudhuri KR, Garcia-Borreguero D, et al. Review of quality of life instruments for the restless legs syndrome/Willis-Ekbom Disease (RLS/WED): critique and recommendations. J Clin Sleep Med. 2014;10(12):1351–7.
20. Gonzalez-Latapi P, Malkani R. Update on restless legs syndrome: from mechanisms to treatment. Curr Neurol Neurosci Rep. 2019;19(8):54.

therapies for RLS and PLMS. Since then, several investigations have been conducted to examine the non-pharmacological treatment for RLS and PLMS.

The Brazilian consensus on sleep physical therapy, published in 2013, stated that exercises, mostly aerobic ones, are an adjunct treatment for RLS and PLMS. For RLS, physiotherapists must promote education about the disease and advice the patients with orientations with the recommended non-drug therapy: to perform physical exercises, to change the periods of inactivity to daytime, to follow a good sleep hygiene program (as sleep deprivation may increase the symptoms substantially), and to avoid nicotine, caffeine, alcohol, and drugs. The usage of some medications (i.e., antidepressants, antihistaminic, anti-nausea, and antipsychotics) should be discussed with the physician, as they also can increase the symptoms. Similarly, attention should be given to iron deficiency populations (i.e., pregnant), peripheral neuropathy, spinal cord, and amputee's rehabilitation [2].

The Brazilian consensus on guidelines for diagnosis and treatment for RLS, published in 2015, stated that there was evidence to support the use of physical exercise, pneumatic compression, and infrared light for RLS, as they were able to reduce the severity of the symptoms. Therefore, acupuncture and enhanced external counterpulsation[1] were considered ineffective for RLS [3].

Two recent systematic reviews bring new evidence on the theme. The first one found that primary RLS severity was improved by complementary and alternative options such as exercise training, pneumatic compression devices, and acupuncture among others. As for secondary RLS (i.e., uremic), intradialytic exercise training showed to be highly efficient in the reduction of RLS symptom severity [1]. In the second systematic review, non-pharmacological interventions including exercise, compression devices, counter-strain manipulation, infrared therapy, acupuncture, cryotherapy, and yoga showed to be complementary to pharmacological managing in individuals with RLS [4]. Vibratory pads, yoga, pneumatic compression devices, acupuncture, and local cryotherapy significantly increased the sleep quality of the participants of those studies but did not change the RLS symptoms severity score [4]. Short-lasting effects were identified with whole-body cryotherapy, repetitive transcranial stimulation, and transcutaneous stimulation. However, despite the relatively few studies included in this last review, most of them had some limitations that reduced their reliability.

A scoping review published in 2020 demonstrated limited evidence for most non-pharmacological treatment options, with scarce studies evaluating each modality. Yet, there is a reliable trend in the findings showing positive results in RLS symptom severity, and most of the non-pharmacologic options did not have any adverse effect [5]. More studies are necessary to investigate the efficacy of yoga, massage, traction straight leg raise, and whole-body vibration. No adverse effects were identified for moderate-intensity exercise, yoga, massage, and pneumatic compression devices [5]. Taken together, these results indicate that there exists insufficient evidence for confidence in resting only in non-pharmacological therapies for RLS and PLMS. Moreover, further exploration with high-quality

[1] The enhanced external counterpulsation treatment compresses the blood vessels in the lower limbs to increase blood flow to the heart. This happens via cuffs attached to air hoses that connect to valves that inflate and deflate the cuffs in accordance to heart beats. This treatment is used in the treatment of patients with angina.

randomized controlled trials is needed, comparing non-pharmacological therapy plus pharmacological treatment with the same pharmacological treatment – to support clinical practice for the treatment plan.

The severity of RLS (and the physiotherapeutic effectiveness) can be assessed using the International RLS Study Group Scale (IRLSSGS), which is a validated questionnaire designed to assess symptom severity, frequency, and impact on daily life [6], before, during, and after treatment (please see more in Chapter "Subjective assessment of Sleep" of this book).

Here we present some therapies and their evidence regarding RLS and PLMS, to build knowledge, and to fundament further investigations on the topic, urgently needed.

1 Intermittent Pneumatic Compression

Pneumatic compression therapy is performed with a device that inflates pressure in bandages placed on the legs. The pressure used in previous studies was 40cmH_2O, for 5 seconds every 1 minute. The patients used the device at home for 1 hour daily and were instructed to activate the device a few moments before they related the onset of the symptoms [7]. The use of the pneumatic compression device for 4 weeks reduced the RLS severity scale score by 12 points, which characterizes an important clinical improvement. It is of value to mention that the patients had been using the medicines for the disease for at least 2 months and the non-pharmacological treatment as adjuvant to the medication. The improvement in symptoms may be explained by the hypothesis that patients with RLS present with venous insufficiency. Tissue hypoxia and ischemia can generate neuronal dysfunction. Compression would stimulate the release of endothelial mediators that modulate the symptoms of the disease, improving local perfusion and lymphatic venous drainage with consequent relief of ischemic symptoms [7].

2 Infrared Light: Light therapy

Infrared light has a wavelength range of about 750–1000 nm. Treatment with near-infrared light with a wavelength between 880 and 890 nm presented increased cutaneous pressure sensation in patients with peripheral neuropathy and increased wound healing and for these reasons started being investigated for RLS. The mechanism of infrared light is its capacity to generate nitric oxide in the endothelium [8] and release it from the red blood cells [9]. Thus, nitric oxide, a neurotransmitter itself, can initiate and maintain vasodilation [10]. In addition, light (i.e., phototherapy) produces changes in the permeability of the membrane, leading to enhanced synthesis of endorphins, increased nerve cell potential, and therefore pain relief [11]. Taken together, infrared light can influence blood flow, neurotransmission, and pain – all factors related to RLS. Infrared light devices were investigated with different frequencies and their impact on RLS symptoms associated with pharmacological treatment in a study showing positive effects [12]. In this study, 25 patients were randomly allocated to near-infrared light devices (either an Anodyne® or HealthLight™, both using a dosage of 650 nm and different frequencies, 292 Hz and 4698 Hz, respectively) treatment for 12 treatments with near-infrared light, 30-minutes, 3 times a week, for 4 weeks, and both frequencies improved significantly the symptoms of RLS, with no significant difference between the two devices [12]. This investigation provided support for the use of infrared light as a noninvasive and non-pharmacological treatment of RLS.

3 Acupuncture

Acupuncture presented insufficient evidence in a systematic review to determine its efficacy for RLS [13]. A Cochrane database systematic review from 2008 brought no evidence for the use of acupuncture solely for RLS [14]. In an objective investigation, participants with RLS used the actigraphy device in the ankles during the evening and night to detect movements before and after treatment. This group was in no pharmacological treatment, neither at the moment of the investigation nor previously, and underwent 6 weeks of acupuncture (i.e., 30 minutes, three times a week) in standard (local) points of traditional Chinese medicine and sham points (randomized and distal points). The authors found improvement in the IRLSRS in the standard group with the use of acupuncture [15]. In the view of traditional Chinese medicine, RLS is considered "(…) a deficiency of 'Yin' and 'Xue' (blood) of the legs, because 'Yin' and 'Xue' are in effect at night and function to relax the mind and body. According to TCM, the activity and function of legs are controlled by liver function, and, thus, the deficiency of 'Yin' and 'Xue' of the liver at night is the main cause of RLS Shenshu (BL23, bilateral), Mingmen (DU4), and Chenshan (BL57, unilateral) have effects on the uncomfortable waist and leg symptoms, Shenshu (BL23, bilateral) and Mingmen (DU4) can also improve 'Shen Qi' (energy and immunity) and increase the 'Yin' of the waist and legs, and Xuehai (Sp10, unilateral) increases 'Xue' (blood) of the body, which means it can tranquilize the legs. Taichun (LR3, bilateral), Zusanli (St36, unilateral), Sanyinjiao (Sp6, bilateral), and Taixi (Ki3, bilateral) increase both 'Yin' and 'Xue' (blood) of the body. If these acupoints are treated properly, the legs should be quiet at night" [15]. The mechanisms of acupuncture in the view of traditional Chinese medicine are not the focus of this book, yet the mechanisms leading to improvement of RLS severity remain to be elucidated. In addition, the dry needling therapy must also be an object of further investigations.

4 Electrical Stimulation

Transcutaneous electrical neural stimulation (TENS) is being investigated for RLS. When the TENS were applied to bilateral legs on a handheld device (3 Hz), the RLS symptom severity decreased in both groups, active group and sham group, revealing a placebo effect of the treatment [16]. Its effect for treating RLS symptoms is used to reduce spinal cord excitability in patients with RLS [17], with short-lasting effect [18]. Recently, some investigations on noninvasive transcutaneous spinal direct-current stimulation emerged, indicating positive effects on the RLS symptoms [19] and providing a rationale for its use [20–22].

5 Whole-Body Vibration

Vibration therapy is an exercise realized through the body vibration platform. The patients are positioned standing on the platform, with semi-flexed knees and feet apart. Whole-body vibration (WBV) applied in healthy individuals resulted in nitric oxide generation, which increased blood flow. The effectiveness of this intervention was investigated in patients with RLS. The patients underwent ten 30-s bouts of WBV at a frequency and amplitude of 26 Hz and 2 mm per bout, and had blood collected for nitric oxide analysis and skin blood flow (flux), as determined by laser Doppler imaging, before and after the sessions, and also compared to a control group. RLS group presented an increase in skin blood flow immediately after the session's bout compared to baseline, in 5-minute post-treatment flux, and also when compared to the control group. These results indicated that the WBV increased the flux in the RLS group. No differences were found in nitric oxide concentration between baseline and after treatment and when compared to controls [23]. Unfortunately, the intervention was performed in the early afternoon and not at evening/night – when symptoms aggravate, as there seems to be circadian rhythmicity of the disease. In addition, the researchers observed an increased skin blood flow in the feet related to controls, and a weakened spatial cooling ability when the environmental temperature was raised [23]. In this sense, patients with RLS have a kind of sympathetic dysfunction as it controls skin microvascular circulation. Furthermore, the length of capillary/perimeter of fiber in the anterior tibialis (indicating a significant remodeling in capillary geometry) has been found to be higher in patients with RLS than in controls [24], as this is one of the hypotheses, as microvessel arrangement are changed, indicating an attempt to counteract local hypoxia in the tissue [24]. Some years later, this same research group investigated the effect of the WBV (i.e., ten 30-s bouts at a frequency and amplitude of 26 Hz and 2 mm) in RLS symptom severity for 2 weeks and found a 5-point decrease in IRLSSG Scale indicating that vibration had a positive effect on symptoms associated with RLS, although it did not normalize skin blood flow in patients with RLS compared to controls [25].

6 Yoga

An Iyengar yoga program was designed for women with RLS: two 90-minute classes per week, and at least 30 minutes of home practice on non-class days, for an overall period of 8 weeks. The yoga postures practice routines were illustrated in a manual

Table 1 Exercise protocols for restless legs syndrome and periodic limb movement disorder

Study	Sample	Protocol	Outcomes
de Mello et al. (2002) [32]	12 patients with complete spinal cord injury between T7 and T12	Chronic aerobic exercise	↓PLMi
de Mello et al. (2004) [33]	13 patients with complete spinal cord injury between T7 and T12	Chronic aerobic exercise	↓PLMi
Aukerman et al. (2006) [31]	41 patients with RLS	Chronic aerobic + resistance exercise	Improvement in RLS symptoms
Sakkas et al. (2008) [34]	14 patients on hemodialysis	Chronic aerobic exercise	Improvement in quality of life
Esteves et al. (2009) [35]	22 patients with PLMS	Acute/chronic aerobic exercise	Acute: ↑TST, ↑SE, ↑ Stage R, ↓WASO, ↓PLMi Chronic: ↑TST, ↑SE, ↑ SL, ↓REM SL, ↓PLMi
Giannaki et al. (2010) [36]	18 patients on hemodialysis with RLS and PLMS	Acute aerobic + resistance exercise	↓PLMi
Esteves et al. (2011) [37]	11 patients with RLS	Chronic aerobic exercise	↓SL ↓SE ↑Stage R ↓PLMi
Cavagnoli et al. (2013) [38]	16 patients with PLMS	Acute aerobic exercise	↑Stage N1 ↓PLMi
Giannaki et al. (2013) [39]	24 patients with CKD	Aerobic exercises	Improved RLS symptoms and depression scales
Giannaki et al. (2013) [40]	32 patients with dialytic CKD + RLS	Aerobic exercises at dialysis	Improvement of RLS symptoms
Mortazavi et al. (2013) [41]	26 patients with CKD + RLS	Aerobic exercises	Improvement of RLS symptoms
Giannaki et al. (2015) [42]	14 dialytic patients with RLS	Aerobic exercises during dialysis	Improvement of RLS symptoms
Aliasgharpour et al. (2016) [43]	33 patients with dialytic CKD	Stretching during dialysis	Relief of RLS symptoms

RLS restless legs syndrome, *PLMS* periodic limb movement of sleep, *CKD* chronic kidney disease, ↑ increased, ↓ decreased, *TST* total sleep time, *SE* sleep efficiency, *Stage R* REM sleep stage, *WASO* wake after sleep onset, *REM SL* REM sleep latency, *PLMi* periodic limb movement index (n°/h)

36° session; stage R increased after both sessions; and, most importantly, PLMi decreased after the 72° session, from 31 n°/h at baseline (moderate) to 14.8 n°/h after chronic exercise (mild) (Fig. 2), indicating the importance of exercise for PLMS.

These data showed that both acute and chronic exercise decreased PLMi and single sessions of intense exercise as well as longer-term regular workouts reduced leg muscle contractions and improved sleep in a small group of people with PLMS

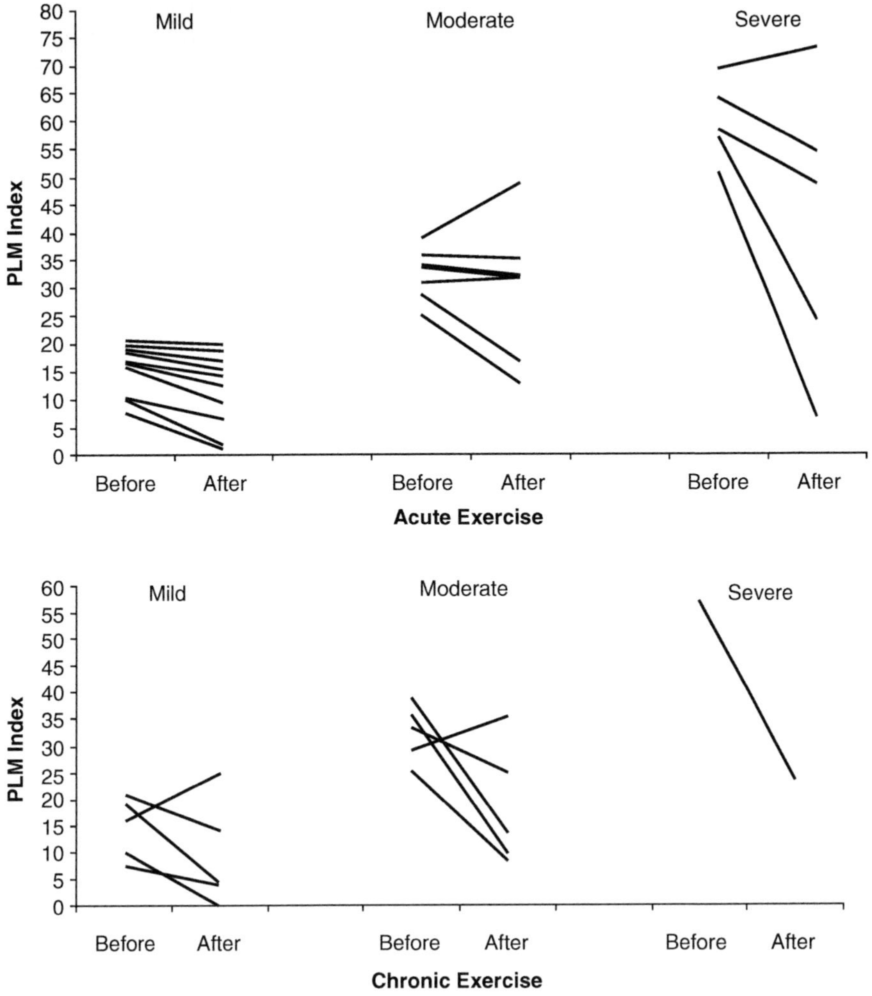

Fig. 2 Above: Changes in the individual PLM index (n°/h) before and after intense acute (1 session) physical exercise using PLMS classification. Below: Changes in the individual PLM index (n°/h) before and after 72 sessions of chronic physical exercise, using PLMS classification (mild, moderate, and severe). (Reprinted with permission from Esteves et al. [35])

[35]. Searching for the mechanisms of which this might happen, the researches investigated the release of ß-endorphin after exercise sessions and found an inverse relationship: more ß-endorphin release and lower PLM indices. Thus, ß-endorphin acted as "a proxy measure", being sufficient to reduce PLMi and to enhance sleep quality. The changes of ß-endorphin were not correlated with the intensity of exercise [35]. Therefore, it is suggested that for individuals with PLMS, physical exercise may be a plausible alternative (or better, complementary alternative) to pharmacological treatment.

There is plenty of evidence on the relationship between the intensity of physical exercise and the release of ß-endorphin, including its mechanisms [44, 45], but not in patients with PLMS. The release of ß-endorphin, which is based on amount and intensity of exercise, affects the dopaminergic system. Conversely, some investigations demonstrated that only chronic physical exercise can lead to these changes [35] and not a single session of physical exercise [38].

Having the dopaminergic system affected, and not knowing completely the role of the opioid and dopaminergic system in the pathophysiology of PLMS, a group of scientists investigated the changes in the dopaminergic system by acute exercise in patients with PLMS. The treatment with pharmacological therapy (such as opioids and dopamine) resulted in an adequate improvement of PLMS severity, so why not?

For acute physical exercise (maximal exercise test), the hypothesis was that a change in dopaminergic dysfunction (known to be present) that occurred in PLMS might happen due to exercise [38]. PLMS symptoms might result from a unbalance of dopaminergic and opioidergic systems in the regions involved in motor actions and/or pain perception, and that is why dopaminergic and opioid compounds are effective in treating RLS/PLMS [46]. Therefore, taking into account that dopamine is a neurotransmitter involved in motor function (and cognitive and emotive responses) [47, 48], dopamine is captured in the synaptic cleft by many different neural receptors, including the dopamine transporter. The dopamine transporter is a molecule located in the presynaptic neuron that modulates the uptake of dopamine using an electrical mechanism coupled to Na^+ and Cl^- [49]. The dopamine transporter regulates the levels of available dopamine in the synaptic cleft [50]. Seventy percent of the dopamine removed from striatal synaptic clefts is mediated by dopamine transporter, which also regulates the levels of available dopamine in the synaptic cleft [50], and its concentrations reflect the homeostatic tone of the dopaminergic system [50, 51]. The researches investigated the dopamine transporter density via SPECT (single-photon emission computed tomography) in patients with PLMS, and found that, despite the reduced symptoms of PLMS after exercise, no changes in dopamine transporter availability occurred. This result showed that physical exercise did not modulate dopamine transporter density - other mechanism might be involved. Curiously, the authors found slightly lower dopamine transporter density in the left putamen region of the PLMS patients compared with healthy participants [38].

Until now, we do not know the exact mechanism of which exercise mediates a decrease, both in symptoms and in objectively measured PLMi. Some well-conducted investigations by a Brazilian group demonstrated that acute exercise statistically significantly reduced PLMi during sleep, measured by PSG, in a sample of athletes with spinal cord injuries [52]. In addition, the effects of aerobic exercise for 45 days in this population were not different from those produced by pharmacological therapy with L-DOPA [33]. Despite the small sample size, both treatments resulted in significant reductions in the PLMi from 35.1 to 19.9 for L-DOPA and from 35.1 to 18.5 for the exercise program [33]. Such studies need reproduction in other PLMS populations. Other investigation was performed to assess the effectiveness of aerobic training in PLMi in individuals with complete spinal cord injury. Using an arm crank ergometer, the physical training program was performed for 44 days, and reduced the PLMi when comparing baseline, 35.1 n°/h, with fifth, 12.7 n°/h, and sixth evaluation, 18.5 n°/h demonstrating objectively (PSG) improvement of PLMS [32].

The message is quite simple, yet it deserves more investigations: any physical intervention is more effective than no treatment or treatment with placebo in abolishing or reducing the occurrence of PLMS and improving the quality of life. There is emerging evidence for providing such suggestions as a more active and comprehensive intervention for exercise program/therapy as part of a treatment for PLMS in physical therapy settings.

9 Final Words

Currently, there is insufficient evidence to evaluate the use of non-pharmacological intervention for RLS and PLMS alone. The interventions presented here appear to be beneficial in improving mainly RLS severity, PLMi and PLMS complaints, and sleep in some individuals. Nevertheless, it is unclear to what extent benefits are because of individual/group interventions, publication bias, or even placebo responses.

Pharmacological treatment is the first line of therapeutic choice for relieving the symptoms of RLS, especially in moderate and severe cases, and non-pharmacological treatment should be considered as an adjunct to pharmacology. The physiotherapist should encourage the patient to maintain the use of his medications, even with the improvement of symptoms with the proposed intervention.

As PTs, many of our daily patients/clients are at risk of having RLS and/or PLMS, such as pregnancy, sleep apnea/snoring, narcolepsy, diabetes mellitus, anemia, iron deficiency, spinal cord injury the ones in use of dopaminergic medications, benzodiazepine or barbiturate withdrawal, drug dependency, and antipsychotic medication. So far, RLS and PLMS have already been handled by programs including aerobic exercises (treadmill bicycles or treadmill) which vary in duration, number of sessions, intensity, and follow-up with favorable outcomes.

Despite no consensus or guidelines on PT management of RLS and/or PLMS, our suggestion, even though more investigations are urgently needed, is that individualized physiotherapy should be considered as a complementary treatment for both diseases, as it has no negative side effects and can contribute to better health overall.

References

1. Aurora RN, et al. The treatment of restless legs syndrome and periodic limb movement disorder in adults--an update for 2012: practice parameters with an evidence-based systematic review and meta-analyses: an American Academy of Sleep Medicine Clinical Practice Guideline. Sleep. 2012;35(8):1039–62.

50. Jaber M, et al. The dopamine transporter: a crucial component regulating dopamine transmission. Mov Disord. 1997;12(5):629–33.
51. Jones SR, et al. Profound neuronal plasticity in response to inactivation of the dopamine transporter. Proc Natl Acad Sci U S A. 1998;95(7):4029–34.
52. de Mello MT, et al. Incidence of periodic leg movements and of the restless legs syndrome during sleep following acute physical activity in spinal cord injury subjects. Spinal Cord. 1996;34(5):294–6.

Circadian Rhythm Sleep-Wake Disorders: An Overview

Melissa Araújo Ulhôa and Claudia R. C. Moreno

Circadian rhythm refers to the biological rhythm that lasts about 24 hours (circa *diem* means "about a day"). The concept of circadian rhythm includes a period that varies from 20 to 28 hours. In humans, the *tau* or circadian rhythm is about 24.2 hours. There are cyclic variations in behavior and physiology, and the sleep-wake cycle is an example of a biological rhythm that is considered circadian. The sleep-wake cycle is the alternation between wakefulness and sleep. There are several other biological rhythms with circadian patterns such as appetite, body temperature, hormone levels, blood pressure, alertness, daily performance, reaction times, etc. The synchronization of the internal rhythms to the external environment is the *circadian phase*.

The regularity and periodicity of biological rhythms are one of the determinants of good organic function and human health. Several circadian rhythms oscillate over 24 hours, and the phase relationship established between these rhythms is important for general well-being. This process is called internal temporal order [1].

The desynchronization (also called circadian rupture, internal desynchronization, or rupture of the internal temporal order) between the internal circadian regulation system and the desired/needed sleep-waking times can result in one of the sleep-wake circadian rhythm disorders and is an important factor to be considered for other sleep disorders [1, 2].

M. A. Ulhôa
Faculty of Medicine of Vale do Aço, School of Health and Education, Centro Universitário Católico do Leste de Minas Gerais; Centro Universitário de Caratinga, Ipatinga, Minas Gerais, Brazil

C. R. C. Moreno (✉)
Department of Health, Life Cycles and Society, School of Public Health, University of São Paulo (USP), São Paulo, SP, Brazil

Stress Research Institute, Psychology Department, Stockholm University, Stockholm, Sweden

C. Frange, F. M. S. Coelho (eds.), *Sleep Medicine and Physical Therapy*,
https://doi.org/10.1007/978-3-030-85074-6_10

1 Physiology of Circadian Rhythm

The intrinsic internal temporal control system modulates several physiological systems, such as body temperature, hormones (e.g., cortisol, melatonin), and digestion. The suprachiasmatic nucleus (SCN) located in the hypothalamus acts as an internal regulator that generates circadian rhythm. Circadian rhythmicity is created endogenously by genetically encoded molecular clocks, whose components cooperate to generate cyclic changes in their activity, with a periodicity of about a day. The SCN is the major circadian pacemaker in humans and helps to maintain alertness by producing alerting signals during the day and maintaining sleep during the night by a reduced signal. If there were no environmental cues, the circadian rhythm would manifest itself for more than 24 hours. However, the earth's axis of rotation generates an important exogenous environmental cue – the dark-light cycle resulted from the alternation between day and night. External cues of luminosity stimulate photoreceptors located in the retina (melanopsin-containing retinal ganglion cells are the major circadian photoreceptors), which communicate the presence of light to the SCN, to the optic nerve, via the retinohypothalamic tract. In turn, this neural pathway synapses with the suprachiasmatic nuclei and generates cues that synchronize endogenous rhythms [2]. In response to the degree of luminosity, the SCN synapses with the pineal gland, thus regulating the release of melatonin. Light (sunlight) is the major *zeitgeber* (German for "time givers") and entrains the SCN into the physical environment. Therefore, light is an important environmental cue that acts to influence the circadian timing system. Environmental factors that can modify biological rhythms are called synchronizing agents or *zeitgebers*. Therefore, exposure to different 24-hour light-dark cycles can shift the circadian rhythm phase. There are peripheral (local) oscillators that are operative in the cells of most organs and tissues such as the thyroid gland, skeletal muscles, pancreas, skin fibroblasts, and others [3, 4]. In addition, the peripheral oscillators serve as input pathways for the SCN. The circadian system in humans is a hierarchical multi-oscillatory network, composed of master pacemaker(s) in the brain and oscillators in peripheral organs [5].

The circadian system has an imperative role in the regulation of the sleep-wake cycle since it influences the duration, continuity, and sleep structure. The mechanisms by which the circadian system interacts with sleep and waking states remain elusive. One of the hypotheses raised refers to the activation of nerve impulses by the circadian system promoting wakefulness during the day and helping to compensate for the progressive increase of sleepiness of the homeostatic sleep system, which accumulates along with prolonged wakefulness and promotes the onset of sleep. After the first half of the sleep episode, this sleep impulse decreases rapidly. This regulatory process takes place under normal homeostatic conditions. A properly aligned circadian system increases the propensity to sleep at night, particularly in the second half of the night, helping to maintain sleep consolidation until the usual time of awakening [6]. Thus, there is an internal order among the rhythms. The core body temperature Variation shows a lower phase during nighttime sleep, and between 3:00 and 4:00 of the night, the melatonin concentration level is at its peak. Subsequently, the core body temperature rises, and the plasma concentration of melatonin begins to fall and finally reaches its lowest rates, which occurs simultaneously to the light (day) phase of the light-dark cycle. In an organism, when the phase shift of the circadian rhythms is altered by any reason, there is a desynchronization, constituting a circadian rhythm sleep-wake disorder (CRSWD).

Therefore, the advent of electric light and technology allowed prolonged exposure to light during the night, anyplace, anywhere, which may desynchronize circadian rhythms due to SCN sensitivity to light [7]. The effect of phase shift from dark to light in the circadian system depends on when light exposure occurs. Exposure to light during the last hours of the typical sleep phase and the early hours of the morning shifts the circadian rhythm to earlier (advanced phase), as physiologically happens with older ones. On the other hand, exposure to light at night and in the first half of the usual sleep phase shifts the circadian rhythm to later (delayed phase), as physiologically happens with adolescents.

The SCN acts on circadian oscillators in peripheral tissues by neural signals from the autonomic nervous system, as well as the secretion of neurohormones. The hypothalamic-pituitary-adrenal axis is important for the hormonal regulation of the circadian system. For example, corticotropin-releasing hormone enters the hypothalamus-pituitary system and stimulates the secretion of adrenocorticotropic hormone (ACTH) by the anterior pituitary gland. ACTH then regulates cortisol production in the adrenal cortex, a hormone with a robust circadian oscillation and important synchronization effects on many peripheral oscillators. Therefore, cortisol peaks when waking up in the morning, while at night its concentration decreases (Fig. 1).

The rhythmic variation of different hormones, as well as of cognitive functions, strength, muscular performance, and dexterity, which occur in 24 hours constitute a predictable time for circadian oscillation of human abilities [9]. In other words, there is variation in alertness, attention, and physical performance according to hormonal and neural variations in a predictable way. In a study with healthy people in which the average sleep period was from 22:30 to 6:30, for example, the peak level of circadian rhythm occurred approximately at the following times: insulin at 16:00 h; triglycerides and cholesterol at 18:00; gastric acid secretion at 22:00; cortisol at 06:00; catecholamines at 07:00; and hemoglobin at 11:00 [10]. In addition, metabolic processes in peripheral oscillators are also modified by nutritional status, and peripheral oscillators relay feedback metabolic information to the hypothalamus. Nowadays, uninterrupted access to food can distort the feeding/fasting cycles that have characterized much of our history and therefore disrupt the circadian system [2]. When the organism is synchronized, the active period is concomitant with the caloric intake during the day (wake). In contrast, inactivity and anabolism occur during the resting phase (sleep). As a result of synchronization, the circadian system ensures a maximum physical performance during the active phase, with predictable circadian changes in blood pressure, heart rate and contractile efficiency of skeletal and cardiac muscles, and substrate oxidation to prepare the body for every day (light, day) activity.

The International Classification of Sleep Disorders (ICSD-3) [11] lists general criteria for CRSWD. The following must be present:

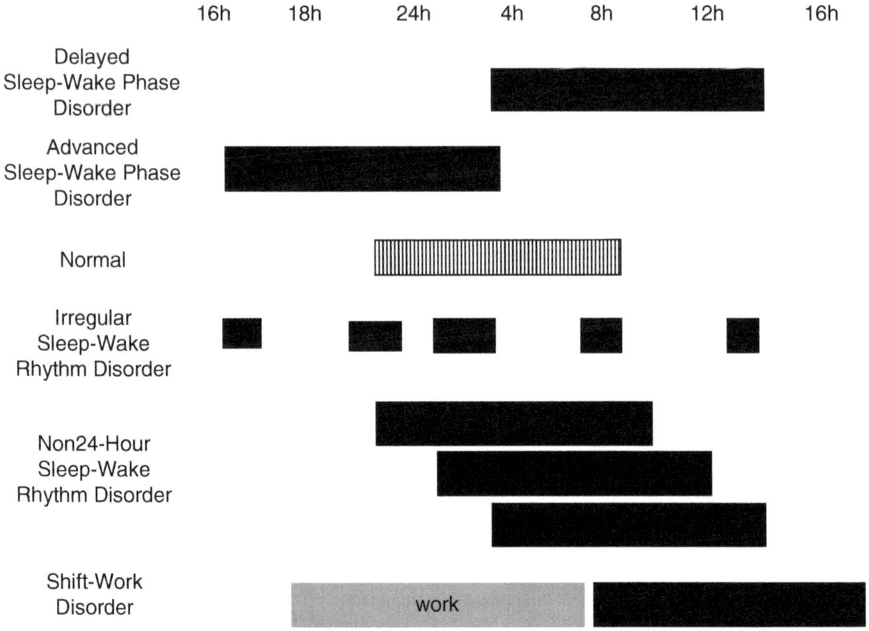

Fig. 2 Schematic representation of the major circadian rhythm sleep-wake disorders including intrinsic and extrinsic causes. Black bars represent sleep periods of circadian disorders; striped bars represent conventional sleep time. (Modified (with permission) from Lu and Zee [12])

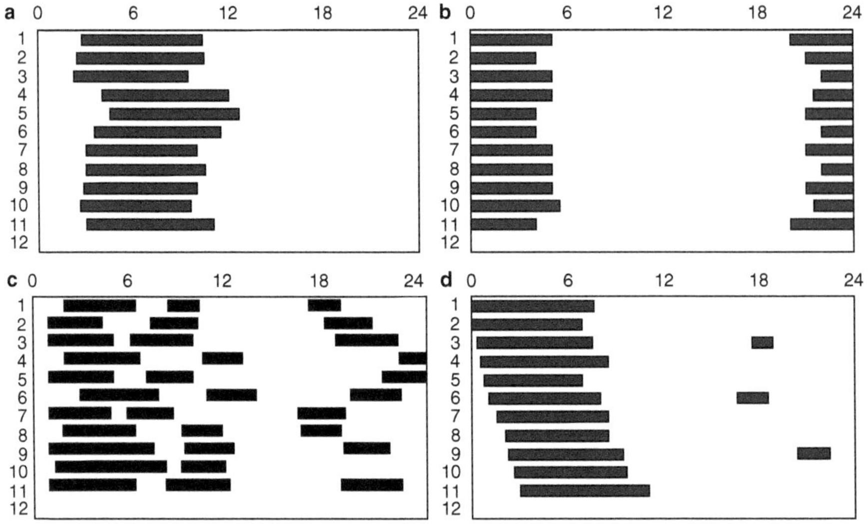

Fig. 3 Example of actograms of clinical manifestations of circadian disorders imposed by intrinsic causes. Each line corresponds to 1 day (12 days in this actograms). Above each graph the 24 hours of a day. The black bars correspond to sleep. (**a**) Individual with delayed sleep-wake phase disorder; (**b**) individual with advanced sleep-wake phase disorder; (**c**) individual with irregular sleep-wake cycle disorder; (**d**) individual with Non-24-hour sleep-wake rhythm disorder or free-running. (Image courtesy from Dr. Claudia Moreno)

encountered in any age group; nonetheless, it is particularly prevalent among adolescents and young adults. Adolescents have a neurodevelopmental feature that promotes changes in sleep-wake rhythm and an extension of the intrinsic circadian period during this age range. Another cause presented in DSWPD is changing in light exposure and altered sensitivity of the circadian system to light [14]. Having this circadian knowledge, school activities should be planned to take into account the biological rhythms for each age range. For instance, pre-adolescents (between 10 and 12 years) usually study in the morning, having classes starting around 7 h/7:30 h. In this age group, the habits have changes to an evening-type, preferring falling asleep and waking up later (night owls) [1]. As a result, school performance in the early morning hours is often compromised. It is important to note that this disorder is part of the neural development in preteens and adolescents and tends to soften with the maturation of the central nervous system in adulthood. Standardized chronotype questionnaires are useful tools to assess circadian preference (morning-, evening-, or intermediate-type) (Chap. 35 of this book).

The advanced sleep-wake phase disorder (ASWPD) happens when there is an advance (early timing) in the phase of the major sleep episode in relation to the desired or required sleep time and wake-up time (Fig. 3b). This must be demonstrated by a chronic or recurrent complaint of difficulty staying awake until the required or desired conventional bedtime, together with an inability to remain asleep until the required or desired time for awakening. Advanced age appears to be a risk factor for ASWPD, in part due to the advancing physiological phase that occurs with aging, combined with the weakening of circadian rhythms and age-related environmental signs. Such phase disorder can be genetically determined in some individuals.

The irregular sleep-wake rhythm disorder (ISWRD) represents a failure of the circadian system to maintain a stable alignment within 24 hours; consequently, the sleep-wake pattern is temporally disorganized (Fig. 3c). In ISWRD patients present with a chronic or recurrent pattern of irregular sleep and wake episodes throughout the 24-hour period, characterized by symptoms of insomnia during the scheduled sleep period (usually at night), excessive sleepiness (napping) during the day, or both. In ISWRD sleep and wake episodes are fragmented, with the longest sleep bout being typically less than 4 hours, but sleep duration across the 24 hours may be normal for age. The risk for ISWRD is increased in neurodegenerative disorders (e.g., Alzheimer's disease, Parkinson's disease, and Huntington disease) and children with developmental disorders. Poor sleep hygiene and lack of exposure to external synchronizing agents (i.e., light, activity, and social cues) may be predisposing as well as precipitating factors involved in the development of ISWRD, particularly in institutionalized older individuals.

Non-24-hour sleep-wake rhythm disorder (Non24 SWD) is characterized by a period lasting 1–2 hours longer than 24 hours, progressively delayed sleep period. Patients with Non24 SWD are not adjusted (entrained) to the 24-hour cycle (Fig. 3d). The disease is also called *free-running* or *non-entrained disorder*. As the biological clock (SCN) continues to operate in *free-running*, appropriate alignment periods may occur eventually, but this resolution is temporary. Symptoms of insomnia or excessive daytime sleepiness can occur because the intrinsic circadian pacemaker is not entrained to a 24-hour light/dark cycle. This disorder can occur in people in which the circadian system loses its ability to synchronize to environmental cues. Blind individuals have an obvious failure to entrain circadian rhythms due to the lack of photic input to the circadian pacemaker. Also, there is an increased incidence of Non24 SWD in psychiatric disorders, and occasionally, the disorder is associated with dementia or developmental intellectual disability.

2.2 *Circadian Disorders Imposed by Extrinsic Causes*

Jet lag and shift work disorders are considered of extrinsic origin. The advent of air travel crossing time zones has led to a disorder called jet lag, since crossing different time zones is associated with the need to sleep and to be awake at times that are misaligned with the circadian system. This change in the time zone modifies the habitual exposure to light, generating a desynchronization of circadian rhythms or a circadian rupture. The severity of the misalignment depends on how many time zones have been crossed and the direction of travel. Because the natural circadian cycle is slightly longer than 24 hours, the journey to the west usually causes fewer interruptions, as it is easier to delay than to advance the circadian cycle. In this case, individuals have difficulty falling asleep at local time in the new zone or keeping awake when necessary. Daytime sleepiness may occur due to sleep deprivation as well as circadian misalignment. These disturbances persist until the circadian system is synchronized to the new destination time zone.

A term used nowadays is "social jet lag," referring to shift work disorder, that is, the desynchronization of circadian rhythms originating from the disorder between the preference of sleep schedules and social obligations (work, school, childcare, domestic and family responsibilities, etc.) [15].

The shift-work disorder manifests by complaints of insomnia or excessive sleepiness that occur in association with work hours that happen during the usual sleep episode – at least in part. There are numerous categories of shift-work agendas, including evening shifts, night shifts, early morning shifts, rotating shifts, split shifts, on-call overnight duty, and long-duration work shifts that include work hours at night. As a result, people accumulate sleep deficit and increase the risk of accidents, mistakes, and other adverse health outcomes in addition to presenting sleep disorders, such as gastrointestinal (stomachache, diarrhea, etc.), cardiovascular (coronary heart disease, hypertension, etc.), and psychosocial disorders (affective and sexual difficulties). The worker cannot rest properly after the shift and cannot participate in social activities [16–19].

Despite the consequences of shift work on workers' health, night work is part of modern society due to the need for services available 24 hours a day. However, night shift work contradicts a biological determination of the human being to perform their waking activities during the day and sleep at night. In this context, shift work can be one of the causes of circadian desynchronization and, therefore, is considered a stressor, causing stress, and can stimulate the HPA axis, thus leading to obesity [20, 21].

The sleep of night or shift workers has a shorter duration compared to day workers. The inversion of the sleep phase (daytime sleep) also generates a higher number of complaints related to sleep and health, since it interferes with sleep structure and results in chronic sleep restriction [22].

For example, truck drivers who worked irregular hours, including during the night, reported worse health conditions and showed higher cortisol concentrations with daily drivers, including the day off, suggesting a more prolonged response to stress [8].

3 Diagnosis and Follow-Up

Several strategies are used to evaluate and monitor the patient with sleep-wake cycle disorder of the circadian rhythm. Some self-reported measures, including sleep diaries/sleep logs, and objective measures such as actigraphy (see Chaps. 35, 36, and 37) have additional benefits to establish a diagnosis. Polysomnography is not normally indicated, except when a sleep disorder is suspected [13, 23] (i.e., obstructive sleep apnea syndrome or narcolepsy).

Regarding melatonin, it can be dosed to determine the circadian phase of an individual. Schedules can be designed with the physician to regulate the release of melatonin and thus help within sleep onset. Melatonin is usually released about 90–120 minutes before the usual bedtime, as long as there is no strong light. Intense light suppresses melatonin production [7]. The dim-light melatonin onset (DLMO) protocol [24] involves intermittent blood or saliva collection every 30–60 minutes, around 6 hours before and 1 hour after bedtime. The time at which melatonin levels rise above the limit provides a valid and reliable indicator of the position of the circadian phase [25]. The DLMO protocol is commonly used in research. It may eventually be used more routinely in clinical practice to help confirm diagnoses in challenging cases and to help identify the ideal time for interventions that aim to change the circadian phase (e.g., exposure to intense light, administration of exogenous melatonin, the practice of physical activity).

4 Final Words

It is very important to recognize the different types of CSWD so that management is as appropriate as possible and patient-centered. In this way, the person will be fully benefited, with improved sleep, health, and quality of life. It is also imperative

Physical Therapy in Circadian Rhythm Disorders: Chrono-rehabilitation?

Cristina Frange

Every circadian sleep-wake disorder requires a specific treatment strategy. For the success of the treatment, the circadian rhythm should be synchronized with the desired/needed sleep-wake cycle. Physiotherapists together with other health practitioners (physicians, psychologists, nutritionist, etc.) treat the patients in order to synchronize the rhythm.

According to the American Academy of Sleep Medicine Clinical Practice Guideline for the Treatment of Intrinsic Circadian Rhythm Sleep-Wake Disorders (CRSWD) [1], and depending on the disorder, useful approaches may include careful adjustments of sleep-wake times, sleep hygiene strategies, behavioral and pharmacological therapies (e.g., administration of melatonin or melatonin receptor agonists), exercise, and bright light therapy.

The physiotherapeutic treatment of CRSWD starts with the clinical picture of the patient: the anamnesis. Questionnaires such as the Munich Chronotype Questionnaire or the Morningness-Eveningness Questionnaire (described in chapter "Subjective Assessment of Sleep") combined with actigraphy and sleep diary for more than 10 days (to have weekdays and weekends sleep-wake cycle) can help to set up the diagnosis (done by a physician), and to follow with the treatment regimen. In case any circadian misalignment is suspected, the physiotherapist (PT) must send the patient to the sleep medicine specialized physician.

Circadian disorders are often presented within sleep disorders. A patient seeking treatment for sleep disorders, or even a patient found to have a sleep disorder,

C. Frange (✉)
Department of Neurology and Neurosurgery, Escola Paulista de Medicina, Universidade Federal de São Paulo, Sao Paulo, SP, Brazil

Certified in Sleep Physiotherapy by the Brazilian Sleep Society (ABS), and The Brazilian Association of Cardiorespiratory Physiotherapy and Physiotherapy in Intensive Care (ASSOBRAFIR), Sao Paulo, SP, Brazil

World Physiotherapy Network for Health Promotion in Life and Work, Sao Paulo, SP, Brazil

C. Frange, F. M. S. Coelho (eds.), *Sleep Medicine and Physical Therapy*, https://doi.org/10.1007/978-3-030-85074-6_11

need to be evaluated regarding his/her routine: at what time he/she goes to bed, what time sleeps, how many times and why he/she wakes up in the night (nocturia? noise? worries? etc.), and at what times he/she wakes up and gets off the bed. Also, daytime repercussions such as waking up refreshed, restored, with lots of energy, or wanting to sleep more and feeling restless, tired and sleepy. In addition, behaviors related to bedtime such as the use of electronic devices (e.g., tv, computer or smartphone) after sleep, light, alarm clock, room temperature, snoring partner, etc., should be taken into consideration to have the most complete "clinical picture" of the patient's routine and behaviors regarding sleep. Having said that, sleep hygiene should be taught, explaining the rationale for each one of the "rules" and implementing it into clinical practice, as the behavior strategies might be used (e.g., stimulus control, sleep restriction therapy, relaxation therapy, cognitive therapy, paradoxical intention) (more on Chapter "Optimizing Behavior Strategies for Sleep".

As diurnal animals, human activity, exercise, and feeding primarily occur during daylight hours, in contrast to sleep, rest, and fasting throughout the night – and we must respect these rhythms, even in the presence of light, technology, and the "avatar" that we became of ourselves in the contemporary life, constantly exposed to light (and specifically to blue bright light). Of course, some preferences, whether determined genetically or by the environment such as chronotype, circadian preferences, and being a shorter, intermediate, or longer sleeper should be taken into account.

1 Morning Larks and Night Owls

Genetically, we can talk about chronotype. The chronotype is associated with an individual's endogenous circadian clock rhythm and determines the circadian preference to realize their activities. The elucidation of molecular clock gene polymorphisms as a genetic basis of chronotype has become a consideration for sports performance, for example. A length polymorphism in the human Per3 gene (along with the gene's endogenous circadian expression) has been associated with altered morning-evening preferences in the general population, the longer allele being linked to morning type, and the shorter allele with evening type [2]. Analysis of elite athletes from both genders, from a variety of sports reveals an overrepresentation of morning types in sports generally taking place in the morning, such as marathon running, cycling, or triathlon [3, 4]. These findings suggest that those with strong morning preferences may be more drawn to sporting activities that take place during the early morning. Alternatively, those with chronotypes that radically oppose the performance schedules of that sport may simply not progress to the very elite level, resulting in a selection bias. Thus, exercise capacity and chronotype may exhibit reciprocal feedback. It's hard to change chronotype; some even say it cannot be changed, but we can learn how to have the best of our genetic predisposed preference, adjusting it in some types of routines, not extreme ones. For example, a morning-type person will always present difficulty to work during the night (e.g., shift work), and PTs can help to ameliorate the difficulties, but no technique/method that PTs make will transition this person to an evening-type.

2 At What Time to Rehab?

Circadian preferences are another fact to be considered, linked to chronotypes. Circadian preferences are the propensity for an individual to sleep at a particular time during 24 hours (classified as morning, evening, or intermediate types). Morning-type people are individuals who prefer to get up early and carry out their activities in the morning; evening-type people are those who prefer to wake up late and carry out their activities during the afternoon or evening, and intermediate ones are those who choose intermediate times between the two extremes and can easily adapt to either one.

Can circadian preferences influence rehabilitation or physiotherapy sessions? Until now, we do not have a consensus on this. Even though clinically (and empirically) I believe that yes, they do have an impact on rehabilitation, no systematic reviews with meta-analysis have been made so far. In a recent investigation, our group examined circadian preferences and sleep quality of stroke rehabilitation. The participants were divided into morning-type, indifferent, and evening-type preferences, according to their responses to the Morningness-Eveningness Questionnaire. All the participants underwent rehabilitation of the upper extremity by the same protocol, performed during the morning (the time that many of the rehabilitation centers work in Brazil). We noticed that evening-type patients demonstrated less improvement in motor skill performance, compared to morning and intermediate types [5], as in other investigations [6, 7]. The influence of circadian preference may help within rehabilitation or may represent a stressor at requesting cognition, strength, memory, and motor learning at non-preferred times, having less cognitive reserve to compensate for additional demands in times of stress. These can lead to fatigue and other physiological, psychological, and environmental factors that affect learning, especially motor abilities.

The time of the day of rehabilitation/physiotherapy session matters, according to the patient's circadian preferences and chronotype. Again, we do not have any evidence to state that the time of rehabilitation should be this or that way. Therefore, some investigations with specific populations are arising. If there is a time of the day (*when*) that we can optimize the session, it means that *what* we do in this session may act as a *zeitgeber*: a rhythmically occurring natural phenomenon that acts as a cue in the regulation of the body's circadian rhythms (German word for time giver). These *zeitgebers* include social contacts, the timing of ingestion of food, the knowledge of time itself, the scheduling of normal rest and activity habits, and, possibly, the participation in regular physical activity and exercise.

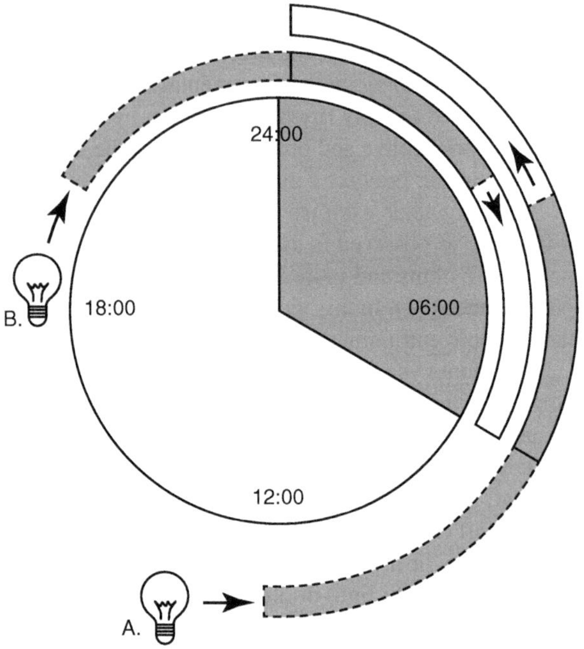

Fig. 1 Schematic representation of light therapy for CRSWD. Bottom, (**a**) morning light therapy will phase advance delayed sleep phase. Left, (**b**) evening light therapy will phase delay advanced sleep phase. Gray pie represents conventional sleep time, and gray bars represent disordered sleep times being phase-shifted. (Reprinted with permission from Lu and Zee [28])

restores the circadian amplitude in sleep-wakefulness [21], and improves restless behavior, enhancing neuronal activity in the suprachiasmatic nuclei [22].

Bright light is a promising non-pharmacological intervention that has been applied therapeutically as a treatment for sleep disorders and for compensating circadian misalignments [23–25]. Some authors suggest the application of bright light at predetermined times to improve sleep, but especially to promote synchronization between biological rhythms (Fig. 1) and working hours in the case of workers undergoing fixed night shifts of work, as well as adapting the content of meals and encouraging the practice of physical activity of these workers [26, 27]. A meta-analysis showed that in general, light therapy is effective in treating sleep problems [24]. Having a routine is a must and will help to reset the internal clocks.

Bright light therapy is offered for the patient by portable units generating about 10,000 lux, and exposure time is about 30–45 min/day [29], and the recommendation is to keep the face directed at the light source, but not to continuously stare into the light. The patient can be eating, reading, or working on a computer while receiving light therapy. Cool color temperatures (blue wavelengths) inhibit melatonin secretion and stimulate the production of cortisol (i.e., alertness and activity hormone), while warm color temperatures stimulate the secretion of melatonin [30]. Hence, treatment must be individualized.

Therefore, there is an urgent need for standardized protocols to allow a comparison between investigations and, further, the writing of a consensus and guideline. Although there is no consensus about the ideal treatment characteristics (duration, frequency, dose, intensity) [31], there is an agreement about the timing of treatment according to the phase response curve to light [29, 32]. This bright light administered in the morning after the lowest point of core body temperature (nadir, around 4 h) shifts the biological clock rhythm to an earlier point in time, having a phase advancing effect, whereas exposure to bright light in the evening (before the nadir of the core body temperature) shifts it to a later time, having a phase delaying effect. Roughly speaking, light in the evening normally causes phase delay, and light in the morning, phase advance. That happens because nocturnal melatonin secretion is suppressed by bright light [21] and therefore can interfere with neuroendocrine hormone production and release timing.

The effectiveness of bright light therapy is supported for the treatment of a variety of diseases: seasonal affective disorder and major depression; sleep disorders [23, 24, 33]; sleep problems related to Alzheimer's disease and dementia [25, 34]; premenstrual dysphoric syndrome [35]; bulimia nervosa [36]; and antepartum and postpartum [37, 38].

5 Circadian Disruption

It has been hypothesized that chronic circadian disruption may be a contributing factor for the increased susceptibility to diseases of the musculoskeletal system [39], including degenerative intervertebral disease and low back pain [40]. Chronic circadian rhythm disruption, as experienced by shift workers, for example, has been associated with an increased risk of various disorders and diseases, including insomnia, obesity, diabetes, hypertension, cardiovascular disease, and cancer [41–43]. The role of the circadian clock within the musculoskeletal system has only recently been studied. In animal studies, evidence shows that disruption of the circadian rhythm acts as a risk factor for the development of osteoarthritis in the mouse knee joint [44], demonstrating a possible link between environmental chronic circadian dysfunction, such as that experienced by night shift workers and frequent travelers moving across time zones, and the development of osteoarthritis over time. Those authors found that phase-shifting activated catabolic signaling and suppressed chondroprotective pathways in the knee joints of the studied animals [44]. Also, mutations in clock genes demonstrated regulation of bone volume [45], suppression of long bone growth [45], and increased vulnerability to rheumatoid arthritis [46], suggesting that the molecular clock is important for proper function within the skeletal system.

CRSWD can result from alterations in the endogenous circadian clock, such as delayed sleep phase, advanced sleep phase, free-running type, and irregular sleep-wake cycle, or from alterations in the physical environment with the endogenous clock, such as shift work disorder and jet lag, as described in the previous chapter of this book. The clinical characteristics and treatment of CRSWD are presented in Table 1.

Even though there is robust evidence that alteration in the circadian timing system is a common etiology of CRSWD, as well as a result of misalignment between endogenous rhythms and the external environment, the specific mechanisms

Table 1 Overview of Clinical Characteristics and Non-pharmacological Treatment of CRSWD

CRSWD	Clinical presentation	Preferred sleep/ wake times	Treatment
Delayed sleep phase	Difficulty falling asleep at night; difficulty waking up in the morning	Bedtime: 02–06 h; wake time: 10–13 h	Bright light therapy: 2000–2500 lux for 2–3 h starting from 06 h Dark goggles from 16 h to dusk (optional)
Advanced sleep phase	Early evening sleepiness; difficulty maintaining sleep in the morning	Bedtime: 6–9 pm; wake time: 2–5 am	Bright light therapy: 2500 lux for 4 h starting from 20 h or 4000 lux for 2–3 h starting from 20–21 h
Free-running type	Alternating periods of insomnia and excessive sleepiness or both, with short asymptomatic periods	Bedtime: delayed each day; wake time: delayed each day	Sleep hygiene
Irregular sleep-wake rhythm	Insomnia or excessive sleepiness	Irregular pattern of sleep and wake times	Increase in social interaction Physical activities Light exposure during the day Bright light therapy: 2500–3000 lux for 2 h in the morning is effective
Shift work disorder	Difficulty falling asleep or maintaining sleep; sleepiness at work	–	Bright light therapy: 5000–10,000 lux beginning early during the night shift and terminating 2 h before the end of shift (continuous or intermittent) Avoidance of morning bright light with dark goggles Wake-promoting agents: caffeine
Jet lag	Sleep initiation and maintenance insomnia; daytime sleepiness; decreased performance	–	Timed light exposure at destination: on eastward flights, minimize morning light and maximize afternoon light; on westward flights, stay awake while there is light outside

Reprinted with permission from Lu and Zee [28]. We have excluded from the original table the melatonin treatment as it only can be prescribed by a physician and was not the scope of this chapter

responsible for most of these disorders are yet unknown. As both behavioral and environmental influences may interfere within CRSWD, physiotherapeutic interventions need to address circadian physiology, along with these influences.

6 Final Words

Circadian rhythmicity of many common diseases and their rehabilitation requires to be explored to establish *chronopreventive* and *chronotherapeutic* strategies, and here we must think about PT practices incorporating these new ideas.

References

1. Auger RR, et al. Clinical practice guideline for the treatment of intrinsic circadian rhythm sleep-wake disorders: advanced sleep-wake phase disorder (ASWPD), delayed sleep-wake phase disorder (DSWPD), non-24-hour sleep-wake rhythm disorder (N24SWD), and irregular sleep-wake rhythm disorder (ISWRD). An update for 2015: an American Academy of Sleep Medicine clinical practice guideline. J Clin Sleep Med. 2015;11(10):1199–236.
2. Archer SN, et al. A length polymorphism in the circadian clock gene Per3 is linked to delayed sleep phase syndrome and extreme diurnal preference. Sleep. 2003;26(4):413–5.
3. Henst RH, et al. A chronotype comparison of South African and Dutch marathon runners: the role of scheduled race start times and effects on performance. Chronobiol Int. 2015;32(6):858–68.
4. Lastella M, et al. The chronotype of elite athletes. J Hum Kinet. 2016;54:219–25.
5. Pereira DD, et al. The influence of sleep quality and circadian preferences on upper extremity rehabilitation in stroke patients after constraint-induced movement therapy. Int J Rehabil Res. 2020;43(1):20–7.
6. Paradee CV, et al. Circadian preference and cognitive functioning among rehabilitation inpatients. Clin Neuropsychol. 2005;19(1):55–72.
7. West A, et al. Impact of naturalistic lighting on hospitalized stroke patients in a rehabilitation unit: design and measurement. Chronobiol Int. 2017;34(6):687–97.
8. Miyazaki T, et al. Phase-advance shifts of human circadian pacemaker are accelerated by daytime physical exercise. Am J Physiol Regul Integr Comp Physiol. 2001;281(1):R197–205.
9. Eastman CI, et al. Phase-shifting human circadian rhythms with exercise during the night shift. Physiol Behav. 1995;58(6):1287–91.
10. Van Reeth O, et al. Nocturnal exercise phase delays circadian rhythms of melatonin and thyrotropin secretion in normal men. Am J Physiol. 1994;266(6 Pt 1):E964–74.
11. Buxton OM, et al. Roles of intensity and duration of nocturnal exercise in causing phase delays of human circadian rhythms. Am J Physiol. 1997;273(3 Pt 1):E536–42.
12. Baehr EK, et al. Circadian phase-shifting effects of nocturnal exercise in older compared with young adults. Am J Physiol Regul Integr Comp Physiol. 2003;284(6):R1542–50.
13. Gill S, Panda S. A smartphone app reveals erratic diurnal eating patterns in humans that can be modulated for health benefits. Cell Metab. 2015;22(5):789–98.
14. Barger LK, et al. Daily exercise facilitates phase delays of circadian melatonin rhythm in very dim light. Am J Physiol Regul Integr Comp Physiol. 2004;286(6):R1077–84.
15. Biello SM, Janik D, Mrosovsky N. Neuropeptide Y and behaviorally induced phase shifts. Neuroscience. 1994;62(1):273–9.
16. Marchant EG, Watson NV, Mistlberger RE. Both neuropeptide Y and serotonin are necessary for entrainment of circadian rhythms in mice by daily treadmill running schedules. J Neurosci. 1997;17(20):7974–87.
17. Lewis P, et al. Exercise time cues (zeitgebers) for human circadian systems can foster health and improve performance: a systematic review. BMJ Open Sport Exerc Med. 2018;4(1):e000443.
18. Buxton OM, et al. Exercise elicits phase shifts and acute alterations of melatonin that vary with circadian phase. Am J Physiol Regul Integr Comp Physiol. 2003;284(3):R714–24.
19. Youngstedt SD, et al. Circadian phase-shifting effects of bright light, exercise, and bright light + exercise. J Circadian Rhythms. 2016;14:2.
20. Martin T, et al. Exploration of circadian rhythms in patients with bilateral vestibular loss. PLoS One. 2016;11(6):e0155067.
21. Lewy AJ, et al. Light suppresses melatonin secretion in humans. Science. 1980;210(4475):1267–9.
22. Swaab DF, Fliers E, Partiman TS. The suprachiasmatic nucleus of the human brain in relation to sex, age and senile dementia. Brain Res. 1985;342(1):37–44.

bowel syndrome, and fibromyalgia, illustrates the complexity in diagnosis and treatment planning of such a condition that requires interdisciplinary collaboration [10–14]. The common clinical belief suggesting that the frequency of sleep bruxism motor activity, a condition further described below, and TMD can be associated or be in a causal relationship is largely debated and not supported by solid evidence at this time [15–18]. Muscle pain dominance over joint one may have different manifestations during sleep [19], a phenotype to be confirmed. A recent consensus study report of the *National Academies of Sciences, Engineering, and Medicine* from the USA published a solid text on many issues related to TMD; it is exploring future directions to improve our understanding and management of such a challenging clinical manifestation (http://nap.edu/25652).

The objective of this chapter is to focus on a sister condition, probably not as well known by a physical therapist, sleep bruxism (SB). It is noteworthy that SB can occur by coincidence or can contribute to exacerbating OFP and TMD, a debated topic well beyond the focus of the present review [15, 17, 18, 20, 21].

It is important to clarify that sleep bruxism (SB) and TMD are not the same entities. Some individuals may have SB without TMD, and some may have OFP and/or TMD for other reasons, such as awake parafunctional habits, acute trauma, and systemic conditions. Also, the physiopathology and mechanisms are most likely different as explained in this chapter.

1 What Is Sleep Bruxism?

Sleep bruxism (SB) is defined, based on an international group of experts, "*as repetitive masticatory muscle activity characterized by clenching or grinding of the teeth and/or by bracing or thrusting of the mandible and specified as either sleep bruxism or awake bruxism*" [22, 23]. SB can be considered a behavioral condition when it is repeated for a non-purposes reason too frequently and/or a motor condition to sleep disorders when its frequency reaches harmful or disrupting level or when SB is associated with comorbidities. Its prevalence is in the range of 5–16% in adults up to 40% in children, again depending on the type of question, methodology used, and duration covered [24–26]. Much higher prevalence is reported for younger age individuals, and it seems the condition runs in families. A study with questionnaire and polysomnography of an adult general population in Sao Paulo City, Brazil, has shown the SB prevalence of 12.4% for reports of SB complaints at least once a week, 5.4% for polysomnography, and 7.3% for both [27].

In the clinic, it is recognized by the following criteria suggested by the ICSD-3 (International Classification of Sleep Disorders), where criteria A and B should meet [28]:

A. Tooth grinding sound awareness has been reported by sleep partner or parents.
B. The presence of one or more of the following clinical signs:

   (i) Tooth wear or damage to a dental restoration

(ii) Complaints of morning jaw muscle pain or fatigue and/or temporal headache and/or jaw locking

SB can also be concomitant to headache, orofacial pain, and temporomandibular disorders and can occur with comorbidities such as obstructive sleep apnea (OSA), gastroesophageal reflux disorder (GERD), insomnia, headache, orofacial pain, periodic limb movement (PLM), REM sleep behavior disorder, and sleep epilepsy [27, 29, 30].

SB can be graded as follows (this is based on the 2018 International consensus) [23]:

(i) **possible** if the individual is aware of tooth grinding or jaw clenching within the sleep period, self-reports
(ii) **probable** if the following is or is not associated with tooth wear, clinical examination
(iii) **definitive (more confirmatory)**, if recording of masseter and/or temporalis muscles activity show a rise in electromyography (EMG) [23]

The EMG recordings are done in the sleep laboratory, polysomnography (PSG), for extensive descriptive research, or in the presence of critical comorbidities or in-home with an ambulatory system using multichannel on only one EMG. The last is mainly a screening or follow-up tool not yet considered for diagnosis. The EMG biomarker is named masticatory muscle activity (MMA), and its frequency can be counted in hours of sleep. Although such index is used in research, their clinical correspondence to clinical severity and manifestations remains to be demonstrated to the therapeutic outcome and presence of sleep comorbidities [29, 31]. Other markers may emerge for such purposes as jaw movement sensors or biomarkers listed in the following section [32, 33].

2 Putative Risk Factors and Mechanism Associated with the Genesis of SB

Even though this is an ongoing area of research with divergent opinions and evidence, few hypotheses have emerged such as emotions, autonomic cardiac and sleep stability, and genetic and other biomarkers with putative mediator roles. So far, none of these could provide a dominant *one-siz-fits-all* explanation. A complex interlaced series of influences probably need to be identified with the use of machine learning analyses and algorithms adapted for age, gender, comorbidities, and cultural differences in the context of personalized medicine.

The role of wake or diurnal emotions as a driver to impede sleep instability is one axis of interest by many investigators. In summary stress and anxiety, although they have different constructs and that their role is debated by some, were shown to be among risk factors [17, 34–36]. Several factors such as mood, concomitant pain, occupational stress (musician), female gender, less sleep duration, and acute vs.

persistent or chronic influences of risk factors must be considered in the analyses [37–39]. In the context of personalized medicine, individual reaction and adaptation are expected. The specificity of emotion, stress, and/or anxiety as a dominant trigger of rising in jaw muscle activity characterizing remains an open research domain for SB [35, 36, 40]. A recent study in TMD individuals reported that "workload and drive to perform" was associated to rise in temporalis muscle activity; such can be a predisposing factor but not a causal one and probably not specific to SB alone [41]. Children and adolescents seem to be more reactive to stress and display a higher rate of reported SB tooth grinding; children of parents under social and emotional pressure seem also at a higher risk to present tooth grinding [42]. Boys with SB tooth grinding with lip-biting habits and poor sleep quality were observed to present more severe SB [43]. Most of these findings are derived from self-reports or parents' reports grading SB as "possible" according to the proposal of the SB international consensus described above [23]. At that moment, caution in the extrapolation of such association is recommended, since parents are not always reliable in reporting awareness of SB for their children's; the concordance of parent reports with studies using EMG is rather weak, and the numbers reported for such prevalence may be influenced by geographical/cultural differences [36, 44–46].

The evidence related to SB and genetic candidates is somehow intricate to interpret. Some studies reported possible association of serotonin and dopamine in adults and others for the muscle fiber gene-related alpha-actinin-3 in children, this with specific but different polymorphism and variant, while some studies did not [47–50]. Genetics of SB is an area of research that will need more attention and probably larger sample size studies, done in a collaborative mode with saliva and/or blood collection with confirmation of definitive SB using standardized methodologies [51, 52]. Furthermore, differentiation of awake from sleep or concomitant type of bruxism was a challenging issue in published studies till now; the sample size of the subgroup was getting small and prevents any firm conclusion since the genetic studies are avid of large sample to prevent false discovery rate [53]. The search for gene candidates for SB and maybe MAD, based on phenotype and endotype, are to come, but this will probably not explain all clinical manifestations. Indeed, as for most conditions, the environment also plays an important role [54].

The role of autonomic cardiac activation in SB individuals has been known for over half a century, but more recently a series of studies have shown that SB-related onset of MMA is associated with a sudden shift in sympathetic dominance over the parasympathetic one resulting in rising in heart rate and blood pressure [55–58]. Such very time-locked activity to SB-MMA events is further supported by a proof-of-concept experimental study using a medication. Clonidine, an alpha agonist, contributes to reducing the surge of sympathetic activity associated with the onset of MMA, this about sleep arousal; such findings have been confirmed by a clinical randomized trial [59, 60]. The effect of clonidine was in part mediated through its action on the cyclic propensity of arousal during sleep, a recurring phenomenon named cyclic alternating pattern, which contributes as a permissive window for MMA onset [61]. Furthermore, a slight reduction in oxygen level was observed in about 25% of otherwise healthy SB individuals, a finding reproduced in older SB patients with concomitant OSA [62, 63].

The role of blood, urine, salivary biomarkers such as hormonal and inflammatory (17-hydroxycorticosteroids, C-reactive protein, and fibrinogen), and also oxidative factors remains to be confirmed, although some preliminary evidence supported that more comprehensive analyses should be performed taking again into account age and comorbidities such as stress, cardiovascular risk (e.g., hypertension), and the possible contribution of sleep breathing disorders [64–67].

3 How to Manage Sleep Bruxism

Although the role of physical therapy is discussed in chapter "Sleep bruxism: physiotherapeutic approach", in this section we elected to overview SB management from a dental and medical perspective. When dentists propose a treatment for SB, first they must establish a differential diagnosis excluding the presence of other health and/or sleep conditions such as sleep apnea, insomnia, gastroesophageal reflux disorders, and rare ones such as sleep epilepsy and REM behavior disorders. Collaboration with a sleep physician is essential [29]. Plus, the clinician needs to assess the role of other conditions such as anxiety, stress, intense lifestyle, smoking, or drug use among exacerbating risk factors.

Management of SB in otherwise healthy individuals is rather straightforward with an oral appliance to act as a tooth protector. But in the presence of comorbidities such as sleep apnea or insomnia, different oral appliance designs or medications are indicated as described below. A recent systematic analysis concluded the following for managing bruxism: "*Although many of the described variables cannot be influenced by prophylactic or therapeutic means, we recommend the following patient-centered approach ('SMS therapy'): self-observation, muscle relaxation, stabilization (Michigan) splint*" [34]. Then the role of physical therapist within a multi-professional team needs to be precise as described below (Table 1) and this more importantly in the presence of sleep comorbidities [1, 68].

Table 1 Route to manage sleep bruxism

After a medical (apnea) and dental (bruxism, orofacial pain) diagnosis, the management should include:
(i) By dentists, oral appliances such as occlusal splint in individuals without sleep breathing condition, otherwise mandibular advancement appliance are recommended
(ii) By a physical therapist, manual therapy, muscle-stretching exercises and education for home exercise, sleep position, sleep hygiene
(iii) By a psychologist, advanced sleep hygiene advice under cognitive behavioral therapies
(iv) By physician medication, if insomnia and prescription of CPAP, sleep positioning devices, oral appliance and/or medication if sleep apnea and proton pump inhibitor if GERD

8 Final Words

In the era of precision medicine, (i) "differential" diagnosis skills with a comprehensive assessment of risk factors, (ii) multidisciplinary/"inter-sector" health management strategies, and (iii) contribution of patients as a partner are essential to achieve clinical success.

The role of physical therapists in the interprofessional management of sleep and pain disorders is essential. However, for SB the lack of evidence supporting the value of physiotherapy suggests caution in differentiating between SB and DTM (or OFP) during the diagnosis and also in choosing the best management therapies.

References

1. Herrero Babiloni A, Lam JTAT, Exposto FG, Beetz G, Provost C, Gagnon DH, et al. Interprofessional Collaboration in Dentistry: role of physiotherapists to improve care and outcomes for chronic pain conditions and sleep disorders. J Oral Pathol Med. 2020;49(6):529–37.
2. Christidis N, Lindström Ndanshau E, Sandberg A, Tsilingaridis G. Prevalence and treatment strategies regarding temporomandibular disorders in children and adolescents-a systematic review. J Oral Rehabil. 2019;46(3):291–301.
3. Bueno CH, Pereira DD, Pattussi MP, Grossi PK, Grossi ML. Gender differences in temporomandibular disorders in adult populational studies: a systematic review and meta-analysis. J Oral Rehabil. 2018;45(9):720–9.
4. Manfredini D, Guarda-Nardini L, Winocur E, Piccotti F, Ahlberg J, Lobbezoo F. Research diagnostic criteria for temporomandibular disorders: a systematic review of axis I epidemiologic findings. Oral Surg Oral Med Oral Pathol Oral Radiol Endod. 2011;112(4):453–62.
5. Pantoja LLQ, de Toledo IP, Pupo YM, Porporatti AL, De Luca CG, Zwir LF, et al. Prevalence of degenerative joint disease of the temporomandibular joint: a systematic review. Clin Oral Investig. 2019;23(5):2475–88.
6. Calixtre LB, Moreira RF, Franchini GH, Alburquerque-Sendín F, Oliveira AB. Manual therapy for the management of pain and limited range of motion in subjects with signs and symptoms of temporomandibular disorder: a systematic review of randomised controlled trials. J Oral Rehabil. 2015;42(11):847–61.
7. Armijo-Olivo S, Pitance L, Singh V, Neto F, Thie N, Michelotti A. Effectiveness of manual therapy and therapeutic exercise for temporomandibular disorders: systematic review and meta-analysis. Phys Ther. 2016;96(1):9–25.
8. Herrera-Valencia A, Ruiz-Muñoz M, Martin-Martin J, Cuesta-Vargas A, González-Sánchez M. Efficacy of manual therapy in temporomandibular joint disorders and its medium-and long-term effects on pain and maximum mouth opening: a systematic review and meta-analysis. J Clin Med. 2020;9(11):3404.
9. Dreweck FDS, Soares S, Duarte J, Conti PCR, De Luca Canto G, Luís Porporatti A. Association between painful temporomandibular disorders and sleep quality: a systematic review. J Oral Rehabil. 2020;47(8):1041–51.
10. Sanders AE, Akinkugbe AA, Fillingim RB, Ohrbach R, Greenspan JD, Maixner W, et al. Causal mediation in the development of painful temporomandibular disorder. J Pain. 2017;18(4):428–36.
11. DKL T, Pang KP. Clinical phenotype of South-East Asian temporomandibular disorder patients with upper airway resistance syndrome. J Oral Rehabil. 2018;45(1):25–33.

12. Peck CC, Goulet JP, Lobbezoo F, Schiffman EL, Alstergren P, Anderson GC, et al. Expanding the taxonomy of the diagnostic criteria for temporomandibular disorders. J Oral Rehabil. 2014;41(1):2–23.
13. Bonato LL, Quinelato V, De Felipe Cordeiro PC, De Sousa EB, Tesch R, Casado PL. Association between temporomandibular disorders and pain in other regions of the body. J Oral Rehabil. 2017;44(1):9–15.
14. Slade GD, Greenspan JD, Fillingim RB, Maixner W, Sharma S, Ohrbach R. Overlap of five chronic pain conditions: temporomandibular disorders, headache, back pain, irritable bowel syndrome, and fibromyalgia. J Oral Facial Pain Headache. 2020. Suppl;34:s15–s28.
15. Ohlmann B, Waldecker M, Leckel M, Bömicke W, Behnisch R, Rammelsberg P, et al. Correlations between sleep bruxism and temporomandibular disorders. Clin Med. 2020;9(2):611.
16. Shimada A, Castrillon EE, Svensson P. Revisited relationships between probable sleep bruxism and clinical muscle symptoms. J Dent. 2019;82:85–90.
17. Smardz J, Martynowicz H, Michalek-Zrabkowska M, Wojakowska A, Mazur G, Winocur E. Sleep bruxism and occurrence of temporomandibular disorders-related pain: a polysomnographic study. Front Neurol. 2019;10:168.
18. Baad-Hansen L, Thymi M, Lobbezoo F, Svensson P. To what extent is bruxism associated with musculoskeletal signs and symptoms? A systematic review. J Oral Rehabil. 2019;46(9):845–61.
19. Santiago V, Raphael K. Absence of joint pain identifies high levels of sleep masticatory muscle activity in myofascial temporomandibular disorder. J Oral Rehabil. 2019;46(12):1161–9.
20. Jiménez-Silva A, Peña-Durán C, Tobar-Reyes J, Frugone-Zambra R. Sleep and awake bruxism in adults and its relationship with temporomandibular disorders: a systematic review from 2003 to 2014. Acta Odontol Scand. 2017;75(1):36–58.
21. Wieckiewicz M, Smardz J, Martynowicz H, Wojakowska A, Mazur G, Winocur E. Distribution of temporomandibular disorders among sleep bruxers and non-bruxers-A polysomnographic study. J Oral Rehabil. 2020;47(7):820–6.
22. Lobbezoo F, Ahlberg J, Glaros AG, Kato T, Koyano K, Lavigne GJ, et al. Bruxism defined and graded: an international consensus. J Oral Rehabil. 2013;40(1):2–4.
23. Lobbezoo F, Ahlberg J, Raphael KG, Wetselaar P, Glaros AG, Kato T, et al. International consensus on the assessment of bruxism: report of a work in progress. J Oral Rehabil. 2018;45(11):837–44.
24. Khoury S, Carra MC, Huynh N, Montplaisir J, Lavigne GJ. Sleep bruxism-tooth grinding prevalence, characteristics and familial aggregation: a large cross-sectional survey and polysomnographic validation. Sleep. 2016;39(11):2049–56.
25. Drumond CL, Ramos-Jorge J, Vieira-Andrade RG, Paiva SM, Serra-Negra JMC, Ramos-Jorge ML. Prevalence of probable sleep bruxism and associated factors in Brazilian schoolchildren. Int J Paediatr Dent. 2018 Oct 30. Online ahead of print.
26. Wetselaar P, Vermaire EJH, Lobbezoo F, Schuller AA. The prevalence of awake bruxism and sleep bruxism in the Dutch adult population. J Oral Rehabil. 2019;46(7):617–23.
27. Maluly M, Andersen ML, Dal-Fabbro C, Garbuio S, Bittencourt L, de Siqueira JTT, et al. Polysomnographic study of the prevalence of sleep bruxism in a population sample. J Dent Res. 2013;92(7 Suppl):97S–103S.
28. American Academy of Sleep Medicine (AASM) - International classification of sleep disorders – Third Edition (ICSD-3). Springer Med; 2014.
29. Mayer P, Heinzer R, Lavigne G. Sleep bruxism in respiratory medicine practice. Chest. 2016;149(1):262–71.
30. Maluly M, Dal Fabbro C, Andersen ML, Herrero-Babiloni A, Lavigne GJ, Tufik S. Sleep bruxism and its associations with insomnia and OSA in the general population of Sao Paulo. Sleep Med. 2020;75:141–8.
31. Manfredini D, Ahlberg J, Wetselaar P, Svensson P, Lobbezoo F. The bruxism construct: from cut-off points to a continuum spectrum. J Oral Rehabil. 2019;46(11):991–7.
32. Okura K, Shigemoto S, Suzuki Y, Noguchi N, Omoto K, Abe S, et al. Mandibular movement during sleep bruxism associated with current tooth attrition. J Prosthodont Res. 2017;61(1):87–95.

33. Martinot JB, Borel JC, Le-Dong NN, Silkoff PE, Denison S, Gozal D, et al. Bruxism relieved under CPAP treatment in a patient with OSA syndrome. Chest. 2020;157(3):e59–62.
34. Kuhn M, Türp JC. Risk factors for bruxism. Swiss Dent J. 2018;128(2):118–24.
35. Manfredini D, Arreghini A, Lombardo L, Visentin A, Cerea S, Castroflorio T, et al. Assessment of anxiety and coping features in bruxers: a portable electromyographic and electrocardiographic study. J Oral Facial Pain Headache. 2016;30(3):249–54.
36. Alfano CA, Bower JL, Meers JM. Polysomnography-detected bruxism in children is associated with somatic complaints but not anxiety. J Clin Sleep Med. 2018;14(1):23–9.
37. Muzalev K, Visscher CM, Koutris M, Lobbezoo F. Long-term variability of sleep bruxism and psychological stress in patients with jaw-muscle pain: report of two longitudinal clinical cases. J Oral Rehabil. 2018;45(2):104–9.
38. Ohlmann B, Bömicke W, Habibi Y, Rammelsberg P, Schmitter M. Are there associations between sleep bruxism, chronic stress, and sleep quality? J Dent. 2018;74:101–6.
39. van Selms M, Kroon J, Tuomilehto H, Peltomaa M, Savolainen A, Manfredini D, Lobbezoo F, Ahlberg J. Self-reported sleep bruxism among Finnish symphony orchestra musicians: associations with perceived sleep-related problems and psychological stress. Cranio. 2020;30:1–8.
40. Smardz J, Martynowicz H, Wojakowska A, Michalek-Zrabkowska M, Mazur G, Wieckiewicz M. Correlation between sleep bruxism, stress, and depression-a polysomnographic study. J Clin Med. 2019;8(9):1344.
41. Schmitter M, Kares-Vrincianu A, Kares H, Malsch C, Schindler HJ. Chronic stress and temporalis muscle activity in TMD patients and controls during sleep: a pilot study in females. Clin Oral Investig. 2019;23(2):667–72.
42. Alves CL, Fagundes DM, PBF S, Ferreira MC. Knowledge of parents/caregivers about bruxism in children treated at the pediatric dentistry clinic. Sleep Sci. 2019;12(3):185–9.
43. Soares JP, Giacomin A, Cardoso M, Serra-Negra JM, Bolan M. Association of gender, oral habits, and poor sleep quality with possible sleep bruxism in schoolchildren. Braz Oral Res. 2020;34:e019.
44. Huynh NT, Desplats E, Bellerive A. Sleep bruxism in children: sleep studies correlate poorly with parental reports. Sleep Med. 2016;19:63–8.
45. Restrepo C, Manfredini D, Castrillon E, Svensson P, Santamaria A, Alvarez C, et al. Diagnostic accuracy of the use of parental-reported sleep bruxism in a polysomnographic study in children. Int J Paediatr Dent. 2017;27(5):318–25.
46. van Selms MKA, Marpaung C, Pogosian A, Lobbezoo F. Geographical variation of parental-reported sleep bruxism among children: comparison between the Netherlands, Armenia and Indonesia. Int Dent J. 2019;69(3):237–43.
47. Abe Y, Suganuma T, Ishii M, Yamamoto G, Gunji T, Clark GT, et al. Association of genetic, psychological and behavioral factors with sleep bruxism in a Japanese population. J Sleep Res. 2012;21(3):289–96.
48. Oporto GH 5th, Bornhardt T, Iturriaga V, Salazar LA. Genetic polymorphisms in the serotonergic system are associated with circadian manifestations of bruxism. J Oral Rehabil. 2016;43(11):805–12.
49. Oporto GH 5th, Bornhardt T, Iturriaga V, Salazar LA. Single nucleotide polymorphisms in genes of dopaminergic pathways are associated with bruxism. Clin Oral Investig. 2018;22(1):331–7.
50. Wieckiewicz M, Bogunia-Kubik K, Mazur G, Danel D, Smardz J, Wojakowska A, et al. Genetic basis of sleep bruxism and sleep apnea-response to a medical puzzle. Sci Rep. 2020;10(1):7497.
51. Belal Bin Heyat M, Akhtar F, Khan MH, Ullah N, Gul I, Khan H, et al. Detection, Treatment planning, and genetic predisposition of bruxism: a systematic mapping process and network visualization technique. CNS Neurol Disord Drug Targets. 2020. Online ahead of print.
52. Manfredini D, Ahlberg J, Aarab G, Bracci A, Durham J, Ettlin D. Towards a Standardized Tool for the Assessment of Bruxism (STAB)-Overview and general remarks of a multidimensional bruxism evaluation system. J Oral Rehabil. 2020;47(5):549–56.
53. Zou G, Zuo Y. On the sample size requirement in genetic association tests when the proportion of false positives is controlled. Genetics. 2006;172(1):687–91.

54. Rintakoski K, Hublin C, Lobbezoo F, Rose RJ, Kaprio J. Genetic factors account for half of the phenotypic variance in liability to sleep-related bruxism in young adults: a nationwide Finnish twin cohort study. Twin Res Hum Genet. 2012;15(6):714–9.
55. Huynh N, Kato T, Rompré PH, Okura K, Saber M, Lanfranchi PA, et al. Sleep bruxism is associated to micro-arousals and an increase in cardiac sympathetic activity. J Sleep Res. 2006;15(3):339–46.
56. Nashed A, Lanfranchi P, Rompré P, Carra MC, Mayer P, Colombo R, et al. Sleep bruxism is associated with a rise in arterial blood pressure. Sleep. 2012;35(4):529–36.
57. Lavigne GJ, Huynh N, Kato T, Okura K, Adachi K, Yao D, et al. Genesis of sleep bruxism: motor and autonomic-cardiac interactions. Arch Oral Biol. 2007;52(4):381–4.
58. Nukazawa S, Yoshimi H, Sato S. Autonomic nervous activities associated with bruxism events during sleep. Cranio. 2018;36(2):106–12.
59. Huynh N, Lavigne GJ, Lanfranchi PA, Montplaisir JY, de Champlain J. The effect of 2 sympatholytic medications--propranolol and clonidine--on sleep bruxism: experimental randomized controlled studies. Sleep. 2006;29(3):307–16.
60. Sakai T, Kato T, Yoshizawa S, Suganuma T, Takaba M, Ono Y, et al. Effect of clonazepam and clonidine on primary sleep bruxism: a double-blind, crossover, placebo-controlled trial. J Sleep Res. 2017;26(1):73–83.
61. Carra MC, Macaluso GM, Rompré PH, Huynh N, Parrino L, Terzano MG, et al. Clonidine has a paradoxical effect on cyclic arousal and sleep bruxism during NREM sleep. Sleep. 2010;33(12):1711–6.
62. Dumais IE, Lavigne GJ, Carra MC, Rompré PH, Huynh NT. Could transient hypoxia be associated with rhythmic masticatory muscle activity in sleep bruxism in the absence of sleep-disordered breathing? A preliminary report. J Oral Rehabil. 2015;42(11):810–8.
63. Suzuki Y, Rompré P, Mayer P, Kato T, Okura K, Lavigne GJ. Changes in oxygen and carbon dioxide in the genesis of sleep bruxism: a mechanism study. J Prosthodont Res. 2020;64(1):43–7.
64. Kara MI, Yanık S, Keskinruzgar A, Taysi S, Copoglu S, Orkmez M, et al. Oxidative imbalance and anxiety in patients with sleep bruxism. Surg Oral Med Oral Pathol Oral Radiol. 2012;114(5):604–9.
65. Minakuchi H, Sogawa C, Miki H, Hara ES, Maekawa K, Sogawa N, et al. Sleep bruxism frequency and platelet serotonin transporter activities in young adult subjects. Sleep Breath. 2016;20(1):271–6.
66. Martynowicz H, Wieckiewicz M, Poreba R, Wojakowska A, Smardz J, Januszewska L, et al. The relationship between sleep bruxism intensity and renalase concentration-an enzyme involved in hypertension development. J Clin Med. 2019;9(1):16.
67. Michalek-Zrabkowska M, Wieckiewicz M, Smardz J, Gac P, Poreba R, Wojakowska A, et al. Determination of inflammatory markers, hormonal disturbances, and sleepiness associated with sleep bruxism among adults. Nat Sci Sleep. 2020;12:969–79.
68. Guaita M, Högl B. Current treatments of bruxism. Curr Treat Options Neurol. 2016;18(2):10.
69. Manfredini D, Ahlberg J, Winocur E, Lobbezoo F. Management of sleep bruxism in adults: a qualitative systematic literature review. J Oral Rehabil. 2015;42(11):862–74.
70. Jokubauskas L, Baltrušaitytė A, Pileičikienė G. Oral appliances for managing sleep bruxism in adults: a systematic review from 2007 to 2017. J Oral Rehabil. 2018;45(1):81–95.
71. Thie NM, Kato T, Bader G, Montplaisir JY, Lavigne GJ. The significance of saliva during sleep and the relevance of oromotor movements. Sleep Med Rev. 2002;6(3):213–27.
72. Gagnon Y, Mayer P, Morisson F, Rompré PH, Lavigne GJ. Aggravation of respiratory disturbances by the use of an occlusal splint in apneic patients: a pilot study. Int J Prosthodont. 2004;17(4):447–53.
73. Nikolopoulou M, Ahlberg J, Visscher CM, Hamburger HL, Naeije M, Lobbezoo F. Effects of occlusal stabilization splints on obstructive sleep apnea: a randomized controlled trial. J Orofac Pain. 2013;27(3):199–205.
74. Wassell RW, Verhees L, Lawrence K, Davies S, Lobbezoo F. Over-the-counter (OTC) bruxism splints available on the Internet. Br Dent J. 2014;216(11):E24.

Sleep Bruxism: Physiotherapeutic Approach

Cinthia Santos Miotto and Amélia Pasqual Marques

There is not much evidence on the role of physical therapy on sleep bruxism (SB) management. Some research has been done showing the results of physiotherapy on the pain control of individuals with temporomandibular disorders (TMD) related possibly to SB [1].

A systematic review published in 2018, which included 24 randomized and non-randomized and controlled and noncontrolled clinical trials and interventions, focused on physical therapy as a treatment for SB or awake bruxism and concluded that there is very low-quality evidence that diverse methods used in physical therapy improve muscle pain and activity, mouth opening, oral health, anxiety, stress, depression, temporomandibular disorder, and head posture in individuals with bruxism. This finding is mainly a result of the poor methodological quality of most of the studies [2].

Although muscle-stretching exercises are a recommended part of several international guidelines for musculoskeletal disorders and may be effective in the management of the jaw muscle activity that gives rise to bruxism, it was shown in a randomized controlled trial using masticatory muscle activity from polysomnography as an outcome measure. Masticatory muscle stretching was not effective in reducing the frequency of SB events in the absence of pain and/or TMD [1–3].

However, most studies of muscle-stretching exercises have mainly focused on their influence on performance (e.g., range of motion, coordination, and muscle strength) of the limb or trunk muscles of healthy individuals or individuals with sports-related injuries. Very few have investigated the stretching of the human

C. S. Miotto
Department of Physiotherapy, Speech Therapy and Occupational Therapy, Faculty of Medicine, University of São Paulo, São Paulo, SP, Brazil

A. P. Marques (✉)
Department of Physical Therapy, Speech Therapy and Occupational Therapy, and Post-Graduate Program in Rehabilitation Sciences, Faculdade de Medicina da Universidade de São Paulo, São Paulo, SP, Brazil

C. Frange, F. M. S. Coelho (eds.), *Sleep Medicine and Physical Therapy*,
https://doi.org/10.1007/978-3-030-85074-6_13

masticatory muscles and non-muscle-stretching exercises in the management of SB. So far there is no prescribed treatment for SB, and conservative and reversible approaches have been used. Among them are physical therapy modalities that focus on reducing the adverse effects of SB on the stomatognathic system and guiding individuals with SB on the importance of awareness of this habit to decrease its frequency and severity [1–3].

The etiology of bruxism is controversial, which makes it difficult to identify a direct cause-effect relationship for its triggering. However, it can be considered a multifactorial disorder, with different factors involved: morphological, psychosocial, and pathophysiological [1–3]. Among the factors related to SB, several investigations highlight that psychosocial factors such as mood disorders and stress play a role in the occurrence, perpetuation, frequency, and severity of SB – especially those based on clinical diagnosis. Although studies based on chin electromyography and/or polysomnography at the sleep laboratory are insufficient to declare that such associations exist in SB, stress and anxiety are related to almost 70% of cases [1–3].

Therefore, it is important to focus on the negative association of the quality of sleep and SB, which can be noticed by the report of the patient having difficulties in sleeping, excessive daytime sleepiness, and insufficient and non-refreshing sleep. They may also complain of insomnia and sleep fragmentation. Sleep duration of fewer than 8 hours, changes in subjective quality, and poor sleep efficiency were associated with SB and suggest impairment of sleep quality, repercussion in daily life activities, and exacerbation of psychosocial factors (e.g., stress, anxiety, and depression), which can consequently contribute to the intensification of SB [1–3].

Among the diagnostic methods for bruxism, polysomnography (PSG) with or without audiovisual recording, performed in the sleep laboratory, and electromyography (EMG) conventional and portable are two of the best ways to establish uniformly and accurately the presence of SB. Clinical diagnosis is a simple, easy-to-apply, affordable, low-cost method and widely used in clinical practice and in studies on bruxism [1–3].

Consequently, anamnesis and clinical examination are used to check for signs, such as the presence of abnormal tooth wear, and specific questionnaires confirm the presence of vigil bruxism (teeth squeezing perceived by the individual himself) and/or sleep (teeth squeaking sound, usually noticed by family members or roommates) in the last six months [1–3].

1 Resources

Despite no consensus or guidelines, some evidence of the physiotherapeutic approach includes resources such as electrotherapeutic transcutaneous electrical nerve stimulation (TENS), microcurrent electrical nerve stimulation (MENS), and biofeedback (BFB) by electromyography (EMG) with visual, sound, and electrical stimuli; postural awareness by movement or Feldenkrais method; muscle relaxation, such as relaxation training and muscle awareness; cognitive behavioral therapy (CBT), such as progressive muscle relaxation and imagination; therapeutic mandibular exercises, muscle stretching, and with facial exerciser; and acupuncture and manual therapy, such as massage therapy [2, 4–21] (Table 1).

Similar to MENS and BFB by visual EMG, TENS improves the pain of the masticatory muscles and generates local relaxation of these muscles respectively [4, 7,

Table1 Evidence on physiotherapeutic treatment for sleep bruxism

	Author	Study	Physiotherapeutic treatment	Parameters (number, duration, and attendance)
Electrical stimulation	Treacy [7]	Blinded RCT	MART/TENS	MART *vs.* TENS *vs.* TENS placebo: 20–30 min session, 20 sessions, 2×/week
	Alvarez-Arenal et al. [4]	Blinded RCT	TENS	TENS: 15 sessions of 45–60 min every 2 days *vs.* Occlusal plaque: 45 days, 24 h/day
	Rajpurohit et al. [11]	Ct	TENS/MENS	TENS *vs.* MENS: 20 min session, 7 sessions
	Jadidi et al. [14]	Blinded cross over RCT	Electrical stimulation	Contingent electrical stimulation: Grindcare® device: 10 weeks
	Jadidi et al. [15]	Pilot study: double-blinded RCT	Electrical stimulation	Contingent electrical stimulation: 5 nights
	Raphael et al. [5]	Ct	Electrical stimulation	Contingent electrical stimulation *vs.* Grindcare®: 6 weeks
	Nishigawa et al. [12]	Pilot study	Electric labial stimulation	Electrical lip stimulation: 5 nights, 1st night: no stimulus, 2nd to 5th night: stimulus every 1 h in the middle of the sleep period
Cognitive behavioral therapy	Restrepo et al. [8]	RCT	CBT	CBT, competency reaction and directed muscle relaxation: 6 months
	Ommerborn et al. [9]	Blinded RCT	CBT	CBT, problem solving + progressive muscle relaxation + night biofeedback + leisure and fun training: 1 h 50 min session,12 sessions *vs.* Occlusal plaque: 12 weeks
Acupuncture	De La Torre et al. [18]	Ct	Acupuncture	acupuncture: 1 session
	Dallanora et al. [10]	Ct	Acupuncture	acupuncture: 1 session

(continued)

and sleep – which justifies the use of physiotherapy interventions concomitant with other treatments for the management of SB.

References

1. Amorim CSM, Espirito Santo AS, Sommer M, Marques AP. Effect of physical therapy in bruxism treatment: a systematic review. J Manipulative Physiol Ther. 2018;41(5):389–404. https://doi.org/10.1016/j.jmpt.2017.10.014.
2. Amorim CSM, Firsoff EF, Vieira GF, Costa JR, Marques AP. Effectiveness of two physical therapy interventions, relative to dental treatment in individuals with bruxism: study protocol of a randomized clinical trial. Trials. 2014;7(15):8. https://doi.org/10.1186/1745-6215-15-8.
3. Amorim CSM, Vieira GF, Firsoff EFO, Frutuoso JRC, Puliti E, Marques A. Symptoms in different severity degrees of bruxism: a cross-sectional study. Fisioter Pesqui. 2016;23(4):423–30. https://doi.org/10.1590/1809-2950/15988723042016.
4. Alvarez-Arenal A, Junquera LM, Fernandez JP, Gonzalez I, Olay S. Effect of occlusal splint and transcutaneous electric nerve stimulation on the signs and symptoms of temporomandibular disorders in patients with bruxism. J Oral Rehabil. 2002;29(9):858–63. https://doi.org/10.1046/j.1365-2842.2002.00923.x.
5. Raphael KG, Janal MN, Sirois DA, Svensson P. Effect of contingent electrical stimulation on masticatory muscle activity and pain in patients with a myofascial temporomandibular disorder and sleep bruxism. J Orofac Pain. 2013;27(1):21–31. https://doi.org/10.11607/jop.1029.
6. Quintero Y, Restrepo CC, Tamayo V, Tamayo M, Velez AL, Gallego G, et al. Effect of awareness through movement on the head posture of bruxist children. J Oral Rehabil. 2009;36(1):18–25. https://doi.org/10.1111/j.1365-2842.2008.01906.x.
7. Treacy K. Awareness/relaxation training and transcutaneous electrical neural stimulation in the treatment of bruxism. J Oral Rehabil. 1999;26(4):280–7. https://doi.org/10.1046/j.1365-2842.1999.00381.x.
8. Restrepo CC, Alvarez E, Jaramillo C, Velez C, Valencia I. Effects of psychological techniques on bruxism in children with primary teeth. J Oral Rehabil. 2001;28(4):354–60. https://doi.org/10.1046/j.1365-2842.2001.00663.x.
9. Ommerborn MA, Schneider C, Giraki M, Schafer R, Handschel J, Franz M, et al. Effects of an occlusal splint compared with cognitive-behavioral treatment on sleep bruxism activity. Eur J Oral Sci. 2007;115(1):7–14. https://doi.org/10.1111/j.1600-0722.2007.00417.x.
10. Dallanora LJFP, Inoue RT, Santos VMA. Acunpucture use in the treatment of patients with bruxism. Rev Gaucha Odontol. 2004;52(5):333–9.
11. Rajpurohit B, Khatri SM, Metgud D, Bagewadi A. Effectiveness of transcutaneous electrical nerve stimulation and microcurrent electrical nerve stimulation in bruxism associated with masticatory muscle pain--a comparative study. Indian J Dent Res. 2010;21(1):104–6. https://doi.org/10.4103/0970-9290.62816.
12. Nishigawa K, Kondo K, Takeuchi H, Clark GT. Contingent electrical lip stimulation for sleep bruxism: a pilot study. J Prosthet Dent. 2003;89(4):412–7. https://doi.org/10.1067/mpr.2003.82.
13. Wieselmann-Penkner K, Janda M, Lorenzoni M, Polansky R. A comparison of the muscular relaxation effect of TENS and EMG-biofeedback in patients with bruxism. J Oral Rehabil. 2001;28(9):849–53. https://doi.org/10.1046/j.1365-2842.2001.00748.x.
14. Jadidi F, Norregaard O, Baad-Hansen L, Arendt-Nielsen L, Svensson P. Assessment of sleep parameters during contingent electrical stimulation in subjects with jaw muscle activity during sleep: a polysomnographic study. Eur J Oral Sci. 2011;119(3):211–8. https://doi.org/10.1111/j.1600-0722.2011.00822.x.

15. Jadidi F, Castrillon EE, Nielsen P, Baad-Hansen L, Svensson P. Effect of contingent electrical stimulation on jaw muscle activity during sleep: a pilot study with a randomized controlled trial design. Acta Odontol Scand. 2013;71(5):1050–62. https://doi.org/10.3109/00016357.2012.741702.
16. Watanabe A, Kanemura K, Tanabe N, Fujisawa M. Effect of electromyogram biofeedback on daytime clenching behavior in subjects with masticatory muscle pain. J Prosthodont Res. 2011;55(2):75–81. https://doi.org/10.1016/j.jpor.2010.09.003.
17. Conti PC, Stuginski-Barbosa J, Bonjardim LR, Soares S, Svensson P. Contingent electrical stimulation inhibits jaw muscle activity during sleep but not pain intensity or masticatory muscle pressure pain threshold in self-reported bruxers: a pilot study. Oral Surg Oral Med Oral Pathol Oral Radiol. 2014;117(1):45–52. https://doi.org/10.1016/j.oooo.2013.08.015.
18. De la Torre Vera RM, Grillo CM, Sousa MLR, Berzin F. La acupuntura puede alterar los patrones musculares del bruxismo. Rev Int Acupuntura. 2012;6(4):144–50. https://doi.org/10.1016/S1887-8369(12)70069-8.
19. Jardini RS, Ruiz LS, Moyses MA. Electromyographic analysis of the masseter and buccinator muscles with the pro-fono facial exerciser use in bruxers. Cranio. 2006;24(1):29–37. https://doi.org/10.1179/crn.2006.006.
20. Needham R, Davies SJ. Use of the Grindcare(R) device in the management of nocturnal bruxism: a pilot study. Br Dent J. 2013;215(1):E1. https://doi.org/10.1038/sj.bdj.2013.653.
21. Makino I, Arai YC, Aono S, Hayashi K, Morimoto A, Nishihara M, et al. The effects of exercise therapy for the improvement of jaw movement and psychological intervention to reduce parafunctional activities on chronic pain in the craniocervical region. Pain Pract. 2014;14(5):413–8. https://doi.org/10.1111/papr.12075.
22. Gomes CAFP, EL-Hage I, Amaral AP, Herpich CM, Politti F, Kalil-Bussadoni S, Gonzalez TO, Gonzalez DAB. Effects of massage therapy and occlusal splint usage on quality of life and pain in individuals with sleep bruxism: a randomized controlled trial. J Jpn Phys Ther Assoc. 2015;18:1–6. https://doi.org/10.1298/jjpta.Vol18_001.

Obstructive Sleep Apnea: An Overview

Fernanda Louise Martinho Haddad, Lia Rita Azeredo Bittencourt, Renato Stefanini, Débora Strose Villaça, and Sônia Maria Guimarães Pereira Togeiro

Obstructive sleep apnea (OSA) is a sleep-related respiratory disorder characterized by intermittent episodes of upper airway collapse during sleep. The events are predominantly obstructive, with partial (hypopnea) or complete (apnea) occlusion of the upper airway (Fig. 1), resulting in reduced oxyhemoglobin saturation and sleep fragmentation [1].

The pathophysiology of OSA is multifactorial and includes reduction of the upper airways, resulting from both anatomical narrowing of the pharynx and functional alterations such as obesity (infiltration of fat in the neck region), maxillofacial injury or structural alterations [3, 4], increased pharyngeal collapsibility due to reduced neuromuscular compensation (decrease of the pharynx dilatory musculature response), lack of protective reflex of the pharynx during sleep [5], reduction of the awakening threshold, increase of the ventilatory response, decreased pulmonary volume and caudal traction of the pharynx, and fluid displacement to the neck

F. L. M. Haddad
Department of Otorhinolaryngology and Head and Neck Surgery, Escola Paulista de Medicina, Universidade Federal de São Paulo, São Paulo, SP, Brazil

R. Stefanini
Otorhinolaryngology and Head and Neck Surgery Department, Escola Paulista de Medicina, Universidade Federal de São Paulo, São Paulo, SP, Brazil

L. R. A. Bittencourt (✉)
Department of Psychobiology, Escola Paulista de Medicina, Universidade Federal de São Paulo, São Paulo, SP, Brazil

D. S. Villaça
Department of Pneumology, Escola Paulista de Medicina, Universidade Federal de São Paulo, São Paulo, SP, Brazil

S. M. G. P. Togeiro
Department of Clínica Médica e Medicina Laboratorial, Department of Pneumology and Department of Psychobiology, Escola Paulista de Medicina, Universidade Federal de São Paulo, São Paulo, SP, Brazil

C. Frange, F. M. S. Coelho (eds.), *Sleep Medicine and Physical Therapy*, https://doi.org/10.1007/978-3-030-85074-6_14

1 General Treatments

Several treatments are available for OSA, but the choice should be based on severity, including symptoms, complications, and polysomnographic findings. In moderate to severe OSA, positive airway pressure (PAP) is the gold standard treatment. Other therapeutic modalities such as behavioral measures, positional therapy, and oral devices are available and involve an interdisciplinary approach. Surgical treatment in well-selected patients may be indicated.

Clinical and behavioral measures should be offered to all patients with OSA even in those treated with other therapies, such as PAP. Obesity is one of the main risk factors for OSA, so weight loss should be strongly recommended, and a nutritionist may be suggested. Studies with dietary intervention for weight loss along with prescription by a physical therapist for an active lifestyle are welcome in patients with OSA. In patients with mild OSA, the prescription of very low calorie together with lifestyle counseling showed an average weight reduction of 10.7 Kg, and for apnea-hypopnea index (AHI) of 4 events per hour, demonstrating that the greater the weight loss, the greater the decrease of AHI [15]. Another investigation assessed whether PAP influenced weight loss in patients with moderate and severe OSA [16]. For that, three types of intervention were instituted for 24 weeks: (i) use of PAP, (ii) management of weight loss, and (iii) combined intervention of PAP plus weight loss. The isolated PAP group did not present weight loss but presented a reduction of insulin resistance. The other two groups showed a significant weight reduction (~5 kg) in addition to decreased triglycerides and insulin resistance in the group with PAP plus weight loss [16]. This study showed that PAP can enhance metabolic improvement of weight loss.

In patients who do not respond to dietary intervention, bariatric surgery may be indicated. Weight loss through bariatric surgery showed a decrease in OSA in 83.6%–88.5% of patients, with an average reduction of the AHI of 34 n°/h, being the most effective gastric bypass [17]. However, even with considerable weight loss, many patients persist with residual OSA [18] and changes in OSA severity, decreasing it. Bariatric surgery may be an adjuvant in the treatment of OSA, except for the risks of perioperative complications due to OSA and recognition of the possibility of residual OSA.

Behavior measures should also be taken together along with OSA treatment. Alcohol, for example, aggravates OSA by having a dose-response effect [19]. Untreated OSA patients should avoid ingestion of alcohol because it leads to increased duration and frequency of apnea aggravating desaturation during sleep. In addition, other effects of alcohol include reducing sleep latency onset and the REM sleep stage.

Some medications may also aggravate OSA, such as benzodiazepines, benzodiazepine agonist receptors, opioids, and barbiturates, and should be avoided especially in those not under treatment. In cases where such medications are necessary, it is important that the monitoring is performed with adjustment in the prescribed treatment (e.g., increased PAP pressure, adequate mandibular advancement in the case of the oral appliance, etc.). Attention should also be given to medications that increase weight and may aggravate OSA such as some antidepressants and antipsychotics.

2 Myofunctional Therapy

It is an alternative therapy indicated in the presence of orofacial myofunctional disorders associated with mild to moderate OSA associated or not with the use of PAP or intraoral device. Studies have demonstrated, in addition to the improvement of the orofacial myofunctional condition, the quality of life with reduction of the AHI and increased saturation of oxyhemoglobin [20]. When concomitant to CPAP theraphy, can improve CPAP adherence, reducing the require pressure. In many countries, myofunctional therapy is provided by speech therapists.

3 Oral Appliance

An oral appliance, or oral device, is like an orthodontic retainer, a noninvasive treatment, and the patient uses it only at sleep, to support the jaw in a forward position, therefore increasing the upper airway space. Research shows that oral appliance therapy is an effective treatment option for snoring and OSA. They are nocturnal oral devices that stabilize the upper airways and increase their diameters, inducing a decrease in the collapsibility of the pharynx. There are many types, such as maxillary expansion; mandibular advancement devices, which induce the advancement and distraction of the lower jaw; and tongue retaining devices that primarily keep the tongue from falling to the back of the upper airway (Fig. 3). They are made by dentists specializing in dental sleep medicine.

Therefore, the practical parameters of the American Academy of Sleep Medicine together with the American Academy of Sleep Dentistry stipulate that oral devices are not indicated for all OSA patients [23] and are indicated for primary snoring, upper airway resistance syndrome (please refer to chapter "Upper Airway Resistance Syndrome: An Overview"), mild OSA, moderate OSA, and severe OSA that are intolerant to PAP therapy. For example, patients with mild OSA showed no difference in the improvement of AHI between oral devices and PAP therapy [24]. However, in those with moderate or severe OSA, PAP was better in reducing AHI and hypoxemia compared to oral devices [24]. A moderate degree of evidence of the effect of the oral devices of the custom adjustable mandibular advancement type was observed in reducing the AHI, increasing oxygen saturation, decreasing nocturnal awakenings, and improving daytime sleepiness and quality of life compared to the condition before the use of the oral device. Therapeutic adherence to oral devices is generally higher, and its discontinuity is lower compared to PAP [25]. The most common adverse effects are dry mouth,

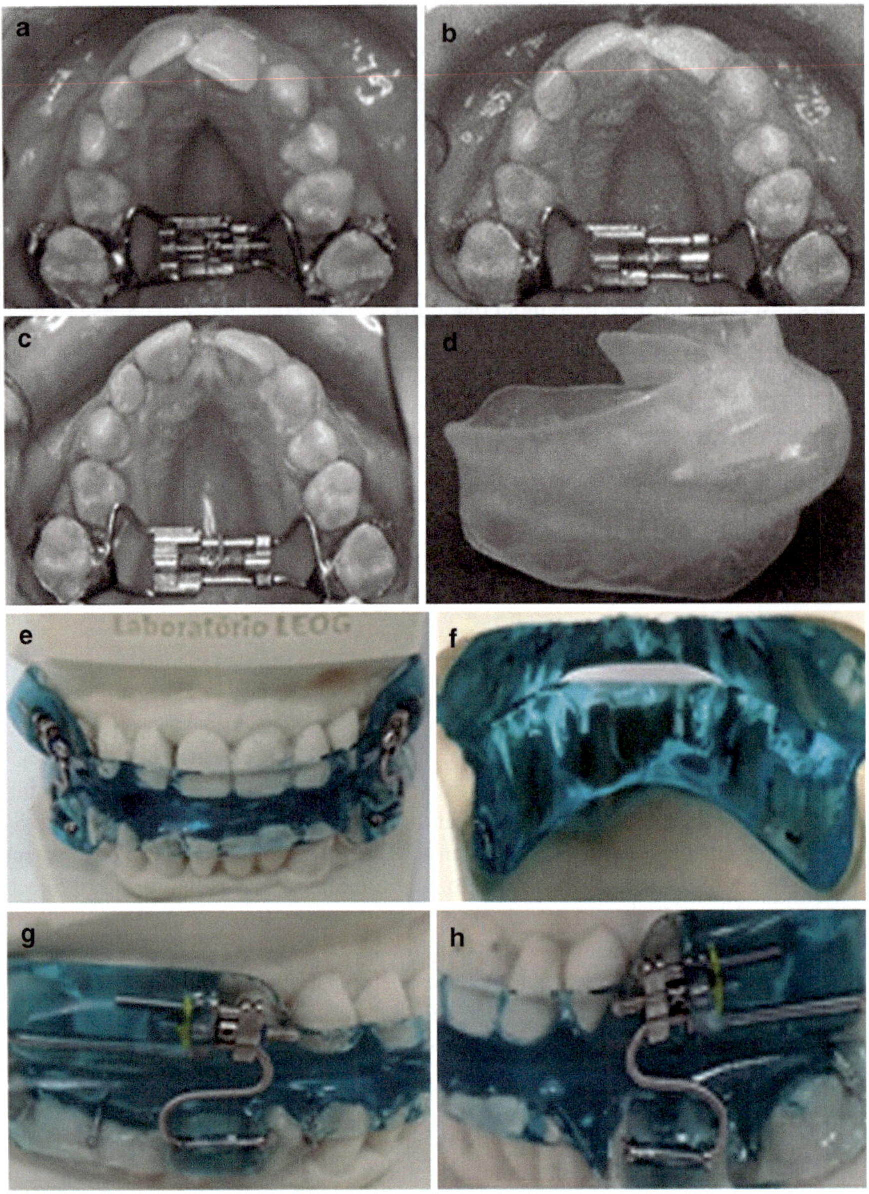

Fig. 3 Oral appliance devices: (**a**–**c**) Occlusal sequence of treatment with rapid maxillary expansion from crowding in the upper central incisors (**a**) to a wide space (**c**); (**e**, **f**) adjustable mandibular repositioning device, front view (**e**), from inside (**f**), right (**g**), and left (**h** sides; and **d**) tongue retaining device, designed to keep the tongue in an anterior position during sleep. This device secures the tongue by means of negative pressure in a soft plastic bulb. A flange, which fits between the lips and teeth, holds the device and tongue anteriorly in the oral cavity. (Reprinted with permission from: (**a**–**c**) Pirelli et al. [21]; (**d**) Higurashi et al. [22]; (**e**–**h**) (Image courtesy from Dr. Eliana Lottenberg Vago (original figure)))

excessive salivation, mandibular discomfort, increased sensitivity to teeth, dental mobility, and occlusal changes. Among the contraindications, we have periodontal disease, acute temporomandibular dysfunction, uncontrolled generalized convulsions, and limited mandibular advancement. Detection of oral device response predictors (positional apnea, BMI, younger patient), as well as accurate determination of the optimal degree of mandibular advancement, may improve the effectiveness of this treatment. It is important to perform follow-up PSG to assess the effectiveness of the oral devices because subjective reports of improvement may not be safe.

4 Surgical Treatment of OSA

The surgical treatment may be indicated with curative purpose, seeking to control the disease, and it may also be indicated as a supporting role, to facilitate adherence to the PAP or oral devices. Recently, studies on different OSA phenotypes started identifying different clusters to try to customize the treatment of OSA and also to understand why surgical treatment has distinct responses in "apparently similar" patients [26]. These different possibilities of responses from the surgical treatment must be presented to the patient at the time of the surgical indication, to suit their expectations within the treatment.

Different surgical modalities and techniques can be performed in the different levels of upper airways, both in the soft parts of the pharynx and in the facial skeleton, such as pharyngoplasty, maxillomandibular advancement and hypoglossal nerve stimulation.

The risks of surgical treatment should be considered, considering the patient's age, the severity of OSA, and the presence of comorbidities such as obesity, diabetes, hypertension, and cardiopathies. The risks of complications are higher in patients with OSA, and care should be taken with pre-anesthetic and anesthetic drugs, orotracheal intubation, extubating in the immediate postoperative period, upper airway edema, and medications prescribed in the postoperative period.

4.1 Nasal Surgeries

The most frequent procedures performed in the nose in the treatment of OSA are septoplasty and partial inferior turbinectomy. They aim to clear the nose to improve nasal breathing. Several studies have shown that nasal surgery, when performed in isolation, has little impact on the improvement of AHI, but there is evidence of improvement in the subjective quality of sleep and may help in the adaptation of PAP [27]. These procedures are often performed in association with other surgical procedures, especially pharyngeal surgeries.

16. Chirinos JA, et al. CPAP, weight loss, or both for obstructive sleep apnea. N Engl J Med. 2014;370(24):2265–75.
17. Sarkhosh K, et al. The impact of bariatric surgery on obstructive sleep apnea: a systematic review. Obes Surg. 2013;23(3):414–23.
18. Lettieri CJ, Eliasson AH, Greenburg DL. Persistence of obstructive sleep apnea after surgical weight loss. J Clin Sleep Med. 2008;4(4):333–8.
19. Issa FG, Sullivan CE. Alcohol, snoring and sleep apnea. J Neurol Neurosurg Psychiatry. 1982;45(4):353–9.
20. de Felicio CM, da Silva Dias FV, Trawitzki LVV. Obstructive sleep apnea: focus on myofunctional therapy. Nat Sci Sleep. 2018;10:271–86.
21. Pirelli P, Saponara M, Guilleminault C. Rapid maxillary expansion in children with obstructive sleep apnea syndrome. Sleep. 2004;27(4):761–6.
22. Higurashi N, et al. Effectiveness of a tongue-retaining device. Psychiatry Clin Neurosci. 2002;56(3):331–2.
23. Ramar K, et al. Clinical practice guideline for the treatment of obstructive sleep apnea and snoring with oral appliance therapy: an update for 2015. J Clin Sleep Med. 2015;11(7):773–827.
24. Lim J, et al. Oral appliances for obstructive sleep apnoea. Cochrane Database Syst Rev. 2003;(4):CD004435.
25. Cistulli PA, et al. Treatment of snoring and obstructive sleep apnea with mandibular repositioning appliances. Sleep Med Rev. 2004;8(6):443–57.
26. Bosi M, et al. Phenotyping the pathophysiology of obstructive sleep apnea using polygraphy/polysomnography: a review of the literature. Sleep Breath. 2018;22(3):579–92.
27. Sufioglu M, et al. The efficacy of nasal surgery in obstructive sleep apnea syndrome: a prospective clinical study. Eur Arch Otorhinolaryngol. 2012;269(2):487–94.
28. Fujita S, et al. Surgical correction of anatomic azbnormalities in obstructive sleep apnea syndrome: uvulopalatopharyngoplasty. Otolaryngol Head Neck Surg. 1981;89(6):923–34.
29. Franklin KA, et al. Effects and side-effects of surgery for snoring and obstructive sleep apnea--a systematic review. Sleep. 2009;32(1):27–36.
30. Pang KP, et al. Palate surgery for obstructive sleep apnea: a 17-year meta-analysis. Eur Arch Otorhinolaryngol. 2018;275(7):1697–707.
31. Friedman M, Ibrahim H, Bass L. Clinical staging for sleep-disordered breathing. Otolaryngol Head Neck Surg. 2002;127(1):13–21.
32. Aurora RN, et al. Practice parameters for the surgical modifications of the upper airway for obstructive sleep apnea in adults. Sleep. 2010;33(10):1408–13.
33. Strollo PJ Jr, et al. Upper-airway stimulation for obstructive sleep apnea. N Engl J Med. 2014;370(2):139–49.
34. Zaghi S, et al. Maxillomandibular advancement for treatment of obstructive sleep apnea: a meta-analysis. JAMA Otolaryngol Head Neck Surg. 2016;142(1):58–66.

Obstructive Sleep Apnea: Physiotherapeutic Approach

Moara Gomes da Rocha Cruz and Rafaela Garcia Santos de Andrade

1 Understanding the General Concept

There are many treatments available for obstructive sleep apnea (OSA) that consider the severity of the disease. Treatment involves simple measures such as weight loss in those overweight or obese individuals, avoiding alcohol or sedatives [1], and sleeping in the lateral position for patients with positional OSA.

The positional therapy (tennis ball technique or vibrating chest belts (Fig. 1)) has great results with an important reduction in the supine sleep time and consequently in the apnea-hypopnea index (AHI) [2]. Mandibular advancement devices are widely used in OSA treatment, with greater benefits in mild and moderate sleep apnea [3]. In some apnea patients, surgical techniques are also available and have good results when appropriately indicated [4]. More recently, myofunctional therapy appears as an option to treat mild and moderate OSA patients. This technique involves oropharyngeal exercises indicated by a speech therapist [5, 6].

The application of positive airway pressure (PAP) during sleep is the "gold standard" for the treatment of patients with moderate (AHI ≥ 15 events/hour) to severe (AHI ≥ 30 events/hour) OSA. Treatment of OSA with PAP was first described by Sullivan et al. in 1981 [7]. The key idea was that PAP applied for nasal route acted

M. G. da Rocha Cruz (✉)
Certified in Sleep Physiotherapy by the Brazilian Sleep Society (ABS), and The Brazilian Association of Cardiorespiratory Physiotherapy and Physiotherapy in Intensive Care (ASSOBRAFIR), Aracaju, Sergipe, Brazil

R. G. S. de Andrade
Department of Pneumology and Heart Institute, Hospital das Clínicas da Faculdade de Medicina da Universidade de São Paulo, São Paulo, SP, Brazil

Certified in Sleep Physiotherapy by the Brazilian Sleep Society (ABS), and The Brazilian Association of Cardiorespiratory Physiotherapy and Physiotherapy in Intensive Care (ASSOBRAFIR), São Paulo, SP, Brazil

C. Frange, F. M. S. Coelho (eds.), *Sleep Medicine and Physical Therapy*,
https://doi.org/10.1007/978-3-030-85074-6_15

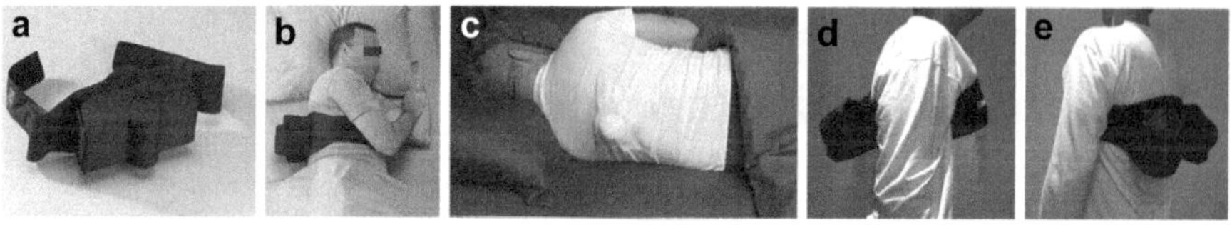

Fig. 1 Devices for positional therapy. (**a**) Chest belts; (**b**) lateral view; (**d** and **e**) inflatable dampers adjusted to provide the best curved positional support around the body. The belt and shock absorbers move with the body and prevent the supine position; and (**c**) tennis ball technique. (Image courtesy from Dr. Rafaela Andrade (**a**, **b**) and from Dr. Vivien Schmeling Piccin (**c**–**e**))

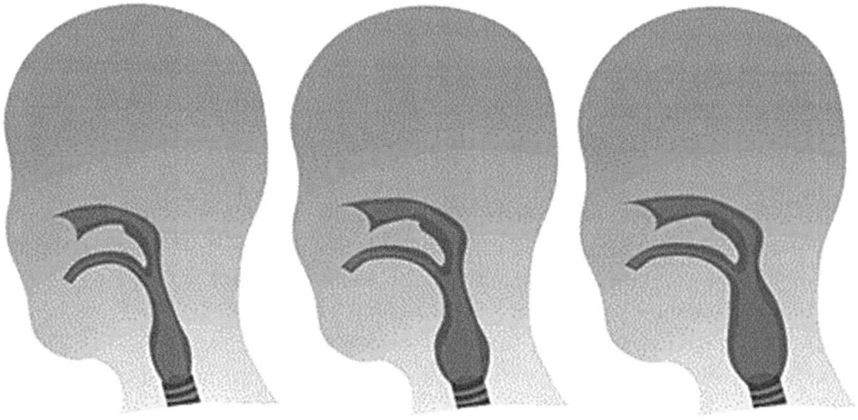

Fig. 2 A schematic illustration of a narrowed upper airway susceptible to collapse without PAP (left). A more open and stable upper airway with a PAP pressure of 5 cmH_2O (center), and with a pressure of 10 cmH_2O we can see a completely open and stable upper airway (right). (Image courtesy from Dr. Rafaela Andrade)

as a pneumatic splint to keep the pharynx stable and open during all sleep time and, consequently, maintain the upper airway patency (Fig. 2). The nasal PAP moves the soft palate and the tongue anteriorly as we can see in Fig. 3.

The reasons for the collapse of the upper airways during sleep in patients with OSA are multiple and not completely understood. The collapse of the upper airways depends on anatomical characteristics, arousal threshold, ventilatory instability during sleep, and neuromuscular control of the upper airway caliber [8]. The Starling resistor model can help to explain this mechanism of collapse and clarify the PAP concept. The Starling resistor consists of two rigid tubes connected by a collapsible tube [9]. The two rigid (bony and cartilaginous) tubes represent the nose and the trachea. The pharynx, which is a collapsible (muscular) part, makes the link (Fig. 4). If we image an overweight man, sleep during the night with complete muscular relaxation, in a supine position with gravitation action, the nasal and tracheal pressure probably was not able to maintain the pharynx open, this tube will be to collapse because of the external forces that will be higher than the nasal and tracheal forces. In this model, the pharyngeal critical pressure is the pressure at which

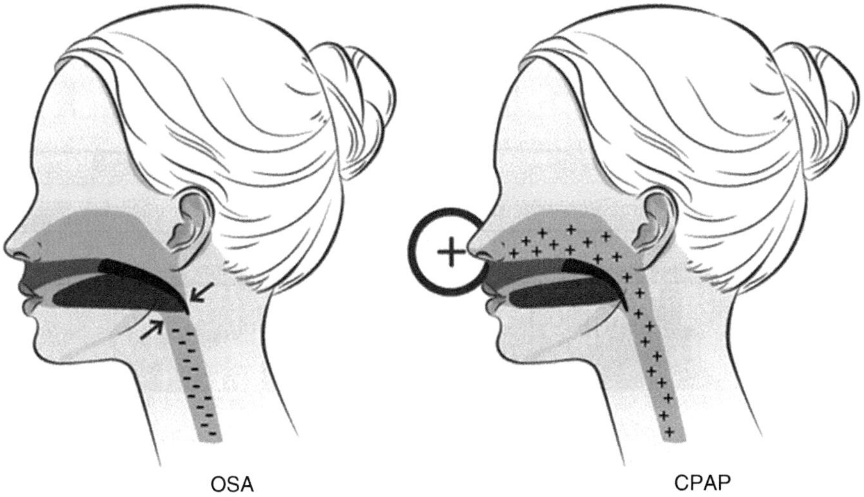

Fig. 3 A schematic illustration of the mechanism of upper airway occlusion and its treatment with PAP. The patient with OSA (left) and then (right) using nasal positive pressure with the upper airway completely open, and the tongue and soft palate anteriorly pushed. (Modified with permission from Sullivan et al. [7])

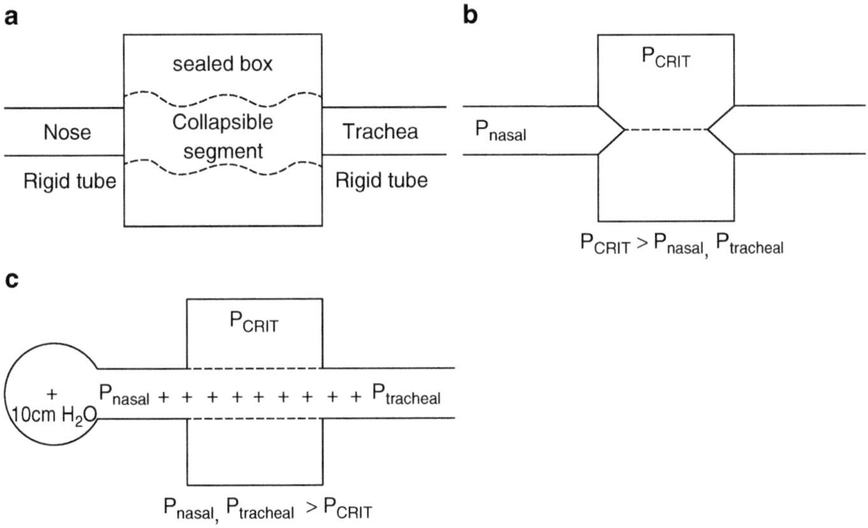

Fig. 4 Schematic illustration of the Starling resistor. (**a**) The nose and the trachea are represented by two rigid tubes connected by a collapsible segment (the pharynx). (**b**) Collapse of the pharynx. (**c**) Illustration of the CPAP mechanism with pressurization of the upper airway. (Image courtesy from Dr. Rafaela Andrade)

3 Comfort Technologies: What Are They and When Should I Use Them

Both CPAP and Bilevel have comfort technologies to improve PAP adherence. They are expiratory relief pressure (a reduction on expiratory pressure during the patient expiration), ramp time (the time in minutes that PAP increases gradually until reaching therapeutic pressure), and heated humidifiers (prevent dryness of the upper airways) [13, 14, 18]. The ramp time can be used to minimize the patient's perception of excessive pressure on the face, favoring sleep induction [13]. The automatic ramp increases the PAP pressure according to the detection of obstructive events or stabilization of the breathing pattern [13, 18]. The sense awake® technologies have recently emerged. Total pressure relief occurs when breathing patterns become unstable, indicating that the patient may be awake, so the PAP pressure is reduced until sleep again and the therapeutic pressure is simultaneously restored. The physiotherapist is the most suitable professional to adapt the patient to PAP as well as to follow in the short, medium, and long terms, solving possible problems and ensuring adherence to treatment [18]. It is important to know when and how using these technologies and know the patient's history and comorbidities.

4 Talking About Adherence

Despite eliminating OSA, the effectiveness of PAP is totally dependent on adherence, which consists of the number of hours of device use per night. Unfortunately, adherence to PAP therapy is extremely variable in the literature (46–80%) [19–22]. The use of the treatment 4 h/night in at least 70% of the nights is considered to be a good treatment adherence [23]. However, in our respiratory physiotherapist clinical practice, we made all the forces to aware the patients to use the PAP device during all time of sleep, this is our goal! The predictive factors for adherence to PAP are multiple and include the severity of OSA [24], the level of excessive daytime sleepiness [25], socioeconomic status [26], the level of understanding of the therapy by the patient (education actions) [27, 28], PAP mode and pressure levels [29, 30], and the interface/mask model [31, 32]. The PAP compliance during the first month and the presence of side effects were the only independent predictors of 12 months PAP adherence [33]. Early PAP adherence had the greatest predictive value for identifying those at the highest risk of nonadherence to long-term PAP [21]. It is so important that the physiotherapist views intensive early interventions to solve the potential side effects and problems with the objective of improving long-term compliance.

For all this reason, it is so important to choose the right interface (mask). Nasal, pillow, and oronasal masks are the most commonly used and are represented in Fig. 7. Silicone, gel, and tissue can be the material used to make these interfaces. We are seeing more frequently masks extremely light and comfortable. In general, they are formed by the fitting of their parts, being easy to handle and clean by patients.

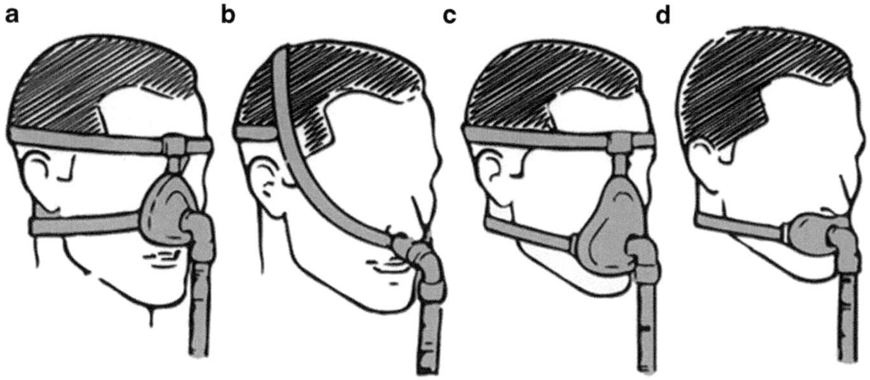

Fig. 7 An illustration of the different types of CPAP interfaces available for the treatment of obstructive sleep apnea: (**a**) nasal mask, (**b**) pillow mask, (**c**) oronasal mask, and (**d**) oral mask. (Modified with permission from Andrade et al. [34])

They are commonly found in sizes small, medium, medium wide and large, and are fixed to the patient's face by adjustable by headgear straps. All the masks have an exhalation port, which prevents the rebreathing of the exhaled carbon dioxide.

The nasal mask covers the nose exclusively and should surround it in such a way that it does not compress the wing of the nose, being immediately above the upper lip and close to the angle of the eye. Some nasal masks have forehead support as a stabilizing component of the mask. This support point allows two parallel tapes to depart from the upper region to fix the mask, and two more tapes from the lower region, composing a fixation in four points. Currently, the nasal mask is becoming increasingly lighter and with minimal contact with the patient's face and nose. The majority of modern interfaces have the tracheal output above the head (Fig. 8).

The nasal pillows consist of two intranasal pillows and emerged as an alternative to the nasal mask. Is a great choice for patients with mustache and claustrophobia because its 2 tapes come out to fix the mask in the upper and posterior region of the head, composing a fixation in 2 points.

The oronasal mask covers the nose and mouth and allows the patient to breathe through both the nose and the mouth. The oronasal interface must be positioned close to the angle of the eye, permeating the entire side of the nose to the mouth and ending below the patient's lower lip, allowing the patient to open the mouth. Oronasal masks, in general, have forehead support as a stabilizing component of the mask. This support point allows two parallel straps from the upper region of the head, and two more straps from the lower region, composing a fixation in four points. Today, a new oronasal mask has been emerging which is increasingly lighter and has minimal patient contact. Oronasal interfaces were initially described in situations of noninvasive ventilation for patients with respiratory failure and high ventilatory demand [35]. However, the oronasal mask has been progressively used in OSA patients that self-report breathing through the nose as an alternative to improve PAP compliance. One study of our group showed that the patients' self-report about

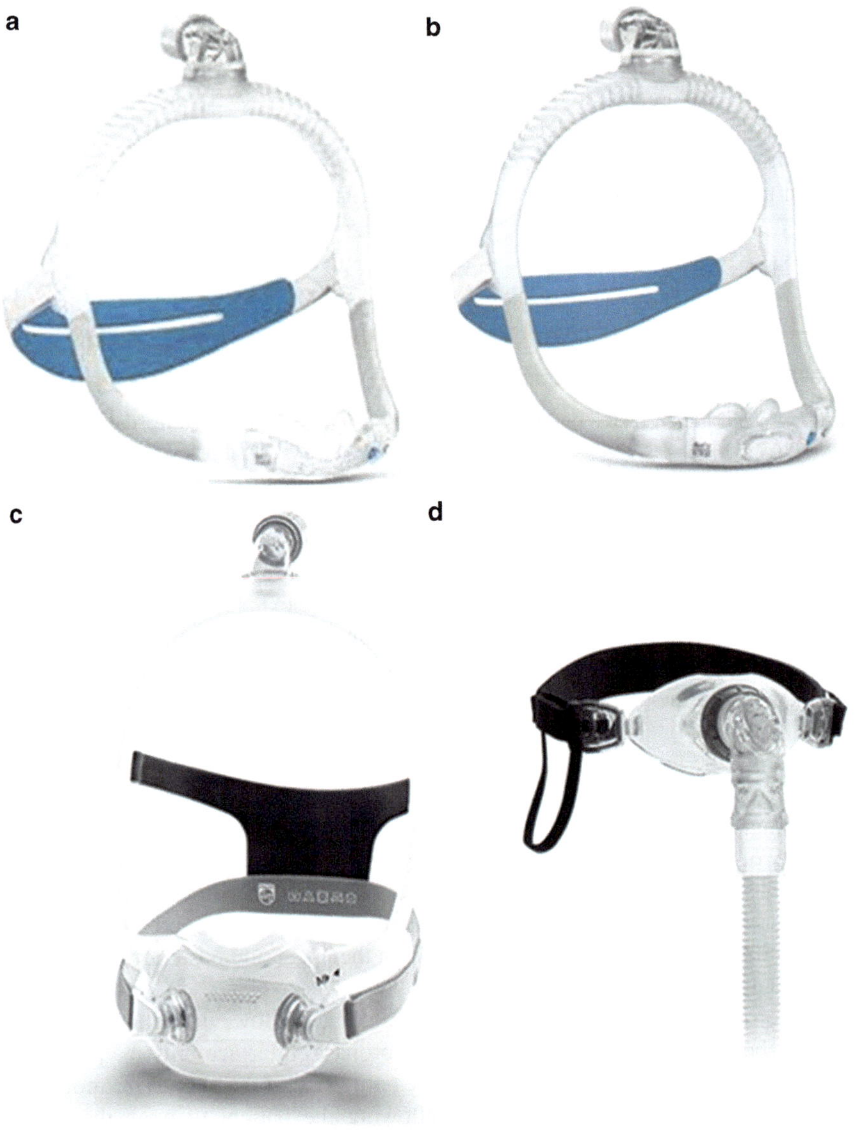

Fig. 8 Examples of masks: (**a**) Nasal mask. (**b**) Pillow mask. (**c**) Oronasal mask and (**d**) oral mask. (Image courtesy from Dr. Rafaela Andrade. (original))

the route (nasal vs. oral) of breathing is different from the real breathing route during sleep [36].

The oral interface is often made of silicone and resembles the shape of a butterfly that is positioned between the lips and the teeth. From the oral mask, two strips come out towards the back of the head to fix it to the patient's face. They have a tongue positioning component, which keeps the tongue stabilized and prevents obstructions to the PAP flow. In clinical practice, they are rarely used.

PAP for OSA treatment was originally designed to be used with a nasal route [7]. In a meta-analysis from our group that compared nasal and oronasal PAP, the oronasal masks were associated with a significantly higher CPAP level (on average, +1.5 cmH_2O) despite a significantly higher residual AHI (+2.8 events/h) and lower adherence (−48 min/night) when compared to nasal mask [31]. In another study, our group evaluated 18 patients with OSA who slept with an oronasal mask with 2 sealed independent compartments (nasal and oral). The acute changes of the CPAP flow route during sleep from nasal to oronasal and oral routes induced obstructive events and narrowing of oropharyngeal dimensions due to a posterior displacement of the tongue as demonstrated by nasendoscopy example (Fig. 9) [37].

During stable flow limitation, oronasal CPAP led to lower peak inspiratory flow, higher driving pressure, higher inspiratory resistance, and lower upper airway dimensions, both at the retropalatal and retroglossal areas [38]. The key to explaining this behavior is the pressure transmitted through the mouth during oronasal CPAP. So, the nasal route (nasal or pillow mask) must be the first choice in the treatment of OSA patients [39]. If the patient has some nasal obstruction, it was preferable to treat the nose after beginning the PAP therapy. If a percentage of mouth breathing persists during nasal PAP use, the use of a chin strap to minimize mouth breathing is indicated (Fig. 10).

In claustrophobic patients, the use of a small mask is recommended as we mentioned above. Claustrophobia is one of the largest side effects of PAP therapy, cited by 63–84% of respondents in previous studies and associated with a greater risk of poor PAP adherence or abandonment [40]. It is characterized by a feeling of being uncomfortable with the PAP mask, positive pressure, or both, causing anxiety, worry, avoidance, and, often, insomnia. This is a delicate patient, and the PAP adaptation process is slower. A lot of studies suggest a desensitization process (graded

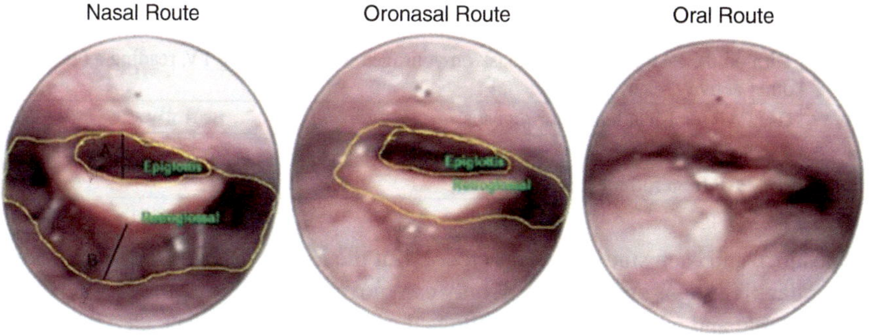

Fig. 9 Image of the upper airway of a patient during the experiment in the retroglossal region during the nasal, oronasal, and oral route. A significant reduction in the retroglossal dimensions was observed. The yellow line delimits the retroglossal and epiglottis areas. (**a**) Distance between the epiglottis and the posterior pharyngeal wall. (**b**) Distance between the epiglottis and the base of the tongue. (Modified with permission from Andrade et al. [37])

(b) Explain the disease, risk factors, types of available treatments for each instance, what to look for, and consequences of the lack of treatment.
(c) Elucidate the importance of weight loss and sleep hygiene (sleep positioning, alcohol addiction, medications and benefits of a physical activity program, etc.).
(d) Mask adaptation and the PAP equipment.

II. *The first, the third, and the sixth month of PAP Use*

(a) Evaluate the treatment adherence
(b) Investigate possible causes of mask and equipment intolerance

III. *After this period, the patient may return every 6 months in order to verify treatment adherence and possible causes of treatment intolerance.*

References

1. Tuomilehto HP, Seppa JM, Partinen MM, Peltonen M, Gylling H, Tuomilehto JO, et al. Lifestyle intervention with weight reduction: first-line treatment in mild obstructive sleep apnea. Am J Respir Crit Care Med. 2009;179(4):320–7.
2. Ravesloot MJL, White D, Heinzer R, Oksenberg A, Pepin JL. Efficacy of the new generation of devices for positional therapy for patients with positional obstructive sleep apnea: a systematic review of the literature and meta-analysis. J Clin Sleep Med. 2017;13(6):813–24.
3. Cuccia AM, Caradonna C. Mandibular advancement devices: indications and predictors of treatment outcome. A review. Minerva Stomatol. 2007;56(9):427–43.
4. Aurora RN, Casey KR, Kristo D, Auerbach S, Bista SR, Chowdhuri S, et al. Practice parameters for the surgical modifications of the upper airway for obstructive sleep apnea in adults. Sleep. 2010;33(10):1408–13.
5. Guimaraes KC, Drager LF, Genta PR, Marcondes BF, Lorenzi-Filho G. Effects of oropharyngeal exercises on patients with moderate obstructive sleep apnea syndrome. Am J Respir Crit Care Med. 2009;179(10):962–6.
6. Ieto V, Kayamori F, Montes MI, Hirata RP, Gregorio MG, Alencar AM, et al. Effects of oropharyngeal exercises on snoring: a randomized trial. Chest. 2015;148(3):683–91.
7. Sullivan CE, Issa FG, Berthon-Jones M, Eves L. Reversal of obstructive sleep apnoea by continuous positive airway pressure applied through the nares. Lancet. 1981;1(8225):862–5.
8. Eckert DJ, Malhotra A, Jordan AS. Mechanisms of apnea. Prog Cardiovasc Dis. 2009;51(4):313–23.
9. Andrade RG, Piccin VS, Nascimento JA, Viana FM, Genta PR, Lorenzi-Filho G. Impact of the type of mask on the effectiveness of and adherence to continuous positive airway pressure treatment for obstructive sleep apnea. J Bras Pneumol. 2014;40(6):658–68.
10. Gold AR, Schwartz AR. The pharyngeal critical pressure. The whys and hows of using nasal continuous positive airway pressure diagnostically. Chest. 1996;110(4):1077–88.
11. Patil SP, Ayappa IA, Caples SM, Kimoff RJ, Patel SR, Harrod CG. Treatment of adult obstructive sleep apnea with positive airway pressure: an American Academy of Sleep Medicine systematic review, meta-analysis, and GRADE assessment. J Clin Sleep Med. 2019;15(2):301–34.
12. Haddad FLM, Gregório LC. Manual do residente: medicina do sono. In: LBM G, editor. Tratamento dos distúrbios obstrutivos com aparelhos de pressão positiva: visão prática. 1st ed. Barueri: Manole; 2017.

13. Martins RB, Santella F, Bagnato MC. Modalidades de aparelhos de pressão positiva no tratamento da SAOS. Sono: série atualização e reciclagem em pneumologia-SPPT. 1st ed. Rio de Janeiro: Atheneu; 2018. p. 65–7.
14. Piccin VS. Aparelhos de pressão positiva: adesão, cuidados e segmento. Sono: série atualização e reciclagem em pneumologia-SPPT. 1st ed. Rio de Janeiro, Atheneu; 2018. p. 73–87.
15. Berry RB, Chediak A, Brown LK, Finder J, et al. Best clinical practices for the sleep center adjustment of noninvasive positive pressure ventilation (NPPV) in stable chronic alveolar hypoventilation syndromes. J Clin Sleep Med. 2010;6(5):491–509.
16. Selim B, Ramar K. Sleep-related breathing disorders: when CPAP is not enough. Neurotherapeutics J Am Soc Exp NeuroTherap. 2021;18:81–90.
17. Patil SP, Ayappa IA, Caples SM, Kimoff RJ, Patel SR, Harrod CG. Treatment of adult obstructive sleep apnea with positive airway pressure: an American Academy of Sleep Medicine clinical practice guideline. J Clin Sleep Med. 2019;15(2):335–43.
18. Nerbass FB, Piccin VS, Peruchi BB. Atuação da fisioterapia nos distúrbios respiratórios do sono. ASSOBRAFIR Ciência. 2015;6(2):13–30.
19. Drager LF, Malhotra A, Yan Y, Pepin JL, Armitstead JP, Woehrle H, et al. Adherence with positive airway pressure therapy for obstructive sleep apnea in developing versus developed countries: a big data study. J Clin Sleep Med. 2020;17:703–9.
20. Pepin JL, Krieger J, Rodenstein D, Cornette A, Sforza E, Delguste P, et al. Effective compliance during the first 3 months of continuous positive airway pressure. A European prospective study of 121 patients. Am J Respir Crit Care Med. 1999;160(4):1124–9.
21. Campos-Rodriguez F, Navarro-Soriano C, Reyes-Nunez N, Torres G, Caballero-Eraso C, Lloberes P, et al. Good long-term adherence to continuous positive airway pressure therapy in patients with resistant hypertension and sleep apnea. J Sleep Res. 2019;28(5):e12805.
22. Lee CHK, Leow LC, Song PR, Li H, Ong TH. Acceptance and adherence to continuous positive airway pressure therapy in patients with obstructive sleep apnea (OSA) in a Southeast Asian privately funded healthcare system. Sleep Sci. 2017;10(2):57–63.
23. Gay P, Weaver T, Loube D, Iber C, Positive Airway Pressure Task F, Standards of Practice C, et al. Evaluation of positive airway pressure treatment for sleep related breathing disorders in adults. Sleep. 2006;29(3):381–401.
24. Baratta F, Pastori D, Bucci T, Fabiani M, Fabiani V, Brunori M, et al. Long-term prediction of adherence to continuous positive air pressure therapy for the treatment of moderate/severe obstructive sleep apnea syndrome. Sleep Med. 2018;43:66–70.
25. Jacobsen AR, Eriksen F, Hansen RW, Erlandsen M, Thorup L, Damgard MB, et al. Determinants for adherence to continuous positive airway pressure therapy in obstructive sleep apnea. PLoS One. 2017;12(12):e0189614.
26. Billings ME, Auckley D, Benca R, Foldvary-Schaefer N, Iber C, Redline S, et al. Race and residential socioeconomics as predictors of CPAP adherence. Sleep. 2011;34(12):1653–8.
27. Olsen S, Smith SS, Oei TP, Douglas J. Motivational interviewing (MINT) improves continuous positive airway pressure (CPAP) acceptance and adherence: a randomized controlled trial. J Consult Clin Psychol. 2012;80(1):151–63.
28. Smith CE, Dauz E, Clements F, Werkowitch M, Whitman R. Patient education combined in a music and habit-forming intervention for adherence to continuous positive airway (CPAP) prescribed for sleep apnea. Patient Educ Couns. 2009;74(2):184–90.
29. Chihara Y, Tsuboi T, Hitomi T, Azuma M, Murase K, Toyama Y, et al. Flexible positive airway pressure improves treatment adherence compared with auto-adjusting PAP. Sleep. 2013;36(2):229–36.
30. Kushida CA, Berry RB, Blau A, Crabtree T, Fietze I, Kryger MH, et al. Positive airway pressure initiation: a randomized controlled trial to assess the impact of therapy mode and titration process on efficacy, adherence, and outcomes. Sleep. 2011;34(8):1083–92.
31. Andrade RGS, Viana FM, Nascimento JA, Drager LF, Moffa A, Brunoni AR, et al. Nasal vs oronasal CPAP for OSA treatment: a meta-analysis. Chest. 2018;153(3):665–74.

32. Mortimore IL, Whittle AT, Douglas NJ. Comparison of nose and face mask CPAP therapy for sleep apnoea. Thorax. 1998;53(4):290–2.
33. Chai-Coetzer CL, Luo YM, Antic NA, Zhang XL, Chen BY, He QY, et al. Predictors of long-term adherence to continuous positive airway pressure therapy in patients with obstructive sleep apnea and cardiovascular disease in the SAVE study. Sleep. 2013;36(12):1929–37.
34. Andrade RG, Madeiro F, Genta PR, Lorenzi-Filho G. Oronasal mask may compromise the efficacy of continuous positive airway pressure on OSA treatment: is there evidence for avoiding the oronasal route? Curr Opin Pulm Med. 2016;22(6):555–62.
35. Barach AL, Martin J, Eckman M, et al. Positive pressure respiration and its application to the treatment of acute pulmonar edema. Ann Intern Med. 1938;12:754–95.
36. Nascimento JA, Genta PR, Fernandes PHS, Barroso LP, Carvalho TS, Moriya HT, et al. Predictors of oronasal breathing among obstructive sleep apnea patients and controls. J Appl Physiol (1985). 2019;127(6):1579–85.
37. Andrade RG, Madeiro F, Piccin VS, Moriya HT, Schorr F, Sardinha PS, et al. Impact of acute changes in CPAP flow route in sleep apnea treatment. Chest. 2016;150(6):1194–201.
38. Madeiro F, Andrade RGS, Piccin VS, Pinheiro GDL, Moriya HT, Genta PR, et al. Transmission of oral pressure compromises oronasal CPAP efficacy in the treatment of OSA. Chest. 2019;156(6):1187–94.
39. Genta PR, Kaminska M, Edwards BA, Ebben MR, Krieger AC, Tamisier R, et al. The importance of mask selection on continuous positive airway pressure outcomes for obstructive sleep apnea. An official American Thoracic Society workshop report. Ann Am Thorac Soc. 2020;17(10):1177–85.
40. Chernyak Y. Improving CPAP adherence for obstructive sleep apnea: a practical application primer on CPAP desensitization. MedEdPORTAL. 2020;16:10963.
41. Edinger JD, Radtk RA. Use of in vivo desensitization to treat a patient's claustrophobic response to nasal CPAP. Sleep. 1993;16(7):678–80.
42. Malhotra A, Crocker ME, Willes L, Kelly C, Lynch S, Benjafield AV. Patient engagement using new technology to improve adherence to positive airway pressure therapy: a retrospective analysis. Chest. 2018;153(4):843–50.
43. Telles SCL, Paiva LBN, Arrais T, Marzola IHT. Brazilian consensus on sleep physiotherapy. Sleep Sci. 2013;6(4):159–74.

Central Sleep Apnea: An Overview

Luciane Impelliziere Luna Mello and Luciana Palombini

Central sleep apnea (CSA) is characterized by the temporary loss of the production of respiratory stimuli from the pacemaker in the pontomedullary region of the central nervous system (CNS). The absence of the central ventilatory stimulus results in loss of movements of the main ventilatory muscles (diaphragm, thorax, and abdomen). The central events are depicted in the polysomnography by the absence of inspiratory effort throughout the entire period of apnea (absent airflow). The CSA is also associated with the absence of abdominal thoracic movement captured by respiratory inductance plethysmography. However, in obstructive sleep apnea, the movements of the respiratory muscles remain in the absence of airflow [1].

1 Methods for the Evaluation of Central Sleep Apnea

1.1 Esophageal Pressure

The esophageal pressure (Pes) is the most accurate method for the differential diagnosis of central and obstructive hypopnea since it directly evaluates intrathoracic pressure when inserted into the esophagus. Because it is invasive, this method of evaluation is rarely used in sleep laboratories.

L. I. L. Mello (✉) · L. Palombini
Sleep Institute, Associação Fundo Incentivo à Pesquisa, São Paulo, SP, Brazil

C. Frange, F. M. S. Coelho (eds.), *Sleep Medicine and Physical Therapy*,
https://doi.org/10.1007/978-3-030-85074-6_16

somnography, with the persistent onset of central events (apnea or hypopnea) associated with PAP therapy. The diagnosis of this disease is made in the PSG of PAP titration, with the appearance of five or more central apnea and/or hypopneas, with the number of central apnea and hypopneas greater than or equal to 50% of the total number of respiratory events and in the absence of CSB [5]. Patients usually present symptoms of daytime sleepiness or disrupted sleep. Also, patients with central emergent apnea associated with treatment (PAP or Bilevel) are thought to have instability in ventilatory control or a sleep state instability that seems to be exacerbated by PAP or Bilevel.

Breathing frequency and deepness are regulated by a negative feedback control system, which *aims* to maintain, at relatively constant levels, the partial PCO_2 and pressures of arterial oxygen (PO_2), even in the presence of hypoxemia, hypocapnia, or hypercapnia caused by lung or chest wall disease [6]. The ventilatory response varies widely between the wake period and the sleep period, as well as between REM sleep and NREM sleep. Central apnea events rarely occur during the wake period, as well as during R sleep stage. However, during NREM sleep changes in the ventilatory pattern are chemically controlled by PCO_2's blood levels. Mild reductions in PCO_2 levels lead to a central ventilatory response with the cessation of breathing (apnea threshold), stimulated by hypocapnia and caught by the central and peripheral chemoreceptors that command this response. NREM sleep respiratory oscillations may be increased by spontaneous sleep awakenings, which promote transient hyperventilation with consequent hypocapnia, initiating central apnea events, primarily during NREM sleep, and which persist until the elevation of PCO_2 above the apnea threshold. The duration and magnitude of hyperventilation will determine the level of hypocapnia and the consequent appearance of central apnea during stable sleep [1].

During sleep, the normal respiratory rhythm is maintained by a complex feedback mechanism best explained by the "loop gain" concept. "Loop gain" can be defined as the magnitude of the ventilatory response to ventilatory disorders with increased or decreased breathing [1]. This term describes the dynamic feedback of several ventilatory stabilizing mechanisms: (i) the ventilatory control center and the chemoreceptors, the ventilatory response to PO_2 and PCO_2 above or below normal values; (ii) lung and respiratory muscles and their effectiveness in the elimination of CO_2 by the ventilatory response; and (iii) delayed circulation between the lungs and peripheral and central chemoreceptors. More on the "loop gain" concept is in the next chapter.

CSA does not occur as an isolated event, occurs in apnea/hypopnea cycles alternated with hyperpnea, and may initiate a cascade of events that perpetuate ventilation instability. This instability may include the inertia of the central ventilatory control system, narrowing of the upper airways, occlusion, hypoxia, hypercapnia, and transient awakening. Consequently, regular rhythmic breathing will only be resumed when PCO_2 levels are 4–6 mmHg above basal PCO_2 [7]. This sequence explains why CSA does not occur as an isolated event, often accompanied by obstructive and mixed events in the same patient [8].

Regarding the pathophysiology of CSA, there are two main mechanisms responsible for the appearance of central events – (a) secondary to alveolar or hypercapnic hypoventilation and (b) secondary to hyperventilation or non-hypercapnic:

(a) *CSA secondary to alveolar hypoventilation (hypercapnic)* – Individuals with marginal ventilatory status or reduction of the ventilatory drive during the waking period may present some degree of diurnal hypercapnia. Inevitably, the ventilatory changes reported during wakefulness, in addition to other behavioral influences, cause hypercapnia by hypoventilation also during sleep [9]. In the presence of hypercapnia, there is an increase in alveolar ventilation, causing a small increase in ventilatory frequency, which results in a large change in PCO_2 values. Thus, the occurrence of a spontaneous awakening of sleep, associated with a small increase in ventilation, may reduce PCO_2 below the threshold of apnea causing central apnea [1]. The different diseases causing diurnal hypercapnia include neuromuscular diseases such as post-polio syndrome, amyotrophic lateral sclerosis, stroke, central alveolar hypoventilation, multiple sclerosis, Arnold Chiari malformation, muscular dystrophy, and abnormalities in ventilatory mechanics, such as kyphoscoliosis, among others.

(b) *CSA secondary to hyperventilation (not hypercapnic)* – The most common mechanism of central apnea is hypocapnia after hyperventilation and is characterized by a transient instability between the ventilatory control system and normal or increased alveolar ventilation. This type of central apnea is commonly observed in patients with heart failure, who may present hypocapnia during the wake period. Patients with heart failure present an increase in circulatory time, which contributes to the conversion of a negative feedback system into a positive one, contributing to the persistence of compensatory hypoventilation and hyperventilation [7].

2 Risk Factors for Central Apnea

Central sleep apnea may occur during the shifts of sleep stages, in normal sleep, associated with increasing age or related to some clinical disease. Physiological and pathological factors may influence susceptibility to the onset of central sleep apnea, such as:

2.1 Sleep Stage

The transition from the waking period to NREM sleep (stages 1 and 2) may be associated with the recurrent appearance of CSA, explained by the oscillation between the wake period and superficial sleep, with a reciprocal oscillation of PCO_2 near the apnea threshold [10]. Transient awakenings cause brief periods of hyperventilation, followed by hypocapnia, which results in CSA. Usually, these events cease with the deepening of sleep and the stabilization of PCO_2 above the apnea threshold. The appearance of CSA in the transition of the sleep-wake period is a normal phenomenon [11]. CSA usually does not occur during REM sleep, and this can be explained by a lower ventilatory response, the presence of hypercapnia, and hypoxia during this sleep stage and thus a reduced "loop gain," in addition to possible inhibition of respiratory accessory muscles. The reduction of the activity of the accessory muscles may worsen the hypoventilation during REM sleep in patients with paralysis or diaphragm dysfunction, with consequent reduction of the current volume to insignificant levels, and may generate a false CSA (pseudo-CSA). Thus, CSA during REM sleep represents transient hypoventilation rather than hypocapnia after hyperventilation [12].

2.2 *Age and Gender*

CSA is more prevalent in older adults than in middle-aged individuals, according to epidemiological studies. The prevalence of CSA is 1.7% in middle-aged adults vs. 12.1% in old-age adults [13]. The physiological oscillations of sleep may precipitate CSA in the older ones, as in this group the susceptibility to the appearance of CSA induced by mechanical ventilation with a nasal mask is greater [14]. The increased prevalence of CSA in the older ones may be associated with the presence of comorbidities such as hypothyroidism, congestive heart failure, and atrial fibrillation [15]. CSA is less common in women, with prevalence around 0.3% compared to 7.8% in men. The female menstrual cycle showed no influence on the appearance of CSA, ruling out progesterone as the cause of the difference between the sexes [16].

2.3 *Clinical Diseases*

Respiratory disorders are common in individuals with congestive heart failure, having a prevalence of 51% [17]. In this study, most patients (40%) had central apnea, and 11% had obstructive sleep apnea [17]. Patients with CSA and congestive heart failure present pulmonary vascular congestion leading to hyperventilation and hypocapnia. In patients with congestive heart failure, the magnitude of hypocapnia needed to induce CSA is small since these patients have a reduced ventilatory reserve [10].

In 40% of patients with stroke, CSA is the most prevalent sleep disorder. Similarly, 30% of chronic methadone users have CSA. Besides, it is also described in patients with hypothyroidism, acromegaly, and renal failure, with improvement after hemodialysis. The presence of spinal cord injury and tetraplegia is also associated with a higher prevalence of CSA. There is a possibility that these patients present undiagnosed metabolic or cardiac diseases [11, 18, 19].

3 Clinical Picture and Diagnosis

The underlying diseases and the occurrence of CSA influence clinical characteristics of hypercapnic CSA. Patients with clinical diseases and concomitant sleep apnea may present both symptoms of the underlying disease (dyspnea and weakness) and complaints related to sleep apnea, such as sleepiness, presence of snoring, morning headache, and poor quality of sleep. Patients with non-hypercapnic CSA may have common symptoms of sleep apnea syndrome, but do not complain of daytime sleepiness. The transitions between the waking period and stage 1 of NREM sleep can cause sleep fragmentation, poor sleep quality, and insomnia complaints [17].

4 Clinical Treatment

The strategy for treating patients with CSA takes into account the clinical condition, comorbidities, and polysomnographic findings. Therapeutic options may include pharmacological therapy, the use of supplemental oxygen, phrenic nerve stimulation, and PAP therapy. Below are described the therapeutic options, except for the PAP for CSA, addressed in the following chapter of this book.

4.1 Pharmacological Therapy

There are no clinical studies with good scientific evidence demonstrating efficacy in the use of pharmacological therapy for CSA. Little evidence supports the use of acetazolamide or theophylline as a treatment. Acetazolamide is a carbonic anhydrase inhibitor diuretic that causes metabolic acidosis with stimulation of the ventilatory center in response to PCO_2 increase during apnea. Theophylline in turn improves sleep respiratory disorder by increasing central ventilatory drive and cardiac contractility; however, its use may also increase the risk of cardiac arrhythmia and sudden death in these patients. In general, respiratory stimulants are not recommended for routine treatment of CSA [20, 21].

4.2 O_2 and CO_2 Supplementation

Many studies have demonstrated the positive effect of using oxygen supplementation in patients with CSA associated with heart failure. Oxygen therapy mitigates CSA by attenuating the magnitude of hypoxemia and consequently reducing the hyperventilation response after the apnea episode. Patients with non-hypercapnic CSA with high chemoreceptor response may benefit from O_2 therapy by the stabilizing effect of

Central Sleep Apnea: Physiotherapeutic Approach

Juliana Arcanjo Lino and Vivien Schmeling Piccin

Central apnea occurs when the pontomedullary pacemaker fails in generating breathing rhythm. Without brainstem inspiratory neural output there is no work of the inspiratory thoracic pump muscles resulting in the loss of inspiratory ventilatory effort, which is characterized polygraphically by the absence of naso-oral airflow and thoracoabdominal excursions. On sleep medicine, the silence of the inspiratory effort should last at least ten seconds to be considered central sleep apnea (CSA) [1].

The International Classification of Sleep Disorders (ICSD-3) identifies eight different forms of CSA: (I) central sleep apnea with Cheyne-Stokes breathing, (II) central sleep apnea due to a medical disorder without Cheyne-Stokes breathing, (III) treatment-emergent central sleep apnea, (IV) central sleep apnea due to high-altitude periodic breathing, (V) central sleep apnea due to a medication or substance, (VI) primary central sleep apnea, (VII) primary central sleep apnea of infancy, and (VIII) primary central sleep apnea of prematurity [2].

Instead of the CSA classification by the ICSD-3, the underlying pathophysiology of central sleep apnea is due to hyperventilation or hypoventilation. According to the pathophysiological mechanisms that trigger specific central breathing patterns, the subtypes of central sleep apnea – hypercapnic, hypocapnic, or

J. A. Lino (✉)
Medical Sciences, Federal University of Ceara (UFC), Fortaleza, Ceará, Brazil

Certified in Sleep Physiotherapy by the Brazilian Sleep Society (ABS), and The Brazilian Association of Cardiorespiratory Physiotherapy and Physiotherapy in Intensive Care (ASSOBRAFIR), São Paulo, Brazil

V. S. Piccin
Sleep Medicine, Pulmonary Division, Heart Institute, São Paulo, SP, Brazil

Certified in Sleep Physiotherapy by the Brazilian Sleep Society (ABS), and The Brazilian Association of Cardiorespiratory Physiotherapy and Physiotherapy in Intensive Care (ASSOBRAFIR), São Paulo, SP, Brazil

C. Frange, F. M. S. Coelho (eds.), *Sleep Medicine and Physical Therapy*,
https://doi.org/10.1007/978-3-030-85074-6_17

normocapnic – are characterized. This knowledge is especially important to determine appropriate treatment strategies [3–5].

Positive airway pressure therapy (PAP) is indicated for the treatment of hypocapnic, hypercapnic, or normocapnic CSA [6]. Other treatment strategies [7] have also been described in the literature, such as the supply of supplemental oxygen [8, 9]; respiratory center stimulants, such as acetazolamide and theophylline [10, 11]; the increase in inspired CO_2 – supplied directly or through the application of dead space [12, 13]; and, more recently, phrenic nerve stimulation [14–16]. Opioid dose reduction and weight loss both are also options that can improve central apnea [4]. Interventions that improve cardiac function can also attenuate central sleep apnea, especially periodic breathing, common in patients with underlying cardiovascular disease [17].

In recent years, the influence of bed positioning on the rostral displacement of fluid to the chest and neck regions has also been reported, contributing to pulmonary congestion, and increased cervical circumference, causing central and obstructive events, respectively. In this case, the simple recommendation to raise the head of the bed has been effective in the treatment of central apneas, especially in patients with cardiovascular disease [18, 19]. In clinical practice, these treatment strategies can be used in a combined way according to the complexity of each case, and, of course, it requires the experience of the physiotherapist to effectively use the different therapeutic techniques.

Close monitoring of patients with CSA using telemonitoring and detailed graphical analysis (i.e., analysis of respiratory flow curves when using PAP or bilevel pressure therapy) is also essential, especially in cases where the establishment of optimal conducts proves to be more difficult [20, 21].

This chapter presents the detailed physiotherapeutic approach in central sleep apnea with Cheyne-Stokes breathing, CSA due to a medical disorder without Cheyne-Stokes breathing, and CSA emerging from treatment, which represents the greatest clinical challenge in routine care of patients with sleep-disordered breathing.

1 Central Sleep Apnea with Cheyne-Stokes Breathing

Cheyne-Stokes breathing (CSB) is probably the most common form of the types of CSA [2]. Characterized by periods of hyperventilation in an increasing-decreasing pattern of tidal volume, alternating with periods of central apnea or hypopnea, with a respiratory cycle duration usually greater than 40 seconds, CSB presents highly prevalent morbidity but unfortunately is still underdiagnosed in cardiovascular diseases [5, 22].

The CSB is associated with arterial oxygen desaturation, episodes of hypercapnia, sleep fragmentation, and activation of the sympathetic nervous system which, chronically, can be harmful to the heart [23]. In fact, several studies have shown that CSB is a strong independent marker of poor prognosis and increased morbidity and mortality in patients with heart failure (HF) [22, 24, 25]. The pathophysiology of CSB in HF is directly associated with instability of respiratory control, which can be explained by a high *loop gain*. High chemosensitivity is responsible for exaggerated ventilatory response secondary to PCO_2 fluctuations. Patients with HF are in a chronic state of hyperventilation, and, consequently, their eupneic PCO_2 level becomes remarkably close to the apnea threshold. Thus, when the patient falls asleep, the PCO_2 does not rise normally, but the apnea threshold is established at a higher level making it easier for an apnea event to be evoked by a minimal increase in ventilation, typically due to spontaneous arousals [26–28].

Among the main elements that contribute to hyperventilation in HF, pulmonary congestion is correlated with increased pulmonary capillary pressure and can be aggravated in the supine position during the night [29]. It partly explains why the CSB is usually observed more expressively at the end of the night [Fig. 1]. Similarly, this overload fluid can be observed also in chronic kidney disease [30]. As renal failure and HF are characterized by fluid overload, these observations suggest that hypervolemia may contribute to the pathogenesis of CSA in both conditions, through the redistribution of fluids during the night from the legs to the lungs, especially into the interstitial lung tissue [19, 31].

In clinical practice, the treatment of CSA with CSB is still controversial and should be individualized according to the clinical history of each patient. The PAP has been studied in the treatment of CSA in recent years [22, 32]. The Canadian Continuous Positive Airway Pressure for Patients with Central Sleep Apnea and Heart Failure trial (CANPAP study) [33], with 258 patients with HF and CSA, showed that continuous PAP (CPAP) was associated with improvement in intermediate outcomes, including the apnea-hypopnea index (AHI), left ventricular ejection fraction (LVEF), and mean oxyhemoglobin saturation at night. However, there was

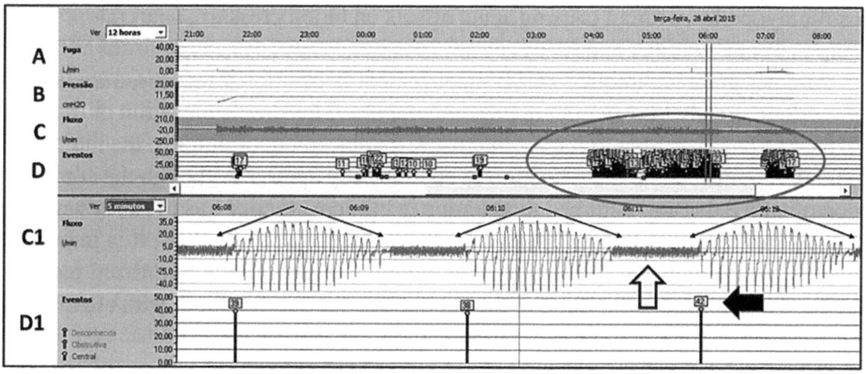

Fig. 1 Screen of a graphical data presentation for the ResScan™ system, extracted from positive pressure equipment by the company ResMed. (**A**) unintentional leak; (**B**) CPAP pressure; (**C**) respiratory flow curve; (**D**) residual respiratory events (obstructive apnea, central apnea, hypopneas, or events of increased airway resistance), during the entire night of CPAP uses; (**C1**) respiratory flow curve; (**D1**) residual respiratory events, in five-minute window of observation. The small arrows highlight the increasing-decreasing breathing pattern (CSB), indicative of respiratory instability; the open arrow shows a central apnea event; the dark arrow shows the marking time of a central apnea event. Circle shows in which moment during the night the increasing-decreasing breathing pattern indicative of CSB (showed at C1) was observed. (Image courtesy from Dr. Juliana Arcanjo Lino (original figure))

Leak l/min	Median:	7.1	Percentile 95%:	29.4	Maximum:	89.8
Events/hour	AI:	6.3	HI:	0.9	➡ AIH:	7.2
Apnea index	⇨ Central:	5.5	Obstructive:	0.3	Unknown:	0.5
RERA index						0.3
Cheyne-Stokes Breathing						49 minutes (9%)
Hours of use						

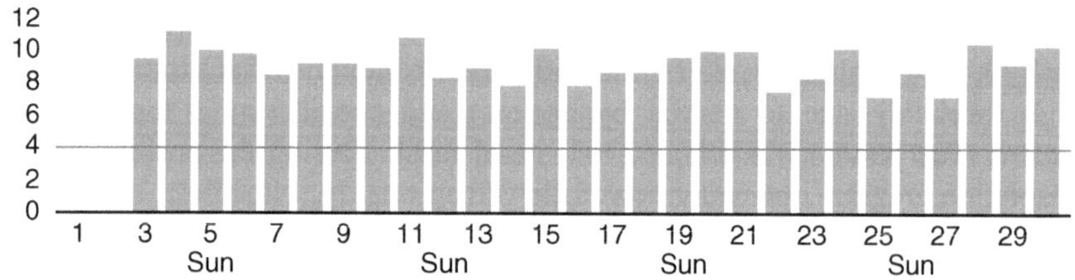

Fig. 2 Screen of the sample report, extracted from AirView – ResMed™. The dark arrow shows total apnea-hypopnea index (AIH); the open arrow shows central apnea index (CAI), Sun, Sunday. (Image courtesy from Dr. Juliana Arcanjo Lino (original figure))

However, these respiratory events have not interfered with the patient's sleep quality, as they report improvement in daytime sleepiness. In addition, we remember that post hoc analysis of the CPAP trial [33] demonstrated that early suppression of central events by PAP for an AHI below 15 per hour appears to be associated with improvement in left ventricular ejection fraction and survival improvement in HF failure patients.

2.1 *Central Apnea Due to a Medical Disorder Without Cheyne-Stokes Breathing*

CSA due to a medical condition without CSB is usually encountered in neurological diseases, in which stroke has been shown to be one of the most common clinical conditions associated with this kind of sleep-disordered breathing (SDB). Forty percent of the patients demonstrate central apnea as the predominant type of sleep disorder after a stroke (Fig. 3) [5, 38]. The mechanism of CSA after stroke has been discussed to be a direct consequence of the injury of central nervous system structures, leading to a lack of central input from the brain to the muscles of respiration [39, 40].

The PAP treatment of CSA without CSB recommends the use of the lowest and effective pressure, capable of treating existing obstructive events and, at the same time, reducing the ventilatory control instability and the central events. In clinical practice, it is not recommended the use of automatic CPAP, as it can trigger an

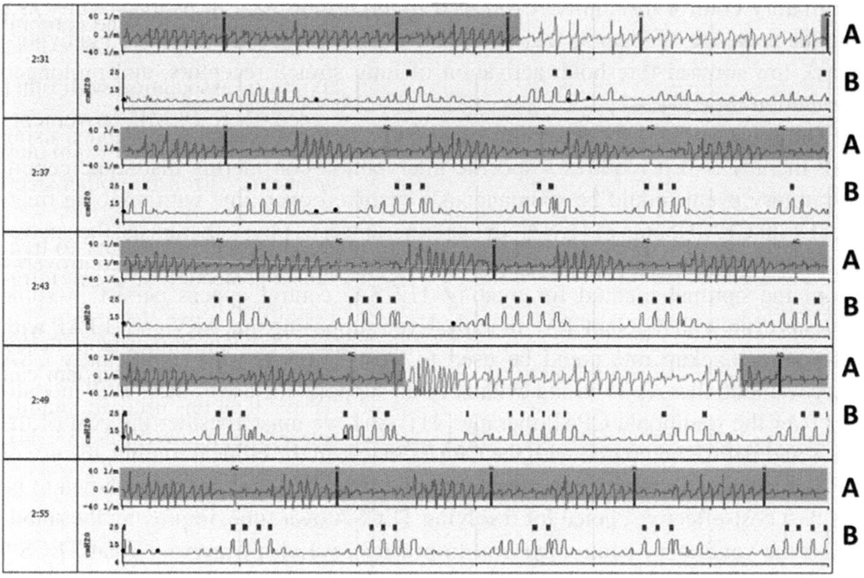

Fig. 3 Screen of a graphical data presentation for the EncorePro 2™ system, extracted from a Philips Respironics servo-ventilator. (**A**) respiratory flow curve; (**B**) pressure support. The gray hatch in (**A**) shows the breathing pattern after a stroke, with an increasing-decreasing respiratory pattern. Note in (**B**) the servo-ventilator sending mandatory breaths in apnea events and considerably decreasing the ventilatory support at central breathing events, to stabilize the patient's breathing pattern. (Image courtesy from Dr. Vivien Schmeling Piccin (original figure))

inhibitory reflex of the respiratory center, and arousals increase at the same time also resulting in periodic breathing events (especially in patients with high loop gain). In practice, the use of expiratory relief and automatic ramp must be avoided whenever possible, as they can also trigger ventilatory control instability precipitating periodic breathing.

3 Treatment-Emergent Central Sleep Apnea

A new addition to the International Classification of Sleep Disorders is the treatment-emergent central sleep apnea (TECSA), a respiratory disorder classified in the recent past as complex sleep apnea syndrome [2]. In TECSA, the patient exhibits predominantly obstructive events during diagnostic sleep testing, but central apneas or central hypopneas emerge or persist during treatment for obstructive sleep apnea. TECSA has been observed after various treatment modalities for OSA, like mandibular advancement device, maxillomandibular advancement surgery, nasal surgery, tracheostomy, or myofunctional therapy, but is more often reported during the initiation of PAP therapy. The potential mechanisms leading to TECSA included ventilatory control instability (expressed by high loop gain in patients with OSA and the presence of upper airway (UA) narrowing during central apneas and hypopneas), low arousal threshold, activation of lung stretch receptors, and prolonged circulation time [41, 42].

The greatest question regarding treatment-emergent central sleep apnea using PAP therapy is if it requires a specific intervention considering that some central respiratory events could be spontaneously resolved over time with ongoing treatment with CPAP therapy [41, 43]. In our experience, as physiotherapists, the answer to this question is yes, principally because, although there is still some controversy about the optimal method for treating TECSA, central apneas persist in some patients even with regular CPAP therapy. Even supposing that ASV and BiPAP with respiratory backup rate could be used to treat TECSA, with significantly CSA improvement, there is no strong evidence that supports the use of these PAP modalities over the traditional CPAP therapy [41]. And we must consider the cost of the ASV and BiPAP compared with the CPAP device. In the clinical routine, the use of CPAP treatment without expiratory relief and fixed pressure has been shown to be the best cost-effective choice for resolving TECSA over time, improving the stability of the ventilatory control system. In practice, we also observe a great TECSA improvement with the addition of traditional physiotherapy techniques to the PAP therapy (especially, positional therapy).

Below we describe a clinical scenario where TECSA was found, discussing our management approach in the context of current guidelines and relevant literature.

4 The Man with Non-restorative Sleep and Difficult Daytime Sleepiness

A 59-year-old male was referred to the PAP therapy adaptation program, complaining of non-restful sleep, nightmares, snoring, and hypersomnia. He had a clinical history of pituitary adenoma. PSG revealed OSA with an apnea-hypopnea index (AHI) of 32/h. Auto-PAP was prescribed at 5.6–13 cmH_2O. Wireless monitoring data during a follow-up visit at 2 weeks of therapy revealed an average hours of CPAP use of 5:14 h. Residual AHI was normal at 3.3/h, but the patient still complained of non-restorative sleep and daytime sleepiness. At the analysis of the respiratory flow curve, we observed some CSA events and a respiratory pattern indicating instability of ventilatory control (Fig. 4).

Considering the respiratory instability observed, the therapeutic model was adjusted to a fixed pressure of 9.0 cmH_2O. Because of a persistent respiratory instability without flow restriction, a gradual decrease in the pressure level up to a pressure of 7.0 cmH_2O was made aiming for the breathing pattern improvement. Despite the increase in the average time of use of CPAP (from 5:14 h to 6:13 h) and the patient's report of better comfort, a more restful sleep sensation, and an improvement in daytime sleepiness, certain periods of respiratory instability during sleep were still noticed (Fig. 5).

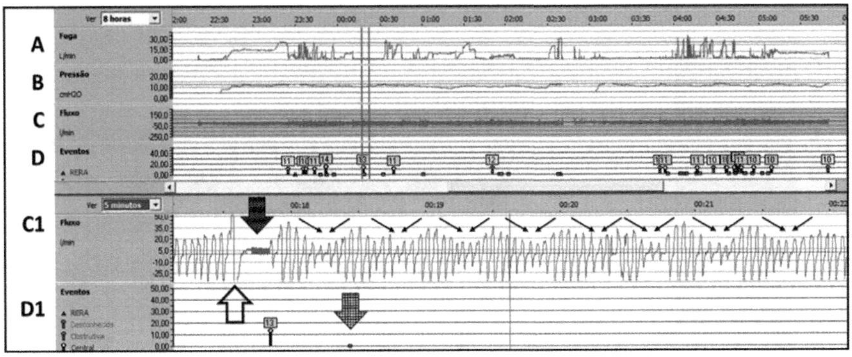

Fig. 4 Screen of a graphical data presentation for the ResScan™ system, extracted from positive pressure equipment by the company ResMed. (**A**) unintentional leak; (**B**) CPAP pressure; (**C**) respiratory flow curve; (**D**) residual respiratory events (obstructive apnea, central apnea, hypopneas, or events of increased airway resistance), during the entire night of CPAP uses; (**C1**) respiratory flow curve; (**D1**) residual respiratory events, in five-minute window of observation. The open arrow shows a physiological sigh event, with a considerable increase in respiratory flow; the dark shaded arrow shows a central apnea event in response to the decrease in the gasometrical level of carbon dioxide caused by the increase in respiratory amplitude in the previous respiratory cycle; the light shaded arrow shows the marking of a hypopnea event; the small arrows highlight the increasing-decreasing breathing pattern, indicative of respiratory instability. Note that this pattern was not detected by the algorithm and was only observed by graphical assessment of the respiratory flow curve (not because there is a problem with the equipment, but because the patient's breathing pattern sometimes has specific characteristics that influence the perception of the breathing pattern by the device's sensors). (Image courtesy from Dr. Vivien Schmeling Piccin (original figure))

Interestingly, the events of respiratory instability were distributed at specific times during the night, raising the hypothesis that they could be associated with an upper airway collapse during REM sleep, by reason of reduced muscular tonus at this sleep phase [44]. However, we could not ignore that these respiratory events could be also associated with positioning during the night, mainly due to palatal prolapse (as the presence of upper airway narrowing in patients with high loop gain or lower arousal threshold can be a possible trigger to CSA events) [45]. Analyzing the patient's data more deeply, we found that the patient had a soft palate elongation (Fig. 6) and a characteristic expiratory flow curve indicating the palatal prolapse (Fig. 7).

These data corroborated a probable palatal prolapse that, added to the hypothesis of high loop gain presented by the patient, could be the factor responsible for the ventilatory disorder, resulting in the emergent central apneas.

According to the Deacon-Diaz et al. [49] study, the product of "control gain (CG)" (represented by the sensitivity of central and peripheral chemoreceptors) versus "plain gain (PG)" (represented by the effectiveness of the lungs to alter blood gases, plus the increase in factors that lead to a collapse of the UA), determines the magnitude of the LG (Fig. 8), and, considering that was not our intention to infer in the CG, the possibility of intervention in the PG was considered. We consider that the PG intervention by adding a positional device could act to decrease the

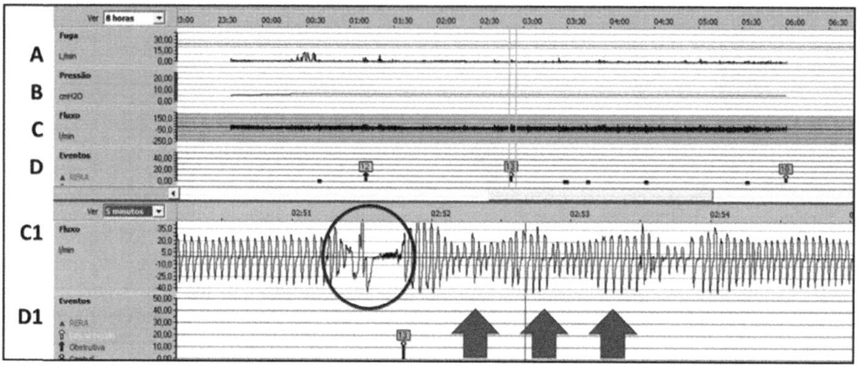

Fig. 9 Screen of a graphical data presentation for the ResScan™ system, extracted from positive pressure equipment by the company ResMed. (**A**) unintentional leak; (**B**) CPAP pressure; (**C**) respiratory flow curve; (**D**) residual respiratory events (obstructive apnea, central apnea, hypopneas, or events of increased airway resistance), during the entire night of CPAP uses; (C1) respiratory flow curve; (D1) residual respiratory events, in five-minute window of observation. The circle shows a sigh. Arrows show that after the sigh, there was an altered ventilatory response, but not an exacerbated ventilatory response. (Image courtesy from Dr. Vivien Schmeling Piccin (original figure))

at 7.0 cmH_2O. After a period of 36 days, we observed a good therapeutic result, with the patient maintaining a median hour of CPAP use of 6:40 h, the percentile 95% hours of use of 7:04 h, and a residual AHI of 6.1 events per hour. The patient was satisfied with the actions implemented for the treatment of OSA, referring a better sleep and significant improvement in daytime sleepiness and quality of life. But unfortunately positional therapy is not easy to maintain during sleep, and PT devices have not been widely adopted in part due to the poor treatment adherence observed [47]. In our case, the residual AHI was contaminated by nights of not using the PT. In the assessment of the respiratory flow curve during sleep when the patient was wearing the positional device, a high LG component was still present, observed by the change in the respiratory pattern after a physiological event of resuscitative sigh, but with a more controlled ventilatory response to the respiratory event (Fig. 9).

Treatment adherence with new vibratory positional devices has been shown to be high, possibly due to enhanced patient comfort with their petite design [47]. Based on our results, we consider that this kind of dispositive must be considered when a treatment-emergent central sleep apnea appears to be due to supine position during the night. In fact, the management strategy of TECSA aims to eliminate abnormal respiratory events, stabilize sleep architecture, and improve comorbidities. Although continuous positive pressure, preferably CPAP, is the standard treatment therapy for these cases, we should evaluate the benefit of therapeutic techniques in addition to pressure therapy. On the other hand, even though insufficient available data support ASV as an early intervention strategy for the treatment of TECSA, if central apneas persist at the follow-up session, changing the mode of PAP to either BiPAP with a back-up rate or ASV could be considered. In part of the cases, the multidisciplinary team needs to evaluate the use of medications (e.g., acetazolamide), oxygen therapy, or carbon dioxide supplementation to improve TECSA, since these methods have been presented in some studies as therapeutic possibilities to improve the ventilatory control stability or raise the arousal threshold for TECSA patients [41, 42, 48].

5 Final Words

Treating central sleep apnea is a challenge. Accurate knowledge of the physiology of sleep and the respiratory system, as well as the pathophysiology of CSA, clinical characteristics, associated morbidities, and polysomnographic findings, is essential for the CSA diagnosis and for the development of the patients' approach. It is also important to know that the treatment of CSA must be multidisciplinary, and more than one treatment strategy can be combined when necessary.

References

1. Javaheri S, Dempsey JA. Central sleep apnea. Compr Physiol. 2013;3(1):141–63.
2. The international classification of sleep disorders (ICSD-3). 3rd ed Darien, American Academy of Sleep Medicine; 2014.
3. Badr MS, Dingell JD, Javaheri S. Central sleep apnea: a brief review. Curr Pulmonol Rep. 2019;8(1):14–21.
4. Eckert DJ, et al. Central sleep apnea: pathophysiology and treatment. Chest. 2007;131(2):595–607.
5. Meir Kryger TR, Dement WC. Principles and practice of sleep medicine. 6th ed. Philadelphia: Elsevier; 2017.
6. Aurora RN, et al. The treatment of central sleep apnea syndromes in adults: practice parameters with an evidence-based literature review and meta-analyses. Sleep. 2012;35(1):17–40.
7. Baillieul S, et al. Diagnosis and management of central sleep apnea syndrome. Expert Rev Respir Med. 2019;13(6):545–57.
8. Javaheri S, et al. Effects of nasal O2 on sleep-related disordered breathing in ambulatory patients with stable heart failure. Sleep. 1999;22(8):1101–6.
9. Sasayama S, et al. Effects of nocturnal oxygen therapy on outcome measures in patients with chronic heart failure and cheyne-stokes respiration. Circ J. 2006;70(1):1–7.
10. Javaheri S. Acetazolamide improves central sleep apnea in heart failure: a double-blind, prospective study. Am J Respir Crit Care Med. 2006;173(2):234–7.
11. Javaheri S, et al. Effect of theophylline on sleep-disordered breathing in heart failure. N Engl J Med. 1996;335(8):562–7.
12. Khayat RN, et al. Cardiorespiratory effects of added dead space in patients with heart failure and central sleep apnea. Chest. 2003;123(5):1551–60.
13. Lorenzi-Filho G, et al. Effects of inhaled carbon dioxide and oxygen on cheyne-stokes respiration in patients with heart failure. Am J Respir Crit Care Med. 1999;159(5 Pt 1):1490–8.
14. Costanzo MR, et al. Transvenous neurostimulation for central sleep apnoea: a randomised controlled trial. Lancet. 2016;388(10048):974–82.
15. Fox H, et al. Long-term efficacy and safety of phrenic nerve stimulation for the treatment of central sleep apnea. Sleep. 2019;42(11):zsz158.

16. Fudim M, et al. Phrenic nerve stimulation for the treatment of central sleep apnea: a pooled cohort analysis. J Clin Sleep Med. 2019;15(12):1747–55.
17. Oldenburg O, et al. Influence of cardiac resynchronisation therapy on different types of sleep disordered breathing. Eur J Heart Fail. 2007;9(8):820–6.
18. Kasai T, Floras JS, Bradley TD. Sleep apnea and cardiovascular disease: a bidirectional relationship. Circulation. 2012;126(12):1495–510.
19. White LH, Bradley TD. Role of nocturnal rostral fluid shift in the pathogenesis of obstructive and central sleep apnoea. J Physiol. 2013;591(5):1179–93.
20. Mello-Fujita, L.I.L.d. and V.S. Piccin, Dispositivos de Terapia com Pressão Positiva (PAP) e Interpretação de Relatórios. In: Manual de Métodos Diagnósticos em Medicina do Sono. Editora Atheneu. Série SONO. 2018.
21. Liu D, et al. Trajectories of emergent central sleep apnea during CPAP therapy. Chest. 2017;152(4):751–60.
22. Terziyski K, Draganova A. Central sleep apnea with Cheyne-stokes breathing in heart failure - from research to clinical practice and beyond. Adv Exp Med Biol. 2018;1067:327–51.
23. Randerath W, et al. Definition, discrimination, diagnosis and treatment of central breathing disturbances during sleep. Eur Respir J. 2017;49(1):1600959.
24. Coniglio AC, Mentz RJ. Sleep breathing disorders in heart failure. Heart Fail Clin. 2020;16(1):45–51.
25. Lanfranchi PA, et al. Prognostic value of nocturnal Cheyne-stokes respiration in chronic heart failure. Circulation. 1999;99(11):1435–40.
26. Drager LF, et al. 1° Posicionamento Brasileiro sobre o Impacto dos Distúrbios de Sono nas Doenças Cardiovasculares da Sociedade Brasileira de Cardiologia. Arq Bras Cardiol. 2018;111:290–340.
27. Flinta I, Ponikowski P. Relationship between central sleep apnea and Cheyne-stokes respiration. Int J Cardiol. 2016;206(Suppl):S8–12.
28. Lorenzi-Filho G, et al. Cheyne-stokes respiration in patients with congestive heart failure: causes and consequences. Clinics (Sao Paulo). 2005;60(4):333–44.
29. Orr JE, Malhotra A, Sands SA. Pathogenesis of central and complex sleep apnoea. Respirology. 2017;22(1):43–52.
30. Lyons OD, Bradley TD, Chan CT. Hypervolemia and sleep apnea in kidney disease. Semin Nephrol. 2015;35(4):373–82.
31. Lin CH, Lurie RC, Lyons OD. Sleep apnea and chronic kidney disease: a state-of-the-art review. Chest. 2020;157(3):673–85.
32. Drager LF, et al. Sleep apnea and cardiovascular disease: lessons from recent trials and need for team science. Circulation. 2017;136(19):1840–50.
33. Bradley TD, et al. Continuous positive airway pressure for central sleep apnea and heart failure. N Engl J Med. 2005;353(19):2025–33.
34. Arzt M, et al. Suppression of central sleep apnea by continuous positive airway pressure and transplant-free survival in heart failure: a post hoc analysis of the Canadian continuous positive airway pressure for patients with central sleep apnea and heart failure trial (CANPAP). Circulation. 2007;115(25):3173–80.
35. Bradley TD, Floras JS, Investigators A-H. The SERVE-HF trial. Can Respir J. 2015;22(6):313.
36. Freitas IG, Togeiro SM, Tufik S. Treatment of Cheyne-stokes respiration in patients with congestive heart failure. Arq Bras Cardiol. 2007;88(3):e68–72.
37. Nerbass FB, et al. Acute effects of nasal CPAP in patients with hypertrophic cardiomyopathy. Chest. 2016;150(5):1050–8.
38. Parra O, et al. Time course of sleep-related breathing disorders in first-ever stroke or transient ischemic attack. Am J Respir Crit Care Med. 2000;161(2 Pt 1):375–80.
39. Blissitt PA. Sleep-disordered breathing after stroke: nursing implications. Stroke. 2017;48(3):e81–4.
40. Mims KN, Kirsch D. Sleep and stroke. Sleep Med Clin. 2016;11(1):39–51.

41. Zhang J, et al. Treatment-emergent central sleep apnea: a unique sleep-disordered breathing. Chin Med J. 2020;133(22):2721–30.
42. Zeineddine S, Badr MS. Treatment-emergent central apnea. Chest. 2021;159(6):2449–57.
43. Stanchina M, et al. Clinical use of loop gain measures to determine continuous positive airway pressure efficacy in patients with complex sleep apnea. A pilot study. Ann Am Thorac Soc. 2015;12(9):1351–7.
44. Alzoubaidi M, Mokhlesi B. Obstructive sleep apnea during rapid eye movement sleep: clinical relevance and therapeutic implications. Curr Opin Pulm Med. 2016;22(6):545–54.
45. Genta PR, et al. The importance of mask selection on continuous positive airway pressure outcomes for obstructive sleep apnea. An official American Thoracic Society Workshop Report. Ann Am Thorac Soc. 2020;17(10):1177–85.
46. Joosten SA, et al. Dynamic loop gain increases upon adopting the supine body position during sleep in patients with obstructive sleep apnoea. Respirology. 2017;22(8):1662–9.
47. Yingjuan M, et al. Positional therapy for positional obstructive sleep apnea. Sleep Med Clin. 2020;15(2):261–75.
48. Kuźniar TJ, Morgenthaler TI. Treatment of complex sleep apnea syndrome. Chest. 2012;142(4):1049–57.
49. Deacon-Diaz N, Malhotra A. Inherent vs. Induced loop gain abnormalities in obstructive sleep apnea. Front Neurol. 2018;9:896.

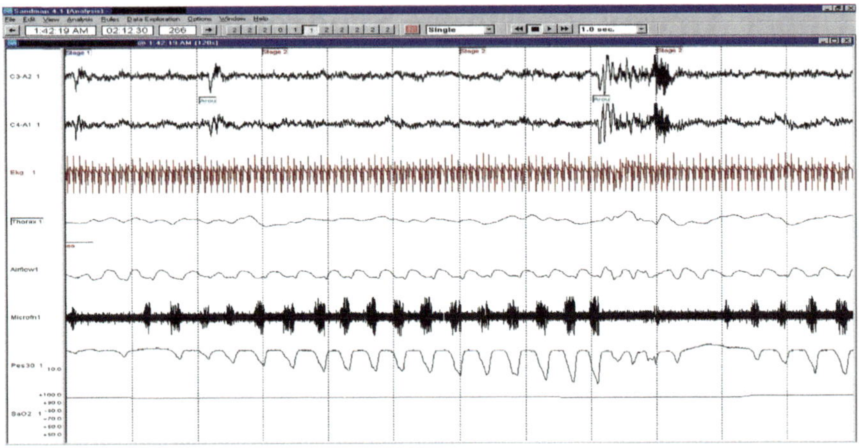

Fig. 1 Respiratory effort-related arousal indicated by esophageal pressure. (Image Courtesy from Dr. Luciana Palombini) (original figure)

research tool not used in clinical polysomnography), a UARS prevalence of 8.4% was observed [4]. However, in a more recent study of a sample from the general population of São Paulo, using the presence of inspiratory flow limitation associated with symptoms to identify UARS, the prevalence was 15% [5].

2 Pathophysiology

UARS pathophysiology is related to partial upper airway obstruction during sleep with OSA. Although the increase in upper airway resistance associated with UARS is not enough to satisfy the criteria of OSA, the increase in upper airway resistance lead to increased respiratory effort and presence of flow limitation, which can lead to significant consequences in sleep architecture and is often undetected by the patient. Individuals with UARS present a higher frequency of oral breathing, abnormalities in the nasal structure, and increased lateral pharyngeal wall volume, compared to individuals with no sleep breathing disorder [6].

UARS is typically observed in younger, thinner individuals and, in some reports, with no male predominance compared to OSA. Patients with UARS present complaints of tiredness and excessive sleepiness. They also present insomnia, restless sleep, depression, and anxiety. An association between UARS and fibromyalgia was described in patients with pain complaints [7, 8]. Other symptoms include dry mouth, excessive sweating at night, and morning headache [7]. UARS has also been described as a triggering factor for sleepwalking in children [9].

It has been demonstrated that those patients with UARS may present worse complaints of poor sleep quality and diurnal consequences compared to patients with OSA, but the mechanism for this finding is not known yet [10]. Different aspects related to specific phenotypes describing individual differences not yet established may be involved [8].

The stress response has been suggested as a mechanism involved in the different clinical manifestations of sleep breathing disorders. Gold et al. demonstrated that sleepiness and fatigue are correlated with the level of somatic arousal, a manifestation of the SNS component of the stress response among UARS patients [8]. However, this aspect needs to be more evaluated, and new studies are necessary to define this factor in the pathophysiology and clinical manifestations of UARS patients.

3 Methods for evaluation

UARS patients can present on physical examination different abnormalities, such as, narrow external nasal valves, internal nasal valve collapse, hypertrophy of the nasal turbinates, and septal deviation. Craniofacial changes in UARS are also described [11]. Cold extremities, postural hypotension, or lower blood pressure have been described in patients with UARS [11, 12].

The first PSG criterion for UARS is absence of OSA criteria. The PSG in the UARS presents events indicative of partial obstruction of the upper airway, including increased respiratory effeort, presence of RERAs [13] and airflow limitation [14]. As mentioned, a quantitative criterion for these events for the diagnosis of UARS is not yet defined.

RERA is currently defined as a sequence of breaths characterized by increased respiratory effort or flattening of the airflow curve of the nasal pressure cannula,

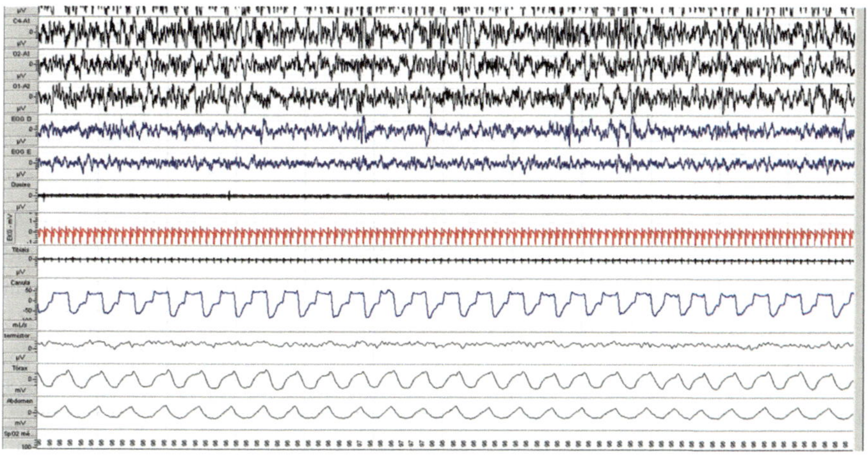

Fig. 2 Polysomnography showing airflow limitation. (Image Courtesy from Dr. Luciana Palombini (original figure))

leading to awakening (that does not reach the criterion for apnea and hypopnea). RERAs have a duration of 10 seconds.

Airflow limitation is defined as an increase in respiratory effort without a proportional increase in airflow. Airflow limitation may be indicated by the flattening flow curve by the nasal pressure cannula (Fig. 2). Periods of airflow limitation are associated with increased respiratory effort, and this event in PSG has been used as an indirect indicator of increased upper airway resistance [13–15]. According to the authors, the nasal pressure cannula can be used instead of esophageal manometry to detect RERA-type events.

The airflow limitation or increased breathing effort, in the absence of awakenings, is not recognized today as a sleep respiratory abnormality by the American Academy of Sleep Medicine (AASM). The presence of airflow limitation has been associated with different consequences, including fibromyalgia, periodic limb movement, somnambulism, preeclampsia, alternating cyclic pattern, changes in systemic blood pressure, and increase of carbon dioxide pressure at the end of expiration [14, 16]. Airflow limitation can also occur in healthy individuals. A study carried out in a sample of the general population showed that up to 30% of the total sleep time of healthy people can have airflow limitation [5]. These findings were not replicated, and possible confounding factors should be considered, such as nasal obstruction.

Other polysomnographic methods have been described to evaluate the increase in upper airway resistance during sleep, among them, the critical pressure technique, but this non-technical technique is also not validated [17].

UARS is associated with sleep fragmentation. Sleep fragmentation may be indicated by an increase in awakenings characterized by fast EEG frequencies, according to standardized definition of AASM [18], but more sensitive methods have been suggested, among these, analysis of the cyclic alternating pattern (CAP). CAP is a marker of instability and sleep fragmentation. CAP includes slow-wave sleep awakenings, EEG synchrony with delta waves, and K-complex [19]. The CAP analysis showed a correlation with sleepiness and fatigue scales in patients with UARS [9].

4 Treatment

Treatment options for UARS include behavioral treatment similar with OSA, including weight loss and nasal evaluation, PAP [20], oral appliances (OA), and surgical treatment. Hypnotic medications, such as zopiclone as adjuvants [21], can also be used to assist in treatment complaints. OA are a therapeutic option for UARS as they anteriorize the jaw and the tongue, in order to reduce the obstruction in the oropharynx. Treatment with OA has shown to reduce the awakening index, lower negative esophageal pressure, increase sleep efficiency percentage and the minimum oxygen saturation, and reduce subjective excessive daytime sleepiness and snoring in UARS patients [22, 23]. The benefits of oral devices in UARS were also demonstrated in a recent double-blind randomized study which improved sleep quality, complaints of depression, and stress symptoms [24, 25].

Surgical treatment of UARS has also been suggested [26]. Surgeries performed include septoplasty, turbinectomy, laser-assisted uvuloplasty, uvulopalatopharyngoplasty, genioglossus advancement, mandibular osteotomy with myotomy, and hyoid suspension. However, it is necessary well designed long term follow up studies to establish surgical treatment in UARS patients [26].

5 Final words

UARS can lead to significant impairment of the sleep quality and consequently quality of life. Although recognized in clinical practice, UARS is still under-diagnosed and under-treated. It is important, however, for the health professional to know that there are different phenotypes of SBD in addition to OSA that needs to be recognized and have appropriate treatment. Studies confirming significant outcomes and effective treatments for the establishment of UARS in sleep medicine are necessary.

References

1. Pépin JL, Guillot M, Tamisier R, Lévy P. The upper airway resistance syndrome. Respiration. 2012;83(6):559–66.
2. Eckert DJ, White DP, Jordan AS, et al. Defining phenotypic causes of obstructive sleep apnea. Identification of novel therapeutic targets. Am J Respir Crit Care Med. 2013;188:996–1004.
3. Guilleminault C, Stoohs R, Clerk A, Cetel M, Maistros P. A cause of excessive daytime sleepiness. The upper airway resistance syndrome. Chest. 1993;104(3):781–7.
4. Kristo DA, Lettieri CJ, Andrada T, Taylor Y, Eliasson AH. Silent upper airway resistance syndrome: prevalence in a mixed military population. Chest. 2005;127:1654–7.
5. Palombini L, Tufik S, Rapoport D, et al. Inspiratory flow limitation in a normal populationof adults in Sao Paolo, Brazil. Sleep. 2013;36:1663–8.
6. Godoy LBM, Palombini LO, Guilleminault C, Dalva Poyares D, et al. Treatment of upper airway resistance syndrome in adults: where do we stand? Sleep Sci. 2015a;8(1):42–8.
7. Gold AR, Dipalo F, Gold MS, Broderick J. Inspiratory airflow dynamics during sleep in women with fibromyalgia. Sleep. 2004;27(3):459–66.
8. Gold AR, Dipalo F, Gold MS, O'Hearn D. The symptoms and signs of upper airway resistance syndrome: a link to the functional somatic syndromes. Chest. 2003;123(1):87–95.
9. Guilleminault C, Lopes MC, Hagen CC, da Rosa A. The cyclic alternating pattern demonstrates increased sleep instability and correlates with fatigue and sleepiness in adults with upper airway resistance syndrome. Sleep. 2007;30(5):641–7.
10. Godoy LBM, Luz GP, Palombini LO, Silva LOE, Hoshino W, Guimarães TM, Tufik S, Bittencourt L, Togeiro SM. Upper airway resistance syndrome patients have worse sleep quality compared to mild obstructive sleep apnea. PLoS One. 2016;11(5):e0156244.
11. Guilleminault C, Poyares D, Rosa A, Huang YS. Heart rate variability, sympathetic and vagal balance and EEG arousals in upper airway resistance and mild obstructive sleep apnea syndromes. Sleep Med. 2005;6(5):451–7.
12. Ayappa I, Norman RG, Krieger AC, Rosen A, O'Malley RL, Rapoport DM. Non-invasive detection of respiratory effort-related arousals (RERAs) by a nasal cannula/pressure transducer system. Sleep. 2000;23(6):763–71.

13. Epstein MD, Chicoine SA, Hanumara RC. Detection of upper airway resistance syndrome using a nasal cannula/pressure transducer. Chest. 2000;117(4):1073–7.
14. Arora N, Meskill G, Guilleminault C. The role of flow limitation as an important diagnostic tool and clinical finding in mild sleep-disordered breathing. Sleep Sci. 2015;8(3):134–42.
15. Mooney AM, Abounasr KK, Rapoport DM, Ayappa I. Relative prolongation of inspiratory time predicts high versus low resistance categorization of hypopneas. J Clin Sleep Med. 2012;8(2):177–85.
16. Calero G, Farre R, Ballester E, Hernandez L, Daniel N, Montserrat Canal JM. Physiological consequences of prolonged periods of flow limitation in patients with sleep apnea hypopnea syndrome. Respir Med. 2006;100(5):813–7.
17. Gold AR, Schwartz AR. The pharingeal critical pressure. The whys and hows of using nasal continuous positive pressure diagnostically. Chest. 1996;110(4):1077–88.
18. Berry RB, Brooks R, Gamaldo C, Harding SM, Lloyd RM, Quan SF, Troester MT, Vaughn BV. AASM scoring manual updates for 2017 (Version 2.4). J Clin Sleep Med. 2017;13(5):665–6.
19. Parrino L, Ferri R, Bruni O, Mario G Terzano MG. Cyclic alternating pattern (CAP): the marker of sleep instability. Sleep Med Rev. 2012;16(1):27–45.
20. Edwards N, et al. Nasal continuous positive airway pressure reduces sleep-induced blood pressure increments in preeclampsia. Am J Respir Crit Care Med. 2000;162:252–7.
21. Lofaso F, Goldenberg F, Thebault C, Janus C, Harf A. Effect of zopiclone on sleep, night-time ventilation, and daytime vigilance in upper airway resistance syndrome. Eur Respir J. 1997a;10(11):2573–7.
22. Loube DI, et al. Successful treatment of upper airway resistance syndrome with an oral appliance. Sleep Breath. 1997;2:98–101.
23. Yoshida K. Oral device therapy for the upper airway resistance syndrome patient. J Prosthet Dent. 2002;87:427–30.
24. Godoy LBM, Sousa KM, Palombini LO, Poyares D, et al. Long term oral appliance therapy decreases stress symptoms in patients with upper airway resistance syndrome. J Clin Sleep Med. 2020;16(11):1857–62.
25. Godoy LBM, Palombini LO, Poyares D, et al. Long-term oral appliance therapy improves daytime function and mood in upper airway resistance syndrome patients. Sleep. 2017;40(12):zsx175.
26. Newman JP, et al. Recognition and surgical management of the upper airway resistance syndrome. Laryngoscope. 1996;106:1089–93.

Upper Airway Resistance Syndrome: Physiotherapeutic Approach

Evelyn Brasil

Upper airway resistance syndrome (UARS) is a syndrome of increased upper airway collapsibility during sleep. The upper airway collapsibility during sleep of patients with UARS is halfway between that of normal subjects and that of patients with mild-to-moderate sleep apnea.

There is a lack of scientific evidence on literature about the treatment of UARS, as most of the research is case series by now. Treatments for UARS range from surgical procedures, oral appliance devices, pharmacological treatment, radiofrequency thermal ablation, and the use of positive airway pressure (PAP) [1]. From the existed investigations, the number of patients treated has been too low and the protocols too limited to be delivered at appropriate outcome recommendations. Still, many of the attempts have shown positive results, suggesting the possibility of several treatment possibilities.

1 Positive Airway Pressure

PAP is one of the most studied treatments for UARS, which can significantly reduce nocturnal awakenings and diurnal clinical symptoms such as excessive daytime sleepiness and fatigue. PAP can also improve sleep consolidation as seen in the example of a hypnogram, decreasing sleep-disordered breathing (Fig. 1), increasing N3 stage as seen in polysomnographic examination (PSG), and reducing SL, as seen in multiple sleep latency test (MSLT).

E. Brasil (✉)
Department of Severe Patients, Hospital Israelita Albert Einstein, Certified in Sleep Physiotherapy by the Brazilian Sleep Society (ABS), and The Brazilian Association of Cardiorespiratory Physiotherapy and Physiotherapy in Intensive Care (ASSOBRAFIR), São Paulo, SP, Brazil

C. Frange, F. M. S. Coelho (eds.), *Sleep Medicine and Physical Therapy*,
https://doi.org/10.1007/978-3-030-85074-6_19

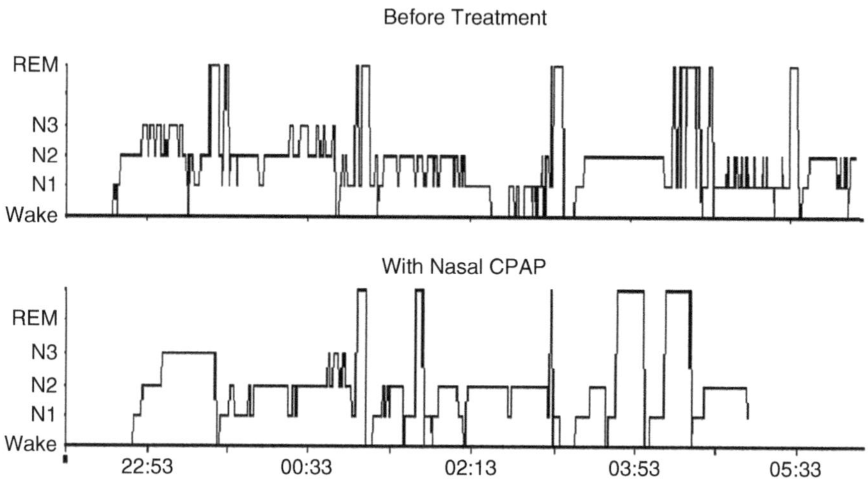

Fig. 1 Hypnograms (plots of sleep stages against time) before and after treatment with positive airway pressure (PAP) that demonstrate increasing sleep consolidation (decreasing sleep stage shifts) for a participant receiving therapeutic nasal continuous PAP (CPAP) (age 43 years; BMI 30 kg/m^2; baseline AHI 5/h; baseline RERA index 23/h). (Abbreviations: *N1* non-rapid eye movement stage 1 sleep, *N2* non-rapid eye movement stage 2 sleep, *N3* slow-wave sleep, *REM* rapid eye movement sleep stage). (Reprinted with permission from Amin et al. [2])

PAP delivered by a nasal route has been effective for UARS, improving daytime symptoms, as evaluated both by objective (PSG) and subjective (questionnaires) measures [3]. An investigation along with participants with idiopathic excessive sleepiness, who had not been diagnosed with other sleep disorders, demonstrated improvement in sleep as seen by the decrease of a number of awakening, increase of N3 stage, and improvement of excessive daytime sleepiness complaints after 4 weeks of treatment with PAP, titrated at a pressure of 7 cmH_2O (±1 cmH_2O). Considering that the individual who has UARS does not have a classically defined amount of apnea and hypopneas, the titration pressure of this investigation was based on the analysis of esophageal pressure measurements [3].

Snoring and excessive daytime sleepiness improve with PAP in patients with UARS [3–5]. Improvement in snoring and systemic arterial hypertension without the use of medication has also been reported in the literature, despite no improvement in subjective symptoms [5].

As for OSA or CSA, there is evidence on the PAP titration for treatment, as the UARS is an entity not fully recognized, and, therefore, no guideline on the treatment exists. But what is the pressure to set up for UARS? The pressure of the regulated PAP must be the lower one as to eliminate the flow limitation and to maintain the upper airway open, as we see in clinical practice. In one study, the mean therapeutic pressure found was 7 cmH_2O with a variation of 4–9 cmH_2O [3]. When comparing fixed PAP (continuous PAP, CPAP) with automatic PAP, another study showed that there was greater adherence to automatic PAP compared to CPAP; however, in both ventilatory modalities, there was an improvement of excessive daytime sleepiness [6].

A pilot study investigated if the change in symptoms correlated with the change in sleep stage shifts after and before treatment with CPAP via nasal route (compared to sham CPAP) and found evidence that sleep-disordered breathing played a role in daytime symptoms of male veterans of war [2]. The change in sleep stage shifts among all participants from pre- to post-treatment PSG examination was well correlated with a positive change in symptoms such as pain, fatigue, sleep quality, and physical and mental components of quality of life [2]. This may have occurred as nasal CPAP is able to splint the pharyngeal airway during sleep, removing stressors such as pharyngeal collapse during sleep and thus decreasing the number of sleep stage shifts.

In women with preeclampsia and flow limitation, an investigation showed that the increase in night blood pressure (that occurs in this population) was eliminated with the use of automatic PAP ranging from 4 to 10 cmH_2O. This range of pressure was sufficient to minimize the increase in night blood pressure [7].

Postmenopausal women with insomnia, treated with hormone therapy, presented frequent awakenings, associated with UARS, tending to worsen the climacteric symptoms. In the investigation, some of the participants were treated with PAP or nasal surgery, both associated with cognitive-behavioral therapy (CBT). The results indicated that PAP associated with CBT improved excessive daytime sleepiness [8].

In clinical practice, due to low adherence, PAP is indicated as a therapeutic test and maintained through adherence and improvement of symptoms. The use of PAP improves the patient's subjective symptoms of UARS; however, adherence to long-term therapy is low. A study demonstrates that although initial acceptance of PAP is high, long-term adherence is low, as about 98% of individuals gave up long-term treatment [9]. In another investigation, the use of PAP in patients with respiratory disturbance index < 5 and awakening rate > 20/hour was evaluated [10]. From the 11 patients assessed, only 19% accepted the use and showed low adherence to PAP therapy (2.8 hours ±1.5 hours) in 6 months [10].

In addition to low adherence to PAP, an American study shows that of the 94 individuals diagnosed with UARS, in a 4-year follow-up, no participant started treatment with PAP. In the United States, this is due to the lack of coverage of treatment with PAP by the health insurance, which considers qualified to receive PAP only individuals with sleep apnea. In Brazil, there is no coverage of the treatment of respiratory sleep disorders by private health insurance or government health insurance [11].

In addition to PAP treatment, there are studies demonstrating the improvement of the airway circumference and symptoms with positional therapy and inspiratory muscle training in cases of sleep apnea [12, 13]. Nevertheless, we still have no investigations evaluating inspiratory muscle training or positional therapy in patients with UARS.

2 Final Words

PAP has been shown to be effective in the treatment of UARS; however, acceptance and adherence to therapy are low, and there is no consensus or guidelines for the use of PAP for UARS. Both for the use of PAP, as for the other therapeutic modalities for UARS, there is an urgent need for randomized controlled studies with follow-up as for new and innovative investigations on treatment.

References

1. de Godoy LB, et al. Treatment of upper airway resistance syndrome in adults: where do we stand? Sleep Sci. 2015;8(1):42–8.
2. Amin MM, et al. The effect of nasal continuous positive airway pressure on the symptoms of Gulf War illness. Sleep Breath. 2011;15(3):579–87.
3. Guilleminault C, et al. A cause of excessive daytime sleepiness. The upper airway resistance syndrome. Chest. 1993;104(3):781–7.
4. Ong KC, Cheng PP, Ong YY. Upper airway resistance syndrome--report of three cases. Ann Acad Med Singap. 2000;29(2):242–5.
5. Watanabe T, et al. Clinical characteristics of upper airway resistance syndrome. Psychiatry Clin Neurosci. 1999;53(2):331–3.
6. Hudgel DW, Fung C. A long-term randomized, cross-over comparison of auto-titrating and standard nasal continuous airway pressure. Sleep. 2000;23(5):645–8.
7. Edwards N, et al. Nasal continuous positive airway pressure reduces sleep-induced blood pressure increments in preeclampsia. Am J Respir Crit Care Med. 2000;162(1):252–7.
8. Guilleminault C, et al. Chronic insomnia, premenopausal women and sleep disordered breathing: part 2. Comparison of nondrug treatment trials in normal breathing and UARS post menopausal women complaining of chronic insomnia. J Psychosom Res. 2002;53(1):617–23.
9. Palombini L, et al. Upper airway resistance syndrome: still not recognized and not treated. Sleep Sci. 2011;4(2):72.
10. Rauscher H, Formanek D, Zwick H. Nasal continuous positive airway pressure for nonapneic snoring? Chest. 1995;107(1):58–61.
11. Guilleminault C, et al. Upper airway resistance syndrome: a long-term outcome study. J Psychiatr Res. 2006;40(3):273–9.
12. Neill AM, et al. Effects of sleep posture on upper airway stability in patients with obstructive sleep apnea. Am J Respir Crit Care Med. 1997;155(1):199–204.
13. Souza AKF, et al. Effectiveness of inspiratory muscle training on sleep and functional capacity to exercise in obstructive sleep apnea: a randomized controlled trial. Sleep Breath. 2018;22(3):631–9.

Narcolepsy: An Overview

Fernando Morgadinho Santos Coelho and Ana Carolina Dias Gomes

Narcolepsy is a sleep disorder that is characterized by excessive daytime sleepiness (EDS) and manifestations of REM sleep disorders such as hallucinations, sleep paralysis, cataplexy, and sleep fragmentation. Narcolepsy is divided into narcolepsy type 1 (NT1), with cataplexy and/or hypocretin-1 (HCRT-1) deficiency, and narcolepsy type 2 (NT2), without cataplexy and normal levels of HCRT-1 [1].

Narcolepsy is prevalent in 0.02–0.18% of the populations of the United States of America and Western Europe. Its prevalence is slightly divergent when different races or ethnicities are analyzed, varying in Japan and other Asian countries between 0.16% and 0.18%. Among Israeli Jews, a prevalence of 0.002% was noted. No epidemiological studies on the disease were found in the Brazilian population, but it is estimated that the rates are similar to those in Western Europe and the United States of America.

There is a bimodal incidence distribution at 15 and 35 years old. The symptoms of narcolepsy can start more rarely in childhood, and in 5% of patients, it starts before puberty. In the third edition of the International Classification of Sleep Disorders (ICSD-3), narcolepsy is part of central disorders of hypersomnolence: NT1, NT2, idiopathic hypersomnia, Kleine-Levin syndrome, insufficient sleep syndrome, and hypersomnia secondary to a clinical illness or medication and associated with psychiatric disorders. It is important to note that EDS is not necessarily caused by comorbid psychiatric illness, they simply need to be diagnosed in the same patient at the same time [1].

F. M. S. Coelho (✉)
Neurology and Neurosurgery Department; Department of Psychobiology, Escola Paulista de Medicina, Universidade Federal de São Paulo, São Paulo, SP, Brazil

A. C. D. Gomes
Psychobiology Department, Escola Paulista de Medicina, Universidade Federal de São Paulo, São Paulo, SP, Brazil

C. Frange, F. M. S. Coelho (eds.), *Sleep Medicine and Physical Therapy*,
https://doi.org/10.1007/978-3-030-85074-6_20

to 2 minutes, usually bilateral and symmetrical, without sleep. If a trigger is maintained, consecutive attacks can follow or appears as a single episode.

The frequency of cataplexy is variable, ranging from less than one attack per month to more than 20 per day. Factors such as the sudden withdrawal of drugs for cataplexy can result in *status cataplecticus*, in which attacks occur continuously [1].

It is often difficult to assess descriptions during the first contact with a patient if a muscle weakness reflects genuine cataplectic episodes or just physiological muscle fatigue associated with laughter or intense physical activity. In a recent epidemiological study, 6.5% of the reported population experienced "sudden and abrupt weakness" in association with laughter or other emotions [2].

Attacks similar to cataplexy are reported after the use of medications (lamotrigine and modafinil) and in a small number of other neurological diseases (Norrie and Niemann-Pick type C disease) [3, 4].

1.3 Fragmented Nighttime Sleep

The nocturnal sleep of these patients can be fragmented due to multiple awakenings, compromising its quality. This is a common finding, and it may even be the main complaint about some of the patients.

1.4 Hypnagogical and Hypnopompic Hallucinations

Hypnagogic hallucinations are defined as vivid dreams that occur in the transition from waking to sleep. Hypnagogic hallucinations occur in the transition from sleep to awakening. Hallucinations usually have a multimodal or "holistic" character, often combining visual, auditory, and tactile phenomena. Hallucinations are more common in people with NT1 (63%–77%), less common in people with idiopathic hypersomnia (25%), and have intermediate rates in people with NT2 (42%).

1.5 Sleep Paralysis

Sleep paralysis describes the disturbing temporary inability to voluntarily move muscles in sleep-wake transitions. Despite being awake and aware of the environment, the affected individual is unable to move his limbs or even open his eyes. The experience can take several minutes and can be very distressing. Other symptoms can include ptosis, blurred vision, and diplopia, probably as a result of drowsiness.

Sleep paralysis is prevalent in NT1 (53%–69%), relatively uncommon in idiopathic hypersomnia (20%), and has intermediate rates to these other two groups in

NT2 (35%). Unlike cataplexy, sleep paralysis is very nonspecific, with approximately 10% of the general population present.

In 2017, a study evaluated patients with NT1 and NT2 to assess exercise tolerance, which is one of the best prognostic markers of all-cause mortality in the general population, and it depends on daily energy expenditure or the amount of daily exercise. The study revealed that patients NT1 and NT2 have less tolerance to exercise and obtained interesting results [5].

Cardiopulmonary fitness is inversely related to the degree of EDS in NT1 and NT2 patients and the number of cataplexy attacks per month in NT1. They concluded that the fact that patients are less physically active (e.g., performing household chores), the day-to-day activities have reduced exercise tolerance with less muscle recruitment [5].

Patients with narcolepsy have several factors that may explain this low tolerance to exercise, such as EDS, episodes of cataplexy triggered by exercise, high fatigue prevalence, and obesity.

These patients are less active, in general, regarding actigraphy in another study, despite treatment with modafinil, a stimulant used to treat EDS. There are also reports that 48% of narcolepsy patients complained of difficulties in playing sports. In another sample of NT1 and NT2, only 19% reported playing any recreational sport. There is still a variable only mentioned in the studies, which is the highest prevalence of depression in NT1, which can also contribute to less physical activity [5].

When compared with controls and NT2, patients with NT1 had lower basal metabolism. It was noted that there was a 35% reduction in strides per day in NT1 when comparing them with the daily activities of a healthy adult non-sedentary [5].

Narcolepsy is associated with a higher cardiovascular risk when registering a greater prevalence of obesity and diabetes [6]. These patients should perform structured physical activities to improve exercise tolerance, as well as potentially improve the overall cardiovascular profile since diagnosis. The physiotherapist and the physical education professional can play a central role in the treatment of these patients by leading the prescription of activities for these patients.

1.6 Diagnosis

The diagnostic criteria based on the ICSD-3 are:

Criteria A and B must be met:

A. The patient has daily periods of irrepressible need for sleep or daytime lapses of sleep occurring for at least 3 months.
B. The presence of one or both:
    1. Cataplexy (as defined in Essential Resources) and an average sleep latency of ≤ 8 minutes and two or more periods of sleep-onset REM periods (SOREMP) in a Multiple Sleep Latency Test (MSLT) performed according

to standard techniques. A SOREMP (within 15 minutes of sleep onset) on PSG the night before MSLT can replace one of the SOREMPs on MSLT.
2. Hypocretin-1 level in the CSF, measured by immunoreactivity, is ≤110 pg/mL or < 1/3 of the mean values obtained in normal subjects with the same standardized test.

The EDS can be graded subjectively by applying scales such as the Epworth Sleepiness Scale (ESS), the Karolinska Sleepiness Scale, and the Stanford Sleepiness Scale. The last two allow the assessment of EDS at the moment of its application, having as a disadvantage the fact that there may be variation in somnolence from one moment to another. ESS, on the other hand, refers to the possibility of napping in everyday situations in the last 30 days [7]. The clinical instruments for quantifying EDS should not be evaluated in isolation, and it is necessary to contextualize the clinical condition of each patient. Recently, a new tool was incorporated to monitor the patients with narcolepsy [8]. The Narcolepsy Severity Scale quantifies the EDS and other symptoms of NT1 patients, and it is useful to follow them [8–10].

The MSLT measures the physiological tendency to fall asleep in monotonous situations, as patients tend to get more sleepy in these situations. The test must be conducted according to the parameters of the American Academy of Sleep Medicine manual. It is recommended that the patient undergo a PSG on the night preceding MSLT.1 The average sleep latency in MSLT below 8 minutes was the best cutoff point in the context of the diagnosis of narcolepsy, with approximately 90% of adult patients with narcolepsy with latency below that level [1].

It is necessary to pay attention to situations that can make differential diagnosis difficult through tests. Sleep deprivation can result in a false-positive result, and, therefore, this test should only be requested for patients who are sleeping well (about 7–9 hours in adults, there is the possibility of individual variations). The assessment of an adequate sleep period before the exam, by an actigraphy or a sleep diary, must be done, at least 1–2 weeks, before polysomnography/MSLT. Several drugs can affect the results of MSLT. Sedative medications that interfere with the average latency for sleep onset or REM sleep suppressant medications, especially serotonergic antidepressants, should be discontinued, if possible, before MSLT. It is necessary to evaluate the half-life of these medications and also if there is an abuse of illicit substances to avoid false-negative results.

For the diagnosis of narcolepsy, the presence of EDS must be confirmed by MSLT, when the average latency for sleep onset is less than 8 minutes and there are two or more periods of REM sleep at the beginning of sleep – SOREMPs. The two SOREMPs must be present in the MSLT and can also be considered in the baseline polysomnography (PSG), performed the night before the MSLT (SOREMP ≤15 minutes in the PSG). PSG and MSLT are objective ways to assess sleep-related parameters [1–11].

In addition to clinical findings, there are markers frequently found in patients with narcolepsy such as the human leukocyte antigen (HLA)-related allele, the HLA-DQB1*0602 allele that may be present in 95% of patients with cataplexy [12].

About 24% of patients without cataplexy will have low levels of HCRT-1 in the CSF, and 10% of patients diagnosed with NT2 will later manifest cataplexy, which will result in a change in diagnosis to NT1.1 There are still 8% of type 2 narcoleptics who present intermediate levels of HCRT-1 in the CSF (> 110 pg/mL and $\leq$ 200 pg/mL) [1].

1.7 Prognosis

Narcolepsy patients have difficulty performing daily life activities and socializing, mainly due to cataplexy attacks and EDS. These patients have a poor quality of life that is similar or inferior to patients with epilepsy or obstructive sleep apnea syndrome [2].

The quality of life of these patients worsens, even more, due to the delay in obtaining a diagnosis and symptom control. The average delay for diagnosis reaches more than 10 years after the onset of symptoms even in Europe, for example. When considering that the majority of patients will present the onset of symptoms in the second decade of life, they would remain untreated during a crucial period of their education and the initial period of their career [2–13].

These patients often have slower responses to external stimuli and varying degrees of difficulty concentrating [13].

2 Narcolepsy and Childhood

The clinical presentation of narcolepsy in childhood is quite different; EDS can be difficult to assess and can be expressed as excessively long night sleep or the recurrence of naps in the previously interrupted daytime period (ICSD-3).

In addition, children may paradoxically exhibit hyperactive behavior, behavioral problems, and worsening school performance. Inattention, lack of energy, insomnia, hallucinations, or a combination of them can lead to an incorrect psychiatric diagnosis of schizophrenia and depression. In this population, the presence of auxiliary symptoms, such as sleep paralysis or hypnagogic hallucinations, can also be difficult to confirm, depending on the child's expression ability.

Early puberty and obesity can also develop near the onset of symptoms. REM sleep behavioral disorder may be present from the beginning as well; it is important to pay attention to the PSG request.

Cataplexy is infrequent before the age of 4 years old with a different phenotype of typical cataplexy triggered by positive emotions. It is common the involvement of the face, eyelids, and mouth, associated with a clear non-association with emotions can occur. Along with the protrusion of the tongue, this characteristic pattern was called cataplectic facies. Children with cataplexy may also have positive motor phenomena, ranging from dyskinetic movements or perioral dystonic movements or

HCRT-1 has a maximum expression during wakefulness, and it is related to muscle tone through the activation of the motor system at the *locus ceruleus* and the *raphe nucleus* by the release of norepinephrine and serotonin, respectively. These neurons are inhibited during REM sleep. The balance between motor excitation and the inhibition generated by an emotional stimulus is altered in the deregulation of this HCRT-1 circuit, generating muscle atony during wakefulness, which is characteristic in NT1 patients. Cataplexy is caused by decreased excitement of noradrenergic neurons and an increased motor inhibition of GABAergic and/or glycinergic neurons. The amygdala and the medial prefrontal cortex contain neural pathways; positive emotions are the triggers for cataplectic phenomena [16].

3.3 Treatment

Non-pharmacological treatment is an essential part of treatment in patients with narcolepsy consisting of taking scheduled naps. Short naps are usually restorative in these patients. Scheduling naps throughout the day and a good night's sleep can have a great benefit to the patient, and this approach should always be associated with pharmacological treatment [2].

Unfortunately, isolated non-pharmacological treatments are generally not sufficient for the treatment of narcolepsy patients. The medications are prescribed to treat EDS- and REM-related symptoms such as cataplexy [18].

4 Pharmacological Treatment of Excessive Daytime Sleepiness

4.1 First-Line Therapy

- Modafinil – several studies with the class of evidence I
  Modafinil is the choice for the pharmacological treatment of EDS in patients with narcolepsy. The mechanism of action is not yet fully understood; the probable mechanism of action is greater presynaptic activation of dopaminergic transmission in some brain regions. It is a non-CNS stimulant with fewer side effects and a lower incidence of tolerance [19].
- Pitolisant – two studies with the class of evidence I
  Pitolisant is an antagonist/agonist inverse to histamine receptor H3. The main action is the presynaptic activation of histaminergic neurons in the brain, promoting wakefulness and improving attention and memory. The effect of pitolisant on EDS in patients with narcolepsy was similar to that of the use of modafinil [20].
- Solriamfetol – one study with a class of evidence I
  Solriamfetol is a selective dopamine and norepinephrine reuptake inhibitor with a similar release of amines to that of amphetamine-type stimulants. Solriamfetol

reduces EDS in patients with narcolepsy, and the main side effects are headache, nausea, decreased appetite, pharyngitis, dry mouth, and anxiety [21].
- Sodium oxybate (GHB) – several studies with the class of evidence I
GHB increases the release of GABA in the hippocampus and the cerebral cortex. Other effects are the modulation of dopaminergic neurotransmission and an increase in tryptophan transport with consequent higher levels of amines and acetylcholine in the brain. The most common side effects are euphoria, amnesia, anabolic effect, aggressiveness, coma, agitation, tremors, and muscle contractions. Studies also demonstrated that GHB improves sleep fragmentation with improved EDS in patients with narcolepsy [22].

4.2 *Second-Line Therapy*

- Methylphenidate – one study with a class of evidence II

  It is a CNS stimulating drug, with characteristics similar to those of amphetamines. It is important to advise the patient not to use the medication on the weekends or for two days during the week to avoid tolerance. Side effects such as insomnia, high blood pressure, irritability, headache, and palpitations are common. Patients being treated with these drugs should be monitored and their complaints assessed [19].

4.3 *Third-Line Therapy*

- Amphetamines – no study with a class of evidence I–IV
Amphetamines are stimulants with a higher prevalence of abuse and risk of adverse cardiovascular events. The use of lisdexamfetamine to treat EDS in patients with narcolepsy has been reported in many cases [23].
- Caffeine – one study with a class of evidence II
Caffeine is a derivative of xanthine which is a selective antagonist of adenosine receptors (A1 and A2a). Possible higher doses necessary to promote wakefulness in patients with narcolepsy can induce anxiety, tremors, headache, and gastrointestinal irritation. However, a recent study demonstrated the benefit of lower doses of caffeine to control EDS in patients with narcolepsy [19].
- L-carnitine – one study with a class of evidence II
L-carnitine is an amine that participates in the metabolism of lipids, playing a fundamental role in the transport of these from the cytoplasm to the mitochondrial matrix to be oxidized. There is a dysfunctional fatty acid beta-oxidation pathway in patients with narcolepsy, and a randomized placebo-controlled study showed the effectiveness of oral L-carnitine in reducing EDS by increasing the action of the enzyme L-carnitine-o-palmitoyl transferase in this population.

Recent findings point to the safe and useful use of L-carnitine during pregnancy in patients with narcolepsy [24].

5 Pharmacological Therapy of Cataplexy

5.1 First-Line Therapy

- Sodium oxybate (GHB) – several studies with a class of evidence I
  GHB is the drug of choice to treat cataplexy. It is an approved drug for the treatment of narcolepsy in children too. There is a higher concentration of sodium in the medication that can elevate blood pressure levels. It should be taken in bed, due to the risk of falls and trauma due to very short sleep latency [22].
- Dual antidepressants – venlafaxine (no study with evidence class)
  Dual antidepressants have double action with an increase in the synapses of both serotonin and norepinephrine. The main side effects are similar to other antidepressants that inhibit serotonin uptake: loss of fine coordination, mental confusion, weight gain, sedation, nausea, insomnia, and altered sexual function; and in rare cases of drug combination, they can cause arrhythmias and death. Venlafaxine is widely used in clinical practice, although there are no studies with a minimum level of evidence [19].
- Pitolisant – one study with a class of evidence I
  Pitolisant is also effective in reducing cataplexy. The use of pitolisant does not seem to lead to abuse and is well tolerated. Common side effects include headache, insomnia, and nausea, especially at the beginning of treatment [20].

5.2 Second-Line Therapy

- Tricyclic antidepressants – clomipramine (one study with a class of evidence IV)
  Tricyclic antidepressants block membrane transport of presynaptic neurons with increased concentration of monoamines in synapses with action on postsynaptic neurons. These drugs have many possible side effects such as dry mouth, impaired vision, intestinal constipation, urinary retention, postural hypotension, weight gain, difficulty concentrating and learning, tachycardia and mania, coma, delirium, cardiac arrhythmias, respiratory depression, and death. The doses used to control cataplexy are lower than those used to treat depression, with a lower prevalence and severity of side effects [19].
- Serotonin reuptake inhibitor antidepressants – fluoxetine (two studies with a class of evidence III) and citalopram (one study with a class of evidence IV)
  Serotonin reuptake inhibitor antidepressants increase the concentration in the serotonin synaptic cleft by inhibiting their reuptake by the presynaptic neuron. The side effects seen are loss of fine coordination, mental confusion, sedation,

weight gain, nausea, insomnia, and altered sexual function and, in rare cases of drug association, can cause arrhythmias and death [19].

5.3 *Third-Line Therapy*

- Monoamine oxidase-B inhibitors – selegiline (one study with a class of evidence II)
  Monoamine oxidase-B inhibitors block the monoamine oxidase-B that degrades serotonin, norepinephrine, and dopamine in the synapse with a consequent higher effect of these neurotransmitters on postsynaptic neurons. Sedation, confusion, tremors, excitement, weight gain, dry mouth, intestinal constipation, urinary retention, and cardiac arrhythmias can all be side effects [19].
- Baclofen – one study with a class of evidence II
  Baclofen is a $GABA_B$ agonist drug, commonly used in neurological patients to control stiffness, pain, and spasticity. There is evidence that baclofen can provide sleep benefits by reducing sleep latency and increasing slow-wave sleep, increasing the total sleep time. There is also a possible benefit of using baclofen to control cataplexy [25].

6 Future Perspectives for the Treatment of Narcolepsy

There is ample evidence of an autoimmune mechanism of NT1. Some studies to modulate the immune system have been made to control the disease. A few series of patients treated with intravenous immunoglobulins have been published, but with negative or transitory results [26].

The improvement in narcolepsy symptoms after the use of steroids and immunomodulatory treatments (alemtuzumab and rituximab) has been described; however, more studies need to be done to define the effectiveness of these immune therapies [26].

The intraventricular infusion of HCRT-1 did not improve symptoms in narcolepsy patients. However, HCRT-1 agonists appear to be promising, as long as these drugs cross the blood-brain barrier [27].

References

1. International classification of sleep disorders – Third edition (ICSD-3). 3rd ed. American Academy of Sleep Medicine; 2014.
2. Trotti LM. Central disorders of hypersomnolence. Continuum (Minneap Minn). 2020;26(4):890–907.

Excessive Daytime Sleepiness: An Overview

Lúcio Huebra Pimentel Filho and Fernando Morgadinho Santos Coelho

Among the daytime symptoms related to sleep disorders, daytime sleepiness is one of the most disabling. This is a frequent reason for seeking medical care on an outpatient basis and sometimes in emergency care units.

Excessive daytime sleepiness or hypersomnia can be conceptualized as difficulty in staying awake and alert with a greater tendency to fall asleep during the day unexpectedly or at inappropriate times. It is important to make it clear that it is not always necessary for sleep to occur, but only this feeling of need for daytime sleep is enough, even if the individual manages to withstand a nap. Thus, daytime sleepiness is primarily a symptom and is directly related to a subjective interpretation. However, as we will see throughout the chapter, there are some strategies to standardize its assessment, whether with subjective clinical scales or with objective neurophysiological parameters.

Patients living with hypersomnia suffer from a very heterogeneous group of syndromes and disorders. It makes its epidemiology very complex. There are several studies in association with age, sex, body mass index, work shift, snoring, obstructive apnea, and among groups of specific comorbidities; however, the prevalence in the general population is little known and varies with the methodology used. An overall prevalence is estimated at around 4–20.6%. A recent prospective study of a Swiss cohort showed an incidence of 5.1% in a 5-year follow-up. Risk factors in this survey, associated with the onset of hypersomnia, were male gender, depressive symptoms, poor subjective quality of sleep, and moderate to severe sleep apnea [1].

L. H. P. Filho (✉)
Neurology and Neurosurgery Department, Escola Paulista de Medicina, Universidade Federal de São Paulo, São Paulo, SP, Brazil

F. M. S. Coelho
Neurology and Neurosurgery Department; Department of Psychobiology, Escola Paulista de Medicina, Universidade Federal de São Paulo, São Paulo, SP, Brazil

C. Frange, F. M. S. Coelho (eds.), *Sleep Medicine and Physical Therapy*,
https://doi.org/10.1007/978-3-030-85074-6_21

Some of the other risk factors also defined in studies of incidence are depression, sleep apnea, obesity, and diabetes [2].

The recognition of hypersomnia becomes very important because it has already been defined that this symptom, in isolation, determines an increase in general morbidity and mortality. A 10-year prospective study of a large cohort showed a mortality all-causes hazard ratio of 1.43, that is, a 43% greater chance of occurring in the group with daytime sleepiness [3]. In addition to higher mortality, it implies economic and social losses.

In this chapter, we will go deeper into the study of hypersomnia, especially in the diagnosis and recognition of its causes and available guidelines for approach and treatment.

1 Diagnosis

Evaluation of patients with excessive daytime sleepiness is generally a clinical challenge. At first, despite being a relatively common complaint in neurology and sleep medicine clinics, the search for medical help in the face of symptoms is still restricted, and, in most cases, it is delayed. The reason for this is diverse and ranges from cultural issues and ignorance about sleep disorders, difficulty in accessing a specialized service, or even prejudices and dysfunctional beliefs in relation to the patient with daytime sleepiness.

The initial step in the management of patients with daytime sleepiness is to better understand the complaint and to know how to precisely identify it. During the consultation, at the initial moment, we can already see if the patient shows signs of drowsiness at that moment. Yawning, little motor activity, difficulty in attention, or even demand for coffee can be indirect signs for the diagnosis. During the interview, it is important to assess whether the patient has daytime episodes when he has difficulty staying awake and how severity is their functional impact, even in social, professional, or school spheres. It is common for the patient, in a simple directed question, to deny having daytime sleepiness, only because he is already accustomed to the symptom or because of not taking daytime naps, but when properly assessed, it is evident that, for several moments, he has some discomfort related to the difficulty of maintaining himself awake.

A distinction that must be made during the clinical interview is whether the patient complains of fatigue and apathy or really daytime sleepiness. Fatigue is referred to as tiredness, lack of energy, and exhaustion. It is usually induced by overactivity and relieves with rest. Daytime sleepiness is referred to as a decreased ability to perform tasks that worsen at rest or in monotonous situations and relieve with sleep or nap.

Some clinical scales support this subjective assessment of the symptom. The Epworth Sleepiness Scale (ESS) is a self-administered questionnaire, a good alternative to quantify the sleepiness of patients with hypersomnia. It is an inexpensive tool, remarkably simple, and quick to execute [4]. The ESS has eight questions that show routine situations in which the patient must graduate the probability of falling asleep, in reference to the symptoms in the last month. Each question is scored from 0 to 3, with 0 being no chance of sleep and from 1 to 3 progressively greater chance of falling asleep. The global score ranges from 0 to 24; the higher the score, the greater the daytime sleepiness. Scores greater than 9 indicates that the patient has excessive daytime sleepiness [4]. The Stanford Sleepiness Scale is also a well-established questionnaire for assessing daytime sleepiness, but it provides little information for assessing outpatients. This scale assesses the patient's state of alert at that precise moment and the propensity to sleep in that momentary situation in which it is applied. The score ranges from 1 to 7; the higher the score, the greater the drowsiness. Scores greater than or equal to 4 show significant drowsiness at that moment [5]. It can be used, in the clinical context, to guide patients with hypersomnia to better recognize and graduate their symptoms, in order to avoid performing risky tasks when at greater drowsiness, thus avoiding work and traffic accidents (please refer to chapter "Subjective assessment of sleep").

In addition to subjective assessments, it is possible, in specific contexts, to use supplementary tests to objectively quantify daytime sleepiness. There are two neurophysiological tests that provide important information for this purpose, the Multiple Sleep Latency Test (MSLT) and the Maintenance of Wakefulness Test (MWT), detailed in chapter "Objective assessment of sleep". MSLT is indicated for the investigation of patients with hypersomnia and is especially important for the diagnosis of narcolepsy and other central origin hypersomnias. MSLT is the multiparametric analysis – electroencephalogram (EEG), electrooculogram (EOG), and chin electromyography (EMG) – of five naps performed during the day. The exam starts two hours after the end of the night polysomnography, and it continues with five opportunities of naps in a calm, dark, and silent environment. The patient is instructed to try to sleep. It is assessed whether the patient falls asleep before 20 minutes of recording, and if it happens, it is observed the first 15 minutes of sleep to assess the sleep stages reached in that period. The most important data used in the interpretation of the result is the mean sleep latency, that is, how long it takes for the patient to start sleeping, from the beginning of the record until the first time of sleep. The mean sleep latency of these five records is suggestive of EDS if it is less than 10 minutes. The lower the average sleep latency, the greater the patient's propensity to nap in monotonous situations [6]. MWT is a neurophysiologic exam very similar to MTLS, especially in data collection, but it has some peculiarities. This exam is not largely used in the diagnosis of hypersomnia, but it can be useful in the clinical follow-up of patients, and it is used in the legal documentation of excessive daytime sleepiness in some countries for labor purposes or vehicular driving. The patient is monitored with EEG, EOG, and EMG of the chin and positioned comfortably in the bed, seated with indirect light in a quiet environment. In this case, the patient is instructed to try not to sleep. Latency to sleep onset is also monitored within four 40-minute opportunities, assessing the mean sleep latency [7].

Once the patient is identified as having hypersomnia, physicians need to identify the cause of this symptom. From this moment on, we will present the main causes of hypersomnia, organized in diagnostic groups with their particular aspects of epidemiology and management.

2.5 Hypersomnia Related to a Circadian Rhythm Disorder

Disorders of circadian rhythm are also common causes of excessive daytime sleepiness. Patients with advanced sleep phase (preferred sleep time earlier than the majority of the population) experience daytime sleepiness in the late afternoon or early evening, and patients with delayed sleep phase experience sleepiness mainly in the early hours of the morning. The diagnostic tip is to assess sleep schedule, their regularity, and especially in the most socially free periods, such as weekends and holidays.

More recently, a new phenomenon related to sleep deprivation and the circadian rhythm has been described, the so-called social jet lag. The "social jet leg" is a time difference between working days and days off. The phenomenon occurs when there is a difference in the midpoint of sleep (bedtime and waking time divided by 2) between working days and rest days greater than 2 hours. Several recent studies show independently higher cardiovascular risk and overall mortality in these patients [10].

The treatment of daytime sleepiness in these cases is dependent on the treatment of the rhythm disorder. Guidance on the regularity of bedtime, searching for a sleep schedule more similar to biological demand, and orientation on times of greater exposure to light can help in the synchronization of the circadian rhythm. The use of melatonin may also be indicated in the treatment of the delayed sleep phase.

2.6 Hypersomnia Due to Sleep Disorder

Various sleep disorders can trigger daytime symptoms such as fatigue, daytime sleepiness, irritability, difficulty concentrating, and learning. Faced with a patient complaining of EDS and signs of poor sleep quality, the investigation should be directed to sleep disorders, and, if indicated, nocturnal polysomnography should be requested.

Polysomnography is a complementary exam that registers several physiological variables during sleep: latency for sleep in minutes, latency for REM in minutes, total recording time in minutes, total sleep time in minutes, sleep efficiency in percentage, sleep stages (N1, N2, N3, and R), arousals per hour of sleep, apnea and hypopnea index, and oxyhemoglobin saturation, as well as body and limb movements. The registration of other variables can also be done depending on the clinical needs of each clinical suspicion. The use of more complex neurological channels in the EEG record, as well as more electrodes for capturing muscle activity in extremities or for detailing bruxism, may be necessary.

Restless legs syndrome, periodical limb movement syndrome, sleep-disordered breathing, bruxism, and parasomnias are part of the differential diagnosis to be excluded [11]. Obstructive sleep apnea (OSA) is a common cause of daytime sleepiness. OSA associated with daytime sleepiness affects 3–7% of the adult male population and 2–5% of adult women. Both sleep apnea and sleepiness secondary to sleep apnea are more common in men; this statistic equalizes when women reach menopause. Some symptoms act as a warning for the diagnosis; the most common are easily recognized such as snoring and apnea. Other less classic symptoms, but very helpful in the diagnosis, especially when the consultation is carried out without the presence of companions, are nocturia, dry mouth, morning headache, non-restorative sleep, night sweating, and sleep fragmentation.

2.7 *Hypersomnia of Central Origin*

Excluding the differential diagnoses mentioned so far, there is a set of rarer hypersomnia named hypersomnia of central origin. Diseases such as narcolepsy, Kleine-Levin syndrome, and idiopathic hypersomnia must be recognized, and the differential diagnoses must be remembered. These diseases lead to a significant reduction in quality of life, as well as a high risk of personal and professional accidents. The delay in diagnosing these diseases is greater than 10 years with a significant impact on the quality of life of these patients [12].

Health professionals need to be well prepared and motivated to make diagnoses of rarer sleep disorders. Efforts by university circles have been made trying to reverse this scenario with continuing education on the topic for patients and health professionals.

Narcolepsy is a chronic neurological disease, with important social, personal, and family repercussions. Narcolepsy is characterized by excessive daytime sleepiness, characterized by short-term recurrent sleep attacks, fragmentation of night sleep, and other REM sleep phenomena, such as cataplexy, sleep paralysis, hypnagogic, and hypnopompic hallucinations. First-degree relatives of narcolepsy patients have a risk of developing drowsiness of central origin about 20–40 times greater than normal individuals in the general population. However, a family pattern for cataplexy alone rarely occurs [13]. Until now, narcolepsy does not have curative treatment. Symptomatic medications are prescribed with the intention of controlling the main symptoms of the disease. Non-pharmacological measures should also be taken with guidance on sleep hygiene, scheduled naps, physical activity, and routine activity regularity [14].

Idiopathic hypersomnia is a sleeping disorder of unknown cause. The diagnosis is defined through neurophysiological evidence of daytime sleepiness, that is, average sleep latency in MLST less than 8 minutes and absence of REM sleep changes. Any other cause of daytime sleepiness should be excluded. Despite being a diagnosis of exclusion, patients with idiopathic hypersomnia have some characteristics that suggest the clinical condition. In general, they are patients with excessive sleepiness with increased total sleep time 24 hours a day. They present permanent sleepiness, different from the sleep attacks characteristic of narcolepsy. Naps of patients with idiopathic hypersomnia are also different from those present in patients with narcolepsy, being generally prolonged, lasting more than 1 hour, and usually not repairing [15]. Another symptom suggestive of idiopathic hypersomnia is sleep inertia. This can be defined as a prolonged difficulty waking up with a frequent return to sleep, irritability, difficulty in performing cognitive tasks, irritability, automatic behavior, and confusion. Autonomic symptoms have been reported, such as orthostatic hypotension, changes in thermal perception, and Raynaud's phenomenon. Treatment must have behavioral and pharmacological approaches. Guidance to family members and the use of stimulants improve the quality of life of these patients.

Kleine-Levin syndrome is a very rare disease, but a classic cause of recurrent hypersomnia, characterized by recurrent-remitting episodes of severe EDS associated with cognitive, psychiatric, and behavioral changes. The duration of the episodes is variable, usually around 10 days, and can last up to 30 days. The episodes have an evident functional impact. Common behavioral symptoms are hyperphagia, hypersexuality, coprolalia, or copropraxia. Patients commonly report a symptom of lack of realization, with difficulty in stating what is real or dream. In the intervals between crises, the patients do not present cognitive or psychiatric symptoms nor sleepiness [16]. There is no specific and effective therapy, and treatment involves medications with different effects. Lithium carbonate and carbamazepine have been used with inconsistent responses to increasing crisis intervals. Usually, there are frequent spontaneous remissions with advancing age.

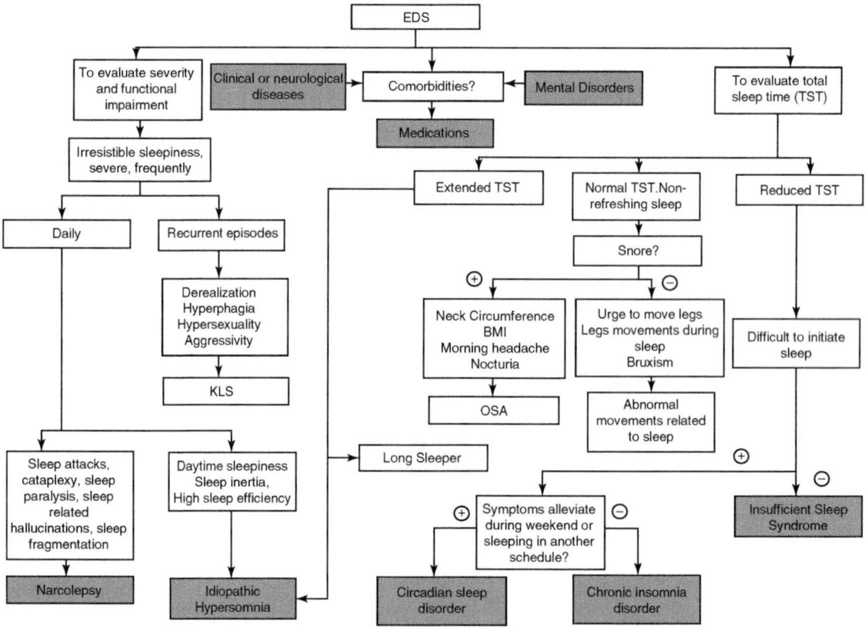

Fig. 1 Proposal for the management of excessive daytime sleepiness and its differential diagnosis. (EDS excessive daytime sleepiness, KLS Kleine-Levin syndrome, TST total sleep time, OSA obstructive sleep apnea)

3 Final Words

Excessive daytime sleepiness is a common sleep complaint, and for its proper management, it is important to understand the groups of causes of hypersomnia to direct the medical interview, the physical and neurological examination, and the complementary investigation. We highlight seven etiological groups to be considered: insufficient sleep syndrome, clinical and neurological diseases, mental disorders, sleep disorders, use of drugs or substances, rhythm disorders, and, more rarely, hypersomnia of central origin (Fig. 1). The treatment of hypersomnia will be directed to its underlying cause, and, in specific cases, when necessary, symptomatic treatment with the use of stimulants may be done.

References

1. Berger M, Hirotsu C, Haba-Rubio J, Betta M, Bernardi G, Siclari F, et al. Risk factors of excessive daytime sleepiness in a prospective population-based cohort. J Sleep Res. 2020;30:e13069.
2. Jaussent I, Morin CM, Ivers H, Dauvilliers Y. Natural history of excessive daytime sleepiness: a population-based 5-year longitudinal study. Sleep. 2020;43(3):e13069.
3. Ng WL, Shaw JE, Peeters A. The relationship between excessive daytime sleepiness, disability, and mortality, and implications for life expectancy. Sleep Med. 2018;43:83–9.
4. Bertolazi AN, Fagondes SC, Hoff LS, Pedro VD, Menna Barreto SS, Johns MW. Portuguese-language version of the Epworth sleepiness scale: validation for use in Brazil. J Bras Pneumol. 2009;35(9):877–83.
5. MacLean AW, Fekken GC, Saskin P, Knowles JB. Psychometric evaluation of the Stanford sleepiness scale. J Sleep Res. 1992;1(1):35–9.
6. Arand DL, Bonnet MH. The multiple sleep latency test. Handb Clin Neurol. 2019;160:393–403.
7. Littner MR, Kushida C, Wise M, Davila DG, Morgenthaler T, Lee-Chiong T, et al. Practice parameters for clinical use of the multiple sleep latency test and the maintenance of wakefulness test. Sleep. 2005;28(1):113–21.
8. American Academy of Sleep Medicine. International classification of sleep disorders. 3rd ed. Darien: American Academy of Sleep Medicine; 2014.
9. Hawley CJ, Gale TM, Sivakumaran T, Paul S, Kondan VR, Farag A, et al. Excessive daytime sleepiness in psychiatric disorders: prevalence, correlates and clinical significance. Psychiatry Res. 2010;175(1–2):138–41.
10. Kayaba M, Sasai-Sakuma T, Inoue Y. Clinical significance of social jetlag in patients with excessive daytime sleepiness. Chronobiol Int. 2018;35(12):1637–46.
11. Slater G, Steier J. Excessive daytime sleepiness in sleep disorders. J Thorac Dis. 2012;4(6):608–16.
12. Dauvilliers Y, Barateau L. Narcolepsy and other central hypersomnias. Continuum (Minneap Minn). 2017;23(4, Sleep Neurology):989–1004.
13. Claudio LA, Bassetti A, Adamantidis D, Burdakov F, Han S, Gay U, Kallweit R, Khatami F, Koning BR, Kornum GJ, Lammers RS, Liblau PH, Luppi G, Mayer T, Pollmächer T, Sakurai F, Sallusto TE, Scammell M, Tafti Y. Dauvilliers Narcolepsy — clinical spectrum aetiopathophysiology diagnosis and treatment. Nature Reviews Neurology 2019;15(9):519–39 https://doi.org/10.1038/s41582-019-0226-9.

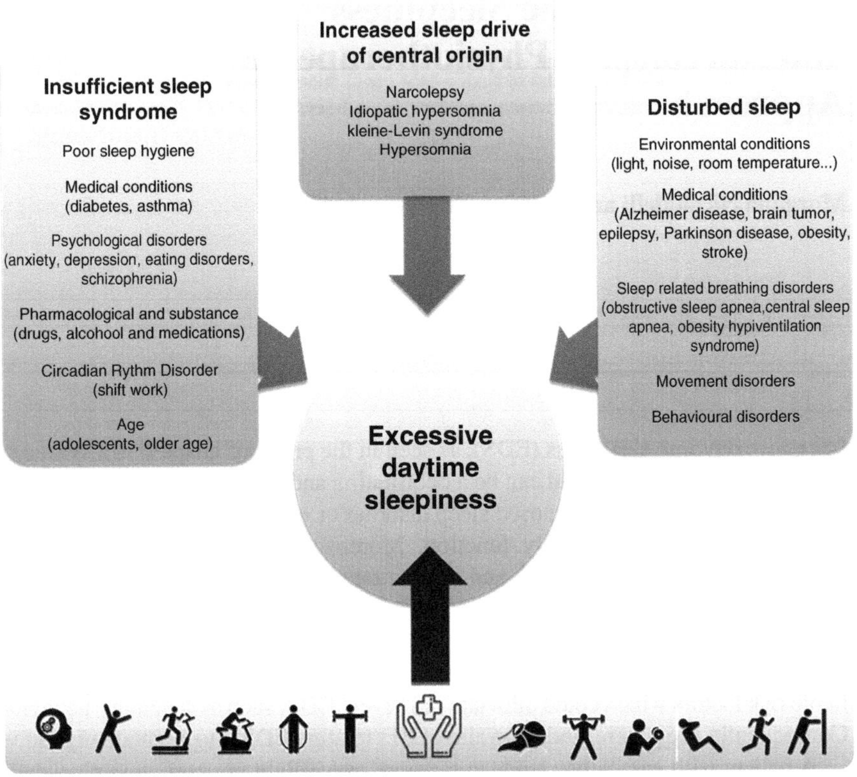

Fig. 1 Excessive daytime sleepiness is a symptom of many diseases and conditions commonly treated by the physical therapist. Physical activity, exercise, and positive airway pressure therapies can act as a countermeasure along with pharmacological treatment

theme, warranting further investigations for both the effectiveness and the mechanisms of physical activity for EDS.

Two epidemiological investigations in general population samples showed that approximately 20–40% of patients with sleep apnea reported EDS with diurnal repercussion [1, 2]. During the PTs initial evaluation of a patient with sleep apnea, there must include an investigation of life habits, sleep perception, pre-bedtime care, stimuli before bed, the sleep environment, and the reporting of the night of sleep. The gathering of this information is quite important for the beginning of treatment, which can also be done using positive airway pressure (PAP) therapy. In clinical practice, many patients do not relate to EDS at the first session, mainly because with daily life, they had not recognized it, because of external stimuli, such as work, movement, use of stimulating beverages, and others that mask the complaint of EDS. It's up to the PT to get to know the EDS, making the patient observe and understand it, in order to treat it. It is important to observe the EDS, as it can affect the predisposition for physical activity and adherence to it. Thus, in addition to the effective treatment with PAP therapy, for the control of obstructive respiratory events and care for the emerging central events that may occur, having the behavioral evaluation of the patient is an important point for the care of the physiotherapy practice. Lack of regular exercise has shown to be a significant predictor for EDS in patients with sleep apnea [3].

1 Exercise and Physical Activity

For EDS exercise might help directly and indirectly. There is no consensus until now on exercise improving EDS neither in an acute (short bout) or chronic (regular) manner. Indirectly, exercise can improve obesity, muscular performance, inflammation, diabetes, metabolic syndrome, and sleep apnea [3, 4], which impact EDS, having it as a symptom.

From observational studies, we know that lack of exercise is associated with increased EDS in children [5, 6], adults [7], and older ones [8, 9]. Lack of exercise has also been known as an independent predictor of EDS in men with sleep apnea, being independent of the degree of apnea [3]. Also, strength training (55 minutes, 3 times a week, for 12 weeks, 3 sets of 10–12 repetitions with a 1-minute rest interval between sets) reduced EDS in adolescents [10].

In addition, evidence on weekly engagement in leisure-time moderate physical activity (e.g., walking) was significantly associated with a 30% lower chance of reporting EDS [11], indicating that a non-sedentary way of life is a choice to prevent many diseases and EDS. The significance of moderate-intensity physical activity cannot be neglected, as moderate-intensity physical activity is associated with numerous health benefits compared with high-intensity physical activity. Nevertheless, for those already engaged in moderate-intensity physical activity, supplementary health benefits may perhaps be achieved with higher intensity and/or duration. One investigation on low-to moderate-intensity physical activity (e.g., tai chi program) performed for 6 months including older adults complaining of sleep demonstrated that tai chi participants reported reduced EDS (assessed by the ESS) compared with controls [12]. With a broad range of age, between 18 and 85 years, another investigation showed that the relative risk of often versus never having EDS decreased by a factor of 0.65 for those meeting physical activity guidelines compared with their counterparts not meeting the guidelines [13]. Taken together evidence points out that meeting physical activity guidelines, including exercise, is of importance for all, and also for sleep and EDS.

The mechanism through which exercise, specifically, improves EDS is not clear and depends on the disease or condition investigated. Regular exercise has anti-inflammatory effects, altering cytokine responses such as C-reactive protein (CRP), tumor necrosis factor-α (TNF-α), and interleukin-6 (IL-6), and in this manner may prevent EDS [14–16]. Another possibility is that exercise improves sleepiness by influencing mood [17]. Furthermore, exercise improves metabolic factors, such as visceral fat and insulin resistance [18, 19], that have been shown to be independently associated with EDS [20, 21].

In patients with sleep apnea, polysomnographic contributing factors of EDS were shorter sleep latency, increased sleep efficiency, and worse nocturnal oxygenation than their counterparts without EDS [22]. In patients with sleep apnea, hypoxemia can be a foremost determinant of EDS. Investigations focused on the possible coexistence of obesity hypoventilation syndrome (OHS), which is a known cause of EDS [23]. The lower nocturnal oxygen saturation and the increased EDS might be due to OHS. Low nocturnal blood oxygen saturation has a fundamental role in EDS, whether or not it is related to OHS [23]. However, EDS is not always associated with low nocturnal blood oxygen saturation in sleep-related breathing disorders, and that other factors are involved. Impaired autonomic cardiac modulation has also been suggested as a mechanism in which it has led to autonomic arousals and might be an additional cause of EDS [24]. Considered together, two independent factors are associated with the pathogenesis of EDS in patients with sleep-disordered breathing: first, a low nocturnal oxygen saturation, probably caused by OHS, and second, an enhanced sympathetic cardiac modulation during the night, probably caused by repeated nocturnal autonomic arousals. In this sense, EDS might be caused by increased sympathetic activity and/or increased nocturnal hypoxemia.

From a clinical standpoint, we suggest that physical activity (including exercise) should be part of the comprehensive clinical assessment of patients with EDS and that regular exercise should be recommended to those patients that are sedentary or have sedentary behavior.

2 Cognitive-behavioral Therapy for Excessive Daytime Sleepiness

Cognitive-behavioral therapy (CBT), discussed in detail in chapter "Optimizing Behavior Strategies for Sleep" of this book, is similarly used in the management of narcolepsy recently. It is proposed that CBT for narcolepsy should have three components:

(i) Behavioral component: begins with specific techniques designed at changing sleep-disordered behaviors or sleep-related disorder variables that are not well-suited (e.g., sleep satisfaction and nap training).
(ii) Cognitive component: intended at modifying beliefs, emotions, and motivations that may play a critical function in maintaining narcolepsy (by this means increasing the frequency of symptoms) and point out the psychosocial effect of the disorder.
(iii) Educational component: instruct the patient about the nature of the disease, the mechanism of pharmacological approach, and precautions regarding the use of medication to accomplish a global awareness of the condition. The acceptance of treatment and the therapeutic relationship becomes important aspects for treatment success, and the use of strategies becomes a type of therapeutic contract [25].

A review on CBT for narcolepsy presents the good effects of the treatment along with pharmacotherapy [25]. Approaches might help with EDS, such as considering having a regular sleep schedule, getting enough sleep during the night according to National

Sleep Foundation Recommendations (see chapter "Normal Sleep: Interindividual Differences and Sleep Variability", Fig. 1), and taking an exercise break to improve alertness. There are behavioral approaches to treat narcolepsy symptoms: (i) structuring nocturnal sleep habits (maintain a regular sleep schedule, avoid changes in sleep time and sleep deprivation, learn relaxation techniques to avoid extreme stimulus before sleep); (ii) planning naps (15- to 20-minute naps after lunch and before 5 PM are highly effective); (iii) diet (avoid caffeine beverages and drinks; healthy eating habits are useful to ensure sleep); (iv) counseling or other assistance (for lifestyle organization, psychotherapy, special considerations at school and work, working during the day) [26].

EDS was one of the variables that determined cardiopulmonary fitness in an investigation with patients with narcolepsy [27]. Cardiopulmonary fitness was inversely related to the degree of sleepiness in patients with narcolepsy type 1or 2. In narcolepsy type 1, cardiopulmonary fitness was also inversely correlated to the number of cataplexy attacks in a month. In addition, the authors found lower cardiopulmonary fitness in patients with narcolepsy compared to the general population [27]. Therefore, one limitation that the authors point out is the fact that the volunteers with narcolepsy of this study were in use of stimulants, which may have influenced the results of cardiopulmonary fitness (prolonging endurance exercise time and reducing the perception of effort, even though the effect of stimulants on cardiovascular function is still controversial). Moreover, the pharmacological state-of-the-art treatment for narcolepsy is the use of stimulants or wake-promoting compounds, and the results were from a treated population of patients with narcolepsy on stable medication. One point that we want to make noticeably clear is the fact that we propose physical therapy as an adjunct therapy for narcolepsy, along with pharmacological treatment.

3 Final Words

Following the possibilities that the physiotherapist can have with the patient with EDS, either by narcolepsy or sleep apnea, more studies are still necessary to prove the evidence of physical activity by itself. Investigations are worth with PAP therapy, its pressure adjustment and relief, control of interface leakage, and thus improvement in sleep fragmentation, as well as its adjuvant orientations, such as sleep hygiene, posture during sleep, and sleep routine, habits and beliefs.

When we score the EDS related to sleep apnea, it is important to remember that in addition to polysomnographic characteristics, the initial clinical evaluation must raise life habits, sleep perception, and behavioral aspects during the day and pre-sleep - all this information may be useful during the evaluation of the evolution of the treatment plan.

References

1. Young T, et al. The occurrence of sleep-disordered breathing among middle-aged adults. N Engl J Med. 1993;328(17):1230–5.

REM sleep parasomnias are more prevalent in the second half of the night, and the chance of spontaneous remission is lower than in NREM sleep parasomnias [3, 4].

1 NREM-Related Parasomnias

1.1 Disorders of Arousal

Confusional arousals are brief episodes of incomplete arousal from sleep, characterized by awakening with mental confusion and often go unnoticed unless reported by the bed partner or parents. It occurs very often in younger children, with almost 2–7% of adults present confusional arousals [5]. Patients don't usually walk out of bed and there is no autonomic arousal (tachycardia, tachypnea, and diaphoresis), and behavior may be inappropriate or actions and responses may be slower than usual. A confusional arousal episode usually lasts up to 5–15 minutes. It is a very common condition in children and usually resolves by the age of 5 years old.

Sleepwalking (somnambulism) consists of a series of complex behaviors that occur during NREM sleep, with evidence of a familial role in the development of sleepwalking. Patients may walk out of bed, with the individual in altered absent consciousness, the eyes are usually open, and may have somniloquy (talking during sleep). In addition to ambulation, the episodes have evidence of persistent sleep, altered consciousness, and impaired judging during ambulation – which can lead to inappropriate behaviors or dangerous ones. Patients are difficult to arouse when sleepwalking. When awakening from such an episode, there are tachycardia, mental confusion, amnesia, and abnormal behaviors. The prevalence varies in children, ranging from 3.5% and 14.5%, and in adults between 0.6% and 34% [6]. Sleepwalking can be calm or agitated, with varying degrees of complexity and duration, and may also be accompanied by sleep terrors.

Sleep terrors (night terrors, *pavor nocturnus*) are sudden arousals from sleep accompanied by loud screams, crying, and the autonomic nervous system and behavioral manifestations of intense fear. There is often intense autonomic discharge (e.g., tachycardia, tachypnea, flushing of the skin, diaphoresis, mydriasis, and increased muscle tone). The patient frequently sits up in bed and does not remember what happened. The sleep terror episode may be accompanied by incoherent vocalizations. Sometimes there is prolonged inconsolability associated with a sleep terror in children or adults. It typically occurs in prepubertal children, diminishes in adolescence, and is uncommon in adulthood [1, 7].

Importantly, a given episode may be a mixture of the mentioned types of disorders of arousal, all of them with confusion during the episode and partial or complete amnesia.

1.2 Sleep-Related Eating Disorder

Recurrent episodes of involuntary eating and drinking during arousals from sleep are called sleep-related eating disorders. They are associated with diminished levels of consciousness and subsequent recall, with problematic consequences. Eating episodes occur involuntarily during partial arousals from sleep with subsequent partial recall. Patients usually don't remember having eaten during the night. This condition can be idiopathic but can be associated with a primary sleep disorder, another clinical condition, or the use of a sedative-hypnotic medication [1].

2 REM-Related Parasomnias

2.1 REM Sleep Behavior Disorder

REM Sleep Behavior Disorder (RBD) is characterized by complex motor activity or vocalization during sleep (i.e., loss of muscle atony during REM sleep) associated with dreaming [1]. *Dream enactment behavior* or *acting out one's dream* is observed when the patient presents motor activity, as "staging, acting" the dream, without suppression or muscle atony [8].

Data on the prevalence of the disease in the population are still scarce and limited since it has a low prevalence and part of the diagnostic criteria requires video polysomnography, which makes the diagnosis expensive and limited. In addition, in many cases, the change is not observed and reported by the patient and/or roommate [9]. For diagnosis, in addition to clinical history, it is necessary to observe, with the video polysomnography the absence of muscle atony during the period of recording REM sleep. In polysomnography (PSG) findings, there are sustained muscle activity in REM sleep on chin electromyography (EMG) and transient muscle activity during REM on chin or limb EMG (Fig. 1).

RBD predominates in males and increases with age. It usually begins in the fifth or sixth decade of life. In younger patients, it may also be related to narcolepsy type 1 and the use of antidepressants. It is also related to the use of alcohol, lower educational levels, depression, anxiety, and posttraumatic stress, among others [10]. An important characteristic of RBD is that it is the greatest prodromal marker of α-synucleinopathies, and it may be present before the development of these diseases. A-synucleinopathies are neurodegenerative diseases in which there is an accumulation of α-synucleins in nerve cells, as Parkinson's disease, Lewi body dementia, and multiple system atrophy [11].

The patient with RBD has a clinical history of complex movements and/or vocalization during the dream, which may include laughing, crying, cursing, singing, clapping, punching, slapping, kicking, gesticulations, and chewing, among others. The movements are often aggressive and can cause physical trauma to the patient and roommate. After waking up, the patient may be alert and able to report the dream, consistent with the motor activity he presented while sleep [1].

RBD can be classified as idiopathic, due to medication or identifiable changes [12], or even secondary, when caused by neurodegenerative diseases, autoimmune diseases, lesions or tumors in the central nervous system, tautopathy associated with anti-IgLON5 antibodies, after stroke, medications (in particular the use of antidepressants) [13], and narcolepsy [14]. RBD has a strong association

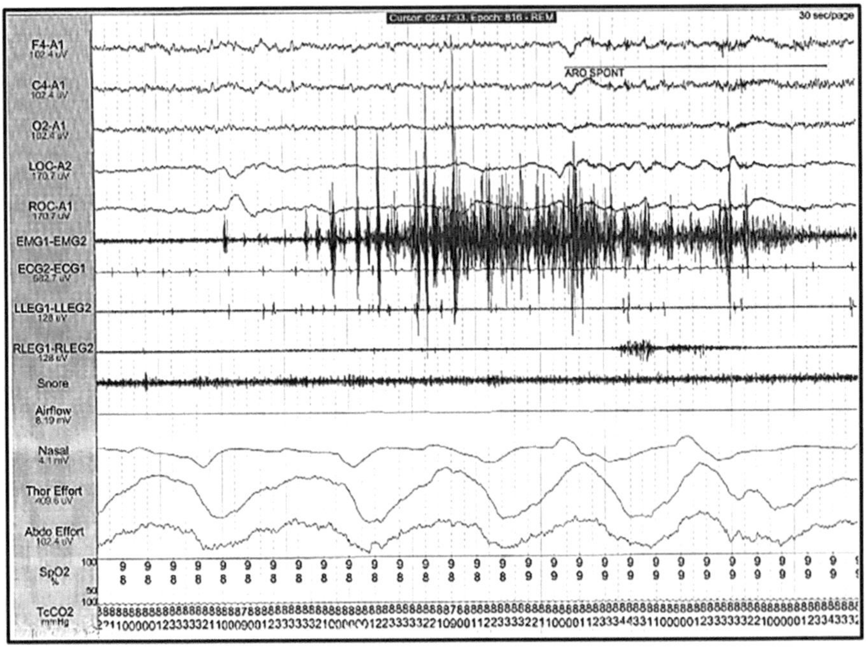

Fig. 1 Thirty-second (epoch) window page of polysomnography showing the loss of muscle atony during REM sleep stage in the arm electromyography (EMG1-EMG2). Note also brief movements in left and right legs (LLEG1-LLEG2 and RLEG1-RLEG2). (Image courtesy from Dr. Fernando Morgadinho Santos Coelho)

with neurodegenerative diseases, and that idiopathic RBD is an important prodromal of α-synucleinopathies. Older patients have a 33% risk of developing a neurodegenerative disease within 5 years, and 91% in 14 years after the onset of RBD [15].

There is no treatment that can prevent the progression to this disease. However, early monitoring and recognition of neurodegenerative disorders can lead to early treatment and monitoring of the patient, and neuroprotective measures, which can be beneficial in the evolution of the disease [16].

2.2 *Recurrent Isolated Sleep Paralysis*

Recurrent sleep paralysis is characterized by an inability to move at sleep onset (hypnogogic) or on awakening (hypnopompic), lasting from a few seconds to minutes. Patients are awake and have full memory of the event. Episodes can cause anxiety and fear of sleep and although the diaphragm is not affected, there may exist a sensation of dyspnea. In sleep paralysis, there is partial memory preservation of the event, and there are no stereotyped movements.

The age of onset of sleep paralysis is variable but is more common in adulthood and middle age. Prevalence can range from 4.7% to 41% of the population

[5], which may have had at least 1 episode during life. Predisposing factors are sleep deprivation, irregular sleep periods, sleep disruption, and stress. Sleep paralysis is common in narcolepsy and idiopathic hypersomnia (and the term *isolated* refers to the absence of these diseases). Treatment is not normally necessary in isolated cases, and sleep hygiene measures are an effective way to control sleep paralysis.

2.3 Nightmare Disorder

Nightmare disorder is characterized by repeated occurrences of extended, dysphoric, and well-remembered dreams. They are disturbing mental experiences that generally occur during REM sleep and that often result in awakening. When awakening the patients quickly are oriented and alerted. Details of the content of nightmares are usually recalled by patients. Patients may also present increased prevalence of mood disorders (persistence of nightmare effect, anxiety, dysphoria), sleep resistance (fear of sleep or subsequent nightmares, bedtime anxiety), cognitive impairment (intrusive nightmare imagery, concentration, impaired memory), behavioral problems (bedtime avoidance, fear of the dark), fatigue, and daytime sleepiness [17].

Nightmares occur in around 60–75% of children. Both sexes are equally affected until adolescence when girls are more affected. In adults, about 2–8% have nightmare disorders (18) being more frequent in psychiatric disorders, including posttraumatic stress disorder, borderline personality, and substance abuse, stress, and anxiety. The posttraumatic stress disorder dreams may occur out of NREM stages N2 and N3, during REM sleep, and at the onset of sleep. Cognitive-behavioral treatments have been used to treat nightmares with success.

3 Final Words

Treatment of parasomnias includes avoiding precipitating factors (e.g., sleep deprivation and medications) environmental precautions and eventually the use of medications to control the presented condition. There is no evidence of physical therapy interventions for these disorders. The treatment of the parasomnias by a physician is important for the reduction of clinical manifestations and protection of the patient and bed partner, yet physiotherapists may refer the patients to a physician in case of suspicious parasomnia.

References

1. International classification of sleep disorders. 3rd ed. Westchester: American Academy of Sleep Medicine, 2014.

Sleep-Wake Disturbances in Childhood and Adolescence

Giuliano da Paz Oliveira and Marcia Pradella-Hallinan

Adequate sleep is essential for the child's growth, development, learning and well-being. Insufficient and/or poor-quality sleep are associated with increased occurrence of mood disorders, behavioral disorders, and learning difficulties due to inattention. Similarly, untreated sleep apnea in childhood is associated with increased irritability, inattention, emotional dysregulation, unsatisfactory academic performance, impairment of growth. Although more rarely, systemic arterial hypertension and pulmonary hypertension can also be related to some sleep-related breathing disorders [1–3].

Sleep disorders are very common in the pediatric population, with a worldwide prevalence ranging from 20 to 40% [4–6]. A Brazilian study using validated child sleep questionnaires estimated an alarming prevalence of sleep disorders of 25.5% among individuals aged 0–19 years [7]. It is also noteworthy that sleep habits of the child are very rarely approached by health-care professionals in order to identify, prevent and treat possible sleep disorders [8].

The American Academy of Sleep Disorders (AASM) developed a consensus published in 2016 with the amount of sleep needed to promote health among children and adolescents, according to each age group [Table 1]. Infants aged less than 4 months were not included in this consensus due to the great variation of normality regarding duration and sleep patterns [9].

G. da Paz Oliveira (✉)
Universidade Federal do Delta do Parnaíba and Instituto de Educação Superior do Vale do Parnaíba, Parnaíba, Piauí, Brazil

Neurology and Neurosurgery Department, Escola Paulista de Medicina Universidade Federal de São Paulo, São Paulo, SP, Brazil

M. Pradella-Hallinan
Treatment Center for Neuromuscular Diseases (TDN-AFIP) and Sleep Medicine Lab of Sirio Libanês Hospital, São Paulo, SP, Brazil

C. Frange, F. M. S. Coelho (eds.), *Sleep Medicine and Physical Therapy*,
https://doi.org/10.1007/978-3-030-85074-6_24

Table 1 Recommendation of AASM consensus (2016) on total sleep time according to each age group in children and adolescents

Age	Total sleep time
4–12 months	12–16 hours (including naps)
1–2 years	11–14 hours (including naps)
3–5 years	10–13 hours (including naps)
6–12 years old	9–12 hours
13–18 years old	8–10 hours

Table 2 Characteristics of sleep biology and ontogenesis according to each age group of childhood and adolescence

Age	Characteristics of sleep
0–6 months	Categories: awake, quiet sleep, active sleep and indeterminate sleep (transitional sleep) At 6 months, begins to consolidate the night sleep Initiates sleep by REM. REM sleep represents 50–60% of total sleep time
6 months–2 years	One or two daytime naps Starts sleep by NREM. REM sleep represents 25–30% of total sleep time
2–6 years	Transition from two naps to one. Nap usually disappears after 5 years. REM sleep is concentrated in the second half of the night
6–12 years	No naps, 9–12 hours of night sleep
12–18 years	Delayed sleep phase syndrome is common during teenage years

1 Sleep States from Newborn to Adolescent

The characterization of the sleep patterns is based mainly on the electroencephalographic tracings and behavioral characteristics [Table 2].

Up to 6 months of life, the child's states of consciousness are classified into 4 categories: awake, quiet sleep, active sleep and indeterminate sleep (transitional sleep) and indeterminate sleep (transitional sleep). The newborn falls asleep in REM sleep and remains in this state of sleep for about 60% of the total sleep time. This percentage can reach 80% preterm neonates.

Around 6 months the baby comes to sleep up to 6 hours uninterrupted, a period in which the longest night sleep begins to consolidate. Still in this phase, infant initiates the sleep cycle in NREM sleep, which is the predominant phase (70–75% of the total sleep time).

Between 2 and 5 years old, the child usually sleeps between 10 and 14 hours a day, with only one nap during afternoon, which usually disappears around 5 years old. In this phase, a predominance of REM sleep occurs in the second half of the night, as observed in adults.

Adolescents after 12 years of age begin to present a typical alteration called delayed sleep phase syndrome, that is characterized by difficulty in falling asleep at a socially acceptable time and by the need to wake up later. Depending on the social demand (e.g., going to school in the morning), this factor can contribute to the occurrence of sleep deprivation and its consequences [10–12].

2 Sleep-Related Breathing Disorders

2.1 Obstructive Sleep Apnea in the Pediatric Population

In the pediatric population, the peak incidence of obstructive sleep apnea (OSA) occurs in preschoolers, a period in which there is an imbalance between the growth of palatine tonsils and adenoid, concerning the growth of the upper airway, that allied to the physiology of sleep/muscle relaxation favors the occurrence of obstructive respiratory events [13, 14].

Unlike the adult, the diagnosis of sleep apnea in the child requires the presence of an apnea index (AHI) greater than 1 event per hour of sleep, often accompanied by multiple awakenings and oxyhemoglobin desaturation. The following table summarizes the indications of polysomnography (PSG) in the pediatric age group [Chart 1] [13].

Adenotonsillectomy is the most widely used treatment for children with OSA. In cases of moderate or severe OSA in which adenotonsillectomy did not show satisfactory results or was contraindicated, the use of continuous positive airway pressure (CPAP) devices should be considered. The greatest limitation of the use of CPAP in children is the low adherence. Also, the chronic use of these devices can lead to facial deformities due to the pressure of the mask on the facial bones. Care with choosing the best mask can minimize these effects [14, 15].

The treatment of the child's OSA should always be multidisciplinary. It is known that about 20% of the children submitted to adenotonsillectomy continue with residual apnea resulting, in its great majority, of the alteration in the relation between the maxilla and mandible, of dental malocclusion. Several studies show the benefit of the use of orthodontic devices and the palatal circuit breakers that make the maxilla

Chart 1 Main indications of PSG in childhood and adolescence. Presence of two or more of the following criteria:

Snoring for at least 4 nights a week associated with restless sleep, frequent awakenings, hyperactive, aggressive, or impulsive behavior, learning difficulties, enuresis, malnutrition, recurrent upper airways infections
Apnea observed by the family
Excessive daytime sleepiness
Laborious breathing during sleep
Polycythemia
Cor pulmonale
Patient will perform any elective surgery and presents suggestive OSA symptoms
Some genetic syndromes and craniofacial malformations

3.2 *Non-pharmacological Treatment of Childhood Insomnia*

The institution of drug treatment aims mainly to interfere in the long period of insomnia to facilitate the performance of behavioral work. Another indication is the presence of neurological, psychiatric, and child comorbidities with marked visual impairment. Melatonin is indicated and mainly used in children with autism spectrum disorders, with global developmental delays and in blind children. Melatonin reduces sleep latency and wake-up frequency and should be ingested 1 to 2 hours before bedtime. Antihistamines such as diphenhydramine, promethazine, and hydroxyzine promote blocking of H1 histaminergic receptors by reducing sleep latency and awakening due to sedation. Benzodiazepine hypnotic drugs (such as clonazepam) act as gamma-aminobutyric acid (GABA) receptor agonists, reducing sleep latency. The effect of muscle relaxation associated with this drug should be considered, especially in the suspicion of sleep-related breathing disorders [30, 31].

4 Sleep-Related Movement Disorders

4.1 *Restless Legs Syndrome (RLS)*

Restless legs syndrome (RLS) is a sensorimotor disorder that affects the sleep and quality of life of the child or adolescent. The affected child describes its symptom as an irresistible need to move the legs, usually accompanied by discomfort, unpleasant feeling, and/or restlessness [32–34].

The clinical course is variable, moderate to severe forms can behave as chronic and progressive. Difficulty in initiating and/or maintaining sleep, feeling that you have not slept enough, tiredness, and weakness are common complaints in children with RLS. Positive family history and the presence of periodic limb movements of the members (identified in PSG) are considered support criteria for RLS, according ICSD-3 [33, 34].

The diagnosis of RLS in the pediatric population, as it occurs among adults, is eminently clinical, as shown below [Chart 2]. If the child cannot describe their discomfort, it must have at least two of these criteria: sleep disorder, a first-degree family member with a diagnosis of RLS and periodic limb movement index (PLMDi) >5/h in polysomnography [13].

Should always be requested. Several studies show an association of RLS symptoms with a ferritin dosage of less than 50 mcg/L and that iron supplementation surprisingly improves symptoms. In addition to iron supplementation in severe RLS, other drugs can be used such as gabapentin, benzodiazepines such as clonazepam and temazepam, clonidine, dopaminergic agonists and *H. perforatum* [33, 34].

Chart 2 Diagnostic criteria for restless legs syndrome (ICSD-3) [13]

Need to move the legs, caused by an unpleasant sensation
Unpleasant feeling worsens in rest periods
Unpleasant feeling is totally or partially relieved by movement
Need for movement and the feeling of discomfort are worse at night
Symptoms cannot be explained by other medical conditions
Report of the child himself describing with his words the unpleasant sensation and/or discomfort in the legs

We did not find studies of the use of physiotherapy techniques for the treatment of RLS; however, as personal experience of the authors it is worth mentioning that the caregivers refer that vigorous massage on the legs and even the placing of cushions or heavy covers on them helps in the conciliation of sleep [33, 34].

4.2 *Periodic Limb Movement Disorder (PLMD)*

PLMD is characterized by repetitive, intermittent, and stereotyped movements that most frequently affect the lower limbs. Often the caregivers complain that the child has restless sleep or drops the covers or kicks, while sleeping. This complaint, to be relevant, should be associated with symptoms associated with nonrestorative sleep such as behavior and/or mood changes and learning difficulties, among others. For the diagnosis, we should request a PSG where muscle movements/contractions will be counted with a duration of 0.5 to 10 seconds and with an increase of the tibial electromyogram of at least 8 mV. A 5/h periodic movement index is considered significant. Likely RLS, blood tests may be necessary to evaluate iron metabolism and its supplementation (when indicated) may improve the symptoms [32–34].

4.3 *Restless Sleep Disorder in Children*

In 2020 a new sleep-related movement disorder was described. It refers to the complaint of restless sleep reported by parents or caregivers and was studied in the pediatric age group, between 6 and 18 years of age. For the diagnosis, all criteria defined by consensus must be present [Chart 3].

The authors found serum ferritin rates even lower than those observed in patients with IPS, but this was reported in oral communication (not yet published). Again, we must emphasize the importance of analyzing the iron profile in these patients.

Chart 3 Diagnostic criteria for child agitated sleep disorder [35]

Complaint of restless sleep
Observed large body movements during sleep (movements should comprise large muscle groups of the whole body, of the four limbs, arms, legs, or head)
Movements occur during sleep or when the child appears to be sleeping
Video-polysomnographic documentation of 5 or more large body movements/hour
Occurrence at least three times a week for at least three months
Restless sleep is associated with daytime behavioral/mood/cognitive complaints
Restless sleep cannot be caused by a clinical or psychiatric or environmental condition or other sleep disorder

4.4 Sleep Bruxism

Sleep bruxism is a rhythmic, involuntary movement of tightening and/or friction of teeth during sleep, associated with repeated contractions of the masseter, temporal, medial and lateral pterygoid muscles, that may or may not produce noises [13].

Polysomnographic studies showed that episodes predominate in NREM sleep. As a result of muscular effort, headache, mandibular pain, tooth wear, pain in the temporal-mandibular joint, and even limitation of mandibular movement may occur. The annual incidence of some episodes of bruxism is 15%, for the age10 group of 20 years, the most affected. Children with intellectual disability, ASD and cerebral palsy have a higher incidence [34].

Bruxism can occur in situations of stress and anxiety or association with other sleep disorders such as snoring, obstructive sleep apnea, RLS, PLMD movements and epilepsy associated with sleep. The diagnosis is clinical, but the PSG exam may be requested to confirm the diagnosis and also evaluate the occurrence of other sleep disorders [33, 34].

Dental evaluation is always recommended because it may be necessary to treat tooth wear, or its prevention, with the placement of resin protection or use of intra-oral devices in children with established permanent dentition [33, 34].

Pharmacological treatment may be used in cases with dental impairment and/or clinical symptoms. Children with severe encephalopathies and sleep bruxism can also benefit from pharmacological management. The medications used are mainly benzodiazepines (clonazepam) and alpha-agonists (clonidine) in low doses [33, 34].

5 Child Neurology and Sleep Medicine Interface

5.1 Cerebral Palsy (CP)

CP is a chronic motor condition secondary to nonprogressive brain damage in a brain during its development [36]. The worldwide prevalence of CP is 2.11 per 1000 live births and obeys an inverse proportion to gestational age and birth weight [37]. The prevalence of sleep disorders in children with CP varies from 23 to 46%. Some variables can influence these high rates, such as: greater occurrence of pain, epileptic seizures, impaired mobility [38, 39]. The presence of sleep disorders impairs cognitive and emotional development of these children and impacting their physical rehabilitation [38].

Horwood et al. observed that the presence of untreated pain was a strong predictor for abnormal scores in the pediatric sleep scale among children with CP, with an odds ratio of 6.5 [39]. The non-pharmacological approach to pain with physical therapy may be an interesting path for the treatment and prevention of sleep disorders in patients with CP, but there are still no studies proving the effectiveness of this type of intervention. A randomized controlled clinical trial involving 142 children diagnosed with CP found that the Cranial Osteopathy technique did not promote sustained improvement in motor function, quality of sleep, and life [40].

5.2 *Autistic Spectrum Disorder*

Autism Spectrum Disorder (ASD) is a neurodevelopmental disorder characterized by impairment of communication and social skills associated with repetitive behaviors. The prevalence of ASD can reach 1 per 59 individuals [41]. 50 to 80% of children with ASD have problems initiating and/or maintaining sleep, and the occurrence of sleep disorders may contribute to the worsening of behavior problems [42].

Preschoolers and schoolers with ASD have a higher prevalence of behavioral insomnia and parasomnia, while adolescents with ASD have a higher occurrence of short-term sleep and excessive daytime sleepiness. Several reasons are proposed to justify the higher prevalence of sleep disorders in this group of children: alteration of endogenous melatonin synthesis, sleep neurotransmitter system dysfunction, sensory dysregulation, gene mutations related to rhythm disorders and also the increased occurrence of comorbidities (epilepsy, attention deficit hyperactivity disorder, anxiety, and mood disorders) [43, 44].

Several systematic reviews have already been carried out to evaluate the effectiveness of pharmacological and non-pharmacological treatments to approach sleep disorders in children with ASD. Unfortunately, the findings were inconclusive and often controversial. It is a clearly heterogeneous group of patients with different clinical picture and comorbidities [45].

The most evident therapeutic modalities in this context were melatonin use (0.75 to 10 mg/day), behavioral intervention (e.g., sleep hygiene, extinction, positive reinforcement, and sleep restriction), and parental education [45]. A study identified that parental massage therapy reduced the occurrence of sleep disorders in ASD patients. Although promising, this study used a sample of only 20 children; therefore it still lacks replication of its results [46]. Therefore, the role of the professional physiotherapist in parental education seems to be an effective option of intervention.

Table 4 Guidance on breath-stacking technique [21]

Position the patient in a seated position
Accommodate the bag valve mask around the patient's nose and mouth
Press the mask firmly (pressure upwards) so that no air escapes
Inflate bag valve mask as many times as necessary to fill the patient's entire lung (usually two to five breaths are required)
After stacking as many bag valve mask inflations as possible, quickly remove the mask, and encourage the patient to hold that amount of air for 6 seconds
In case of flu or pulmonary secretion, help the patient in the expiration (assisted cough that is performed with chest pressure during expiration)
Insist on assisted coughing as often as necessary until the patient can eliminate all lung secretion
Exercise as many times as necessary during the day, that is, every time the patient has secretion and cannot cough without help

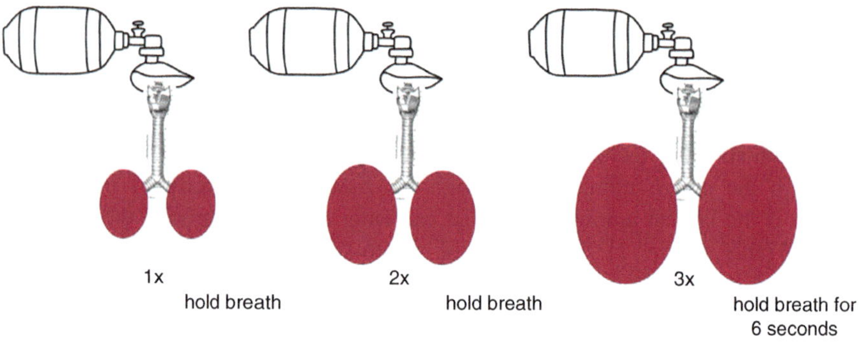

Fig. 1 Schematic drawing on breath-stacking using bag valve mask [21]

References

1. Beebe DW. Neurobehavioral morbidity associated with disordered breathing during sleep in children: a comprehensive review. Sleep. 2006;29(9):1115–34.
2. Carter KA, Hathaway NE, Lettieri CF. Common sleep disorders in children. Am Fam Physician. 2014;89(5):368–77.
3. Chervin RD, et al. Sleep-disordered breathing, behavior, and cognition in children before and after adenotonsillectomy. Pediatrics. 2006;117(4):e769–78.
4. Owens J. Classification and epidemiology of childhood sleep disorders. Prim Care. 2008;35(3):533–46, vii
5. Romeo DM, et al. Application of the sleep disturbance scale for children (SDSC) in preschool age. Eur J Paediatr Neurol. 2013;17(4):374–82.
6. Simola P, et al. Sleep problems and daytime tiredness in Finnish preschool-aged children-a community survey. Child Care Health Dev. 2010;36(6):805–11.
7. Almeida GMF, Nunes ML. Sleep characteristics in Brazilian children and adolescents: a population-based study. Sleep Med. 2019;1:1–7.
8. Honaker SM, Meltzer LJ. Sleep in pediatric primary care: a review of the literature. Sleep Med Rev. 2016;25:31–9.
9. Paruthi S, et al. Recommended amount of sleep for pediatric populations: a consensus statement of the American Academy of sleep medicine. J Clin Sleep Med. 2016;12(6):785–6.

10. Canani S, Silva FA. Sleep evolution from fetal life to adulthood: respiratory and neurologic aspects. J Pediatr. 1998;74(5):357–64.
11. Geib LT. Develpment of sleep stages in childhood. Rev Bras Enferm. 2007;60(3):323–6.
12. Iglowstein I, et al. Sleep duration from infancy to adolescence: reference values and generational trends. Pediatrics. 2003;111(2):302–7.
13. American Academy of Sleep Medicine. International classification of sleep disorders. 3rd ed. Darrien: Diagnostic and coding manual (ICSD-3); 2014.
14. Tan HL, Gozal D, Kheirandish-Gozal L. Obstructive sleep apnea in children: a critical update. Nat Sci Sleep. 2013;5:109–23.
15. Kaditis AG, Alonso Alvarez ML, Boudewyns A, Alexopoulos EI, Ersu R, Joosten K, et al. Obstructive sleep disordered breathing in 2- to 18 year-old children: diagnosis and management. Eur Respir J. 2016;47:69–94.
16. Barbisan BN. Ronco e apnéia obstrutiva do sono. In: Medicina do Sono – atualizações pediátricas. Coord. Beatriz Neuhaus Barbisan, Cristiane Fumo dos Santos, Emiliana Holzhausen Gonçalves da Motta. 1ª ed. Rio de Janeiro: Atheneu; 2019. p. 97–104.
17. Santos CF, Diaferia G, Juliano ML. Apneia obstrutiva do sono:tratamento. In: Medicina do Sono – atualizações pediátricas. Coord. Beatriz Neuhaus Barbisan, Cristiane Fumo dos Santos, Emiliana Holzhausen Gonçalves da Motta, 1ª. Ed, Atheneu, Rio de Janeiro, 2019; pg 105–111.
18. Carvalho GD. Atitudes posturais do Respirador Bucal. In: S.O.S. Respirador Bucal, editor. Uma visão functional e clínica da amamentação. São Paulo: Editora Lovise Ltda; 2003. p. 145–59.
19. Arens R, Muzumdar H. Sleep, sleep disordered breathing, and nocturnal hypoventilation in children with neuromuscular diseases. Paediatr Respir Rev. 2010;11:24–30.
20. Berry RB, Chediak A, Brown LK, Finder J, Gozal D, Iber C, et al. Best clinical practices for the sleep center adjustment of noninvasive positive pressure ventilation (NPPV) in stable chronic alveolar hypoventilation syndromes. J Clin Sleep Med. 2010;6:491–509.
21. Ferraz EC, Grossklaus LF, Akamine RT, Moreira GA, Pradella-Hallinan M. Folheto institucional de orientação aos pacientes portadores de Doenças Neuromusculares tratados na TDN-AFIP, São Paulo, 2017.
22. Owens JA, Mindell JA. Pediatric Insomnia. Pediatr Clin N Am. 2011;58(3):555–69.
23. Mindell JA, Owens JA. A clinical guide to pediatric sleep: diagnosis and management of sleep problems. Philadelphia: Lippincott Williams & Wilkins; 2003. p. 156–62.
24. Meltzer LJ, Mindell JA. Behavioral sleep disorders in children and adolescents. Sleep Med Clin. 2008;3:269–79.
25. Pradella-Hallinan M, Alves RSC. Meu filho não dorme – insônia comportamental. In: Medicina do Sono – atualizações pediátricas. Coord. Beatriz Neuhaus Barbisan, Cristiane Fumo dos Santos, Emiliana Holzhausen Gonçalves da Motta, 1ª. Ed, Atheneu, Rio de Janeiro, pg 27–33, 2019.
26. Arboledas GP. Insomnia in children and adolescentes. A consensus document. Anales de Pediatría (Barcelona). 2017;86(3):165.e1–165.e11.
27. Alves RC, Pradella-Hallinan M, Sander HH, Almeida LA. Insônia na Infância In: Insônia: do diagnóstico ao tratamento. Coord. Andrea Bacelar e Luciano Ribeiro Pinto Jr. Difusão Editora, São Caetano do Sul, São Paulo, pp 141–158, 2019.
28. Nunes ML, Bruni O. Insomnia in childhood and adolescence: clinical aspects, diagnosis, and therapeutic approach. Jornal de Pediatria (Rio J). 2015;91(6 Suppl 1):S26–35.
29. Halal CSE, Nunes ML. Education in children's sleep hygiene: which approaches are effective? A systematic review. J Pediatr. 2014;90:449–56.
30. Dosman C, Witmans M, Zwaigenbaum L. Iron's role in paediatric restless legs syndrome - a review. Paediatr Child Health. 2012;17(4):193–7.
31. Economou NT, Ferini-Strambi L. Sleep-related drug therapy in special conditions: children. Sleep Med Clin. 2018;13:251–62.
32. Walters AS. Simple sleep related movement disorders of childhood including benign sleep myoclonus of infancy, rhythmic movement disorder, and childhood restless legs syndrome and periodic limb movements in sleep. Sleep Med Clin. 2007;2:419–32.

33. Pereira JrJC, Pradella-Hallinan M, Alves RSC. Distúrbios dos movimentos relacionados ao sono. In: Pessoa JH, Pereira JrJC, Alves RS, editores. Disturbios do sono na criança e no adolescente. 2nd ed. São Paulo: Atheneu; 2015.p 169–188.
34. Pereira JJC, Alves RSC, Pradella-Hallinan M. Distúrbios dos movimentos relacionados ao sono. In: Medicina do Sono – atualizações pediátricas. Coord. Beatriz Neuhaus Barbisan, Cristiane Fumo dos Santos, Emiliana Holzhausen Gonçalves da Motta. 1ª ed. Rio de Janeiro: Atheneu; 2019. p. 69–75.
35. DelRosso LM, Ferri R, Allen RP, Bruni O, Garcia-Borreguero D, Kotagal S, Owens JÁ, Peirano P, Simakajornboon N. Consensus diagnostic criteria for a newly defined pediatric sleep disorder: restless sleep disorder (RSD). Sleep Med. 2020;75:335–40.
36. Jan MM. Cerebral palsy: comprehensive review and update. Ann Saudi Med. 2006;26(2):123–32.
37. Oskoui M, et al. An update on the prevalence of cerebral palsy: a systematic review and meta-analysis. Dev Med Child Neurol. 2013;55(6):509–19.
38. Dutt R, Roduta-Roberts M, Brown CA. Sleep and children with cerebral palsy: a review of current evidence and environmental non-pharmacological interventions. Children (Basel). 2015;2(1):78–88.
39. Horwood L, et al. Prevalence of sleep problems and sleep-related characteristics in preschool- and school-aged children with cerebral palsy. Sleep Med. 2018;50:1–6.
40. Wyatt K, et al. Cranial osteopathy for children with cerebral palsy: a randomised controlled trial. Arch Dis Child. 2011;96(6):505–12.
41. Baio J, et al. Prevalence of autism spectrum disorder among children aged 8 years - autism and developmental disabilities monitoring network, 11 sites, United States, 2014. MMWR Surveill Summ. 2018;67(6):1–23.
42. Malow BA, et al. A practice pathway for the identification, evaluation, and management of insomnia in children and adolescents with autism spectrum disorders. Pediatrics. 2012;130(Suppl 2):S106–24.
43. Hyman SL, et al. Identification, evaluation, and management of children with autism spectrum disorder. Pediatrics. 2020;145(1):e20193447.
44. Souders MC, et al. Sleep in children with autism spectrum disorder. Curr Psychiatry Rep. 2017;19(6):34.
45. Cuomo BM, et al. Effectiveness of sleep-based interventions for children with autism spectrum disorder: a meta-synthesis. Pharmacotherapy. 2017;37(5):555–78.
46. Escalona A, et al. Brief report: improvements in the behavior of children with autism following massage therapy. J Autism Dev Disord. 2001;31(5):513–6.
47. Diaz-Roman A, Hita-Yanez E, Buela-Casal G. Sleep characteristics in children with attention deficit hyperactivity disorder: systematic review and meta-analyses. J Clin Sleep Med. 2016;12(5):747–56.
48. Tsai MH, Hsu JF, Huang YS. Sleep problems in children with attention deficit/hyperactivity disorder: current status of knowledge and appropriate management. Curr Psychiatry Rep. 2016;18(8):76.
49. Nozoe KT, Moreira GA, Tolino JR, Pradella-Hallinan M, Tufik S, Andersen ML. The sleep characteristics in symptomatic patients with Duchenne muscular dystrophy. Sleep Breath. 2015;19:1051–6.
50. Moreira GA. Hipoventilação e ventilação não invasiva. In: Medicina do Sono – atualizações pediátricas. Coord. Beatriz Neuhaus Barbisan, Cristiane Fumo dos Santos, Emiliana Holzhausen Gonçalves da Motta. 1ª ed. Rio de Janeiro: Atheneu; 2019. p. 119–28.
51. Berry RB, Chediak A, Brown LK, et al. Best clinical practices for the sleep center adjustment of non invasive positive pressure ventilation (NPPV) in stable chronic alveolar hypoventilation syndromes. J Clin Sleep Med. 2010;6:491–509.

Sleep and Aging

Ligia Mendonça Lucchesi and Ronaldo Delmonte Piovezan

Life expectancy increased by 30 years from the beginning to the end of the twentieth century worldwide and was one of the greatest social achievements of the last century, with longevity becoming the norm for most people. One of the greatest challenges of the twenty-first century will be to guarantee the quality of life of the two billion people aged over 60 who the World Health Organization (WHO) forecast to be alive in 2050, with more than 80% of them living in developing countries [1]. One of the most important factors that will determine the quality of life of this population will be sleep and its disorders, which currently affect about 50% of the population aged 60 and above and two-thirds of those who live in nursing homes [2].

Sleep undergoes a continuous process of change from birth throughout life, a process that is called sleep ontogenesis. However, studies on the changes in the need for sleep over the lifetime have not shown clear and consistent results. The changes observed during adulthood impact both the quantity and quality of sleep, as well as the distribution of each sleep stage and phase during the night. Thus, further studies on sleep ontogenesis are still required to elucidate how changes in the central nervous system (CNS) during the aging process affect sleep. These studies will also need to provide information on the social, physiological, and public health aspects, relevant to maintaining a healthy aging population.

When analyzing sleep changes throughout life, the main difficulty is to establish which changes are the consequences of normal aging, and which are due to the greater morbidity of some older subjects [3]. In fact, if we exclude the influence of pathologies, sleep should be quite similar across different age groups during adult life [4, 5]. Nevertheless, as people get older, it becomes more difficult to find individuals without any kind of disease. It is, therefore, unrealistic to aim for older adults to continue to have the same sleep patterns they did when they were younger, as the majority of individuals do not age optimally, that is, without any health

L. M. Lucchesi (✉) · R. D. Piovezan
Sleep Institute, Associação Fundo Incentivo à Pesquisa, São Paulo, SP, Brazil

C. Frange, F. M. S. Coelho (eds.), *Sleep Medicine and Physical Therapy*,
https://doi.org/10.1007/978-3-030-85074-6_25

Moreover, men and women showed similar trends, but with different effect sizes. The reduction in the percentage of REM sleep significantly correlated with age in women, whereas the reduction in the percentage of SWS correlated with age in men. The periodic limb movement (PLM) index increased with age in both genders [10].

1 Impact of Sleep on Morbidity and Mortality of Older Adults

In advanced age, indicators of good sleep also can positively affect markers of cardiovascular risk. A study carried out with older adults (over 85 years old) showed that regular sleep patterns, maintenance of SWS, and a favorable lipid profile are important in respect of longevity in humans [11]. This study pointed out the importance of a strictly regular sleep pattern in both young (20–30 years) and older (60–70 years) groups. The same study also found that some older individuals showed high levels of adaptation to the age-related effects of sleep. Taken together, these results indicate the importance of sleep not only for the quality of life but also in respect of human longevity [11].

Another study investigated the association of sleep duration with the risk of all-cause mortality among older Brazilians using data from a 9-year population-based cohort study, the Bambui Health and Aging Study, undertaken in southeastern Brazil. In the multivariate analysis, using sleep duration as a categorical variable and controlling for various sociodemographic and health status measures, those who slept 9 hours or more per night had a higher risk of mortality than those who slept 7 hours (risk ratio (RR), 1.53; 95% confidence interval (95% CI), 1.12–2.09). This study highlights the fact that it is not only short sleep duration that should be considered to have possible negative outcomes [12].

On the other hand, a study in a Japanese community that associated the risk of mortality and dementia with sleep duration showed that the incidence rates of dementia and mortality from all causes (adjusted for age and sex) were significantly higher in individuals who slept less than 5.0 hours or more than 10.0 hours per day [13].

In a meta-analysis carried out with 27 cohort studies comprising 70,000 older people with follow-ups between 3.4 and 35 years, short- and long-term sleep was associated with increased all-cause mortality (RR, 1.33; 95% CI, 1.24–1.43, and RR, 1.07; 95% CI, 1.03–1.11, respectively), compared with the reference category. For cardiovascular mortality, the pooled relative risks grouped were 1.43 (95% CI: 1.15–1.78) for a long sleep and 1.18 (95% CI: 0.76–1.84) for a short sleep. Daytime napping ($\geq$30 min) was associated with the risk of all-cause mortality (RR, 1.27; 95% CI, 1.08–1.49), compared with no daytime sleep [14].

2 Sleep Characteristics in Older Adults

2.1 Sleep Complaints

Older adults suffer from a range of sleep complaints [8], with women tending to report more than men. The symptoms most commonly related to aging are waking up too early, interrupted or very light sleep, increased periods of wakefulness during the night, and reduced total sleep time. As a result of the poor-quality sleep, there are also complaints of non-restorative sleep, waking up tired, and excessive daytime sleepiness [15].

The frequent interruption of sleep can be the result of an age-dependent change in sleep homeostasis and/or in the maintenance of wakefulness. Awakenings are often more frequent and more prolonged, lasting more than 30 minutes [7]. Older adults tend to characterize sleep as lighter and more fragile than young adults, and there may be greater responsiveness to environmental and other stimuli during sleep that previously did not lead to awakenings [7]. In respect of gender, older women have less fragmented objective-measured sleep than men; however, they are more likely to have subjective sleep problems [8].

2.2 Circadian Rhythm Changes with Aging

Age-related disorders of the sleep-wake cycle are part of complex chronobiological changes in physiological systems that accompany the aging process [8]. Changes in circadian body temperature control and the sleep-wake cycle [10] are probably associated with brain modifications including atrophy of the suprachiasmatic hypothalamic nucleus [5]. Body temperature circadian rhythmicity in aged individuals has reduced amplitude and an advanced phase in comparison to young adults [16, 17]. Although demonstrating greater flexibility than younger subjects to sleep deprivation, older subjects show less tolerance to changes in work shift patterns, a fact that may be related to both social factors and their lower homeostatic capacity [16].

Additionally, the reduction in nocturnal melatonin secretion that takes place in older adults can result in a disruption in circadian rhythm, particularly in relation to phase advancement, which is linked to a less pronounced, but an earlier, decline in body temperature in the evening, as well as an earlier increase in the morning. This can result in less time in bed, less total sleep time, and, therefore, greater daytime sleepiness [8].

2.3 Excessive Daytime Sleepiness and Naps

Excessive daytime sleepiness (EDS) directly impacts the quality of life in older adults and should not be part of normal aging. Epidemiological research has shown that older people without sleep disorders do not have EDS [15]. Daytime sleepiness in older individuals is a common consequence of a number of sleep disorders, as well as neurological and respiratory problems [5, 15]. Although some controversy remains as to whether regular napping in older adults is healthy, it has been reported to have a negative impact on the night-time sleep quality of older people without sleep disorders [18]. However, the question remains whether napping may be a favorable compensating behavior in chronic insomniacs [4].

3 Etiological Factors

Sleep complaints and sleep disorders are frequently persistent and multifactorial in origin older patients. In addition to age-related physiological changes in circadian rhythm and sleep homeostasis, other risk factors in relation to sleep impairment can be classified as follows: (a) medical and psychiatric comorbidities, such as cardiovascular disease, arthritis, gastroesophageal reflux, depression, and the medications used to treat them; (b) social, environmental, and behavioral factors, which can compromise an individual's quality of sleep; (c) primary sleep disorders that can affect mainly the older; and (d) a combination of the factors above mentioned [6, 18].

4 Main Sleep Disorders Affecting Older Adults

With regard to the presence of sleep disorders in older people, an increase in the prevalence of insomnia; sleep-disordered breathing (SDB), including obstructive sleep apnea (OSA); movement disorders; and REM sleep behavior disorder has been reported.

4.1 Insomnia

The prevalence of insomnia in the general population has been estimated at between 10% and 20%, but some studies in older adults report higher frequencies [19]. An epidemiological study including individuals over the age of 65 showed that 42% of the participants complained of difficulties in falling asleep or staying asleep. Higher prevalences are observed in individuals with clinical and mental conditions, those using medications [15], retired or inactive individuals, or in people who are taking care of another older person [20]. Possible consequences of insomnia are depression, anxiety, cognitive decline, increased suicide attempts, clinical diseases (cardiovascular and cancer), increased fragility, and sarcopenia [19–21].

Insomnia in older subjects is related to increased mortality, risk of falls, lower quality of life, depression, and increased anxiety [19]. Insomniacs are more likely to present chronic pain, cancer, chronic obstructive pulmonary disease, and cardiovascular diseases as associated factors [20]. Nocturia, despite being very common in both male and female older individuals, is underestimated as a potential risk factor for insomnia. Many age-related factors contribute to nighttime urinary symptoms, including sleep-disordered breathing such as OSA [15, 22], and these symptoms are related to sleep fragmentation and excessive daytime sleepiness [15]. Menopause also contributes to worse sleep quality, causing nocturia, increased airway resistance, and obesity, in addition to night sweats [23]. On the other hand, the treatment of menopausal symptoms promotes a reduction in subjective insomnia and an increase in sleep efficiency [23].

Additionally, environmental and psychological factors contribute to the increased incidence of insomnia in older people. A large part of the population over the age of 65 years old often experiences social isolation (which has increased with the onset of COVID-19), financial problems, lack of exposure to sunlight, and anxiety due to fear of death and illness. Insomnia in this age group is often treated without a careful assessment of its causes, and self-medication is also frequent [23]. Additional predisposing factors for insomnia are female gender, divorce and widowhood, low education level, drug abuse, physical inactivity, and difficulties in social relationships [20, 24]. As precipitating factors, we have disabilities, the acute beginning of physical and psychiatric illnesses, and the use of medications. As for perpetuating factors, these include immobility, naps, excessive daytime sleepiness, and behavioral changes [20].

Cognitive-behavioral therapy (CBT) has shown long-term efficacy for the treatment of chronic insomnia in older adults [25]. A study confirmed that CBT not only improves sleep quality but reduces acute or long-term pain in patients with insomnia and osteoarthritis. This fact suggests that impaired sleep is not only a symptom of the painful syndrome and that improved sleep can also relieve comorbid disease [26].

4.2 Sleep-Disordered Breathing

In an analysis based on the literature, a high worldwide prevalence of obstructive sleep apnea was reported and was highlighted by country and region [27]. The authors concluded that there is a clear association between OSA and several adverse clinical results, including morbidity and mortality from cardiovascular disease [27]. The estimated prevalence of OSA ranged from 5% to 80% and was generally higher in older people [28]. In the epidemiological study conducted in the city of São Paulo mentioned previously, the prevalence of OSA in the 60–70 age group was 60.2% (55.9% for men and 63.4% for women) and 86.9% above 70 years (88.7 for men and 85.8 for women) [22]. In younger adults, there is a higher prevalence of OSA in of restless sleep, which can occur every day, often at the end of the night when REM sleep predominates. PSG can usually confirm the diagnosis by detecting excessive motor activity during REM sleep, and audio-visual monitoring can show abnormal body movements and vocalizations [48].

RBD is generally considered to be associated with synucleinopathies, such as Parkinson's disease, dementia with Lewy bodies, and multiple system atrophy that usually appear years before the first symptoms of these diseases. RBD is believed to predict neurodegeneration in synucleinopathy. However, growing evidence has shown that it is also found in non-synucleinopathy neurodegenerative diseases, including Alzheimer's, Huntington's diseases, and amyotrophic lateral sclerosis, among other conditions. It can be an early sign of neurodegeneration in these diseases, and also serve as an assessment of non-cognitive symptoms prior to cognitive impairments [49, 50].

The most common treatments used for RBD are clonazepam, melatonin, and ramelteon. It should be noted that drugs used to treat neurodegenerative diseases, such as monoamine oxidase inhibitors and antidepressants, can induce or aggravate RBD symptoms [50].

5 Treatment of Sleep Disorder in Older Adults: Physical Therapy and Exercise

The varied clinical presentations of sleep complaints require a multidisciplinary treatment response. The symptoms and the presence of comorbidities should be used to guide the therapeutic decision. The treatments used to manage sleep disorders include:

- The prevention and treatment of musculoskeletal pathologies using stretching exercises, muscle strengthening, proprioception, and joint mobilization to reduce stiffness and contractures. The current treatment options for sarcopenia include specific physical exercises (sometimes combined with nutritional recommendations). In addition, therapeutic approaches to normalize circadian rhythms and sleep homeostasis strategies can be used to preserve or recover muscle health in older adults [51].
- The treatment of respiratory pathologies using breathing exercises to strengthen the muscles participating in breathing, thereby increasing vital capacity. Although PAP is the most effective treatment in the complete resolution of OSA and in improving saturation rates during sleep [52], physical training, used as an additional option, can help to significantly reduce excessive daytime sleepiness [53]. Furthermore, the use of myofunctional therapy together with PAP has been shown to produce an increase in adherence to PAP [38].
- Fall prevention and treatment of older people with a history of falls: walking and balance training, proprioception, muscle strengthening, and home guidance.

Although this type of therapy is not directly related to sleep, it can also have a positive effect on it.

As a result of these treatments, there is an improvement in physical capacity and quality of life. Also, physical exercises can bring pain relief in older patients [50]. All of these results lead to an improvement in sleep quality.

6 Final Words

Aging can be associated with a decline in motor function, cognitive ability, and functionality. Sleep plays an essential role in all these processes, and its improvement can reduce negative outcomes in older individuals. With aging, changes occur in sleep patterns, which can become more fragmented, less efficient, and susceptible to clinical, mental, and sleep disorders. The sleep disorders that most commonly affect older adults, including insomnia, respiratory disorders, RLS, PLMD, and RBD, can be associated with the risk of geriatric syndromes, such as dementia, depression, delirium, falls, frailty, and sarcopenia.

Recent advances in physiotherapeutic approaches mean that we can improve the quality of sleep of individuals in this age group, as well as reduce the risk of falls, and the impact of other age-related conditions, with a consequent improvement in the quality of life brought about by the relief from symptoms and increased independence.

References

1. Kalache A. Envelhecimento: é urgente repensar o Brasil. Folha de São Paulo. 2006:A3.
2. Barthlen GM. Sleep disorders. Obstructive sleep apnea syndrome, restless legs syndrome, and insomnia in geriatric patients. Geriatrics. 2002;57(11):34–9; quiz 40.
3. Bachman DL. Sleep disorders with aging: evaluation and treatment. Geriatrics. 1992;47(9):53–6, 9-61.
4. Vitiello M. Recent advances in understanding sleep and sleep disturbances in older adults: growing older does not mean sleeping poorly. Current Directions in Psychological Science CurrenCt Directions in Psychological Science Current Directions in Psychological ScienceCu Current Directions in Psychological Science Current Directions in Psychological Science. 2009;6:4.
5. Bliwise D. Normal aging. In: Principles and practice of sleep medicine. 5th ed. Philadelphia: Elsevier Saunders; 2011.
6. Lucchesi L, Moraes W. Características do sono no idoso. O Sono e a Medicina do Sono. 1st edn. Minha Editora; 2014.
7. Ohayon MM, Carskadon MA, Guilleminault C, Vitiello MV. Meta-analysis of quantitative sleep parameters from childhood to old age in healthy individuals: developing normative sleep values across the human lifespan. Sleep. 2004;27(7):1255–73. https://doi.org/10.1093/sleep/27.7.1255.

8. Crowley K. Sleep and sleep disorders in older adults. Neuropsychol Rev. 2011;21(1):41–53. https://doi.org/10.1007/s11065-010-9154-6.
9. Dos Santos SM, Bazzana CM, de Souza AL, Ramos LR, Tufik S, Lucchesi LM, et al. Relationship between perceived sleep and polysomnography in older adult patients. Sleep Sci. 2015;8(2):75–81. https://doi.org/10.1016/j.slsci.2015.04.002.
10. Moraes W, Piovezan R, Poyares D, Bittencourt LR, Santos-Silva R, Tufik S. Effects of aging on sleep structure throughout adulthood: a population-based study. Sleep Med. 2014;15(4):401–9. https://doi.org/10.1016/j.sleep.2013.11.791.
11. Mazzotti DR, Guindalini C, Moraes WA, Andersen ML, Cendoroglo MS, Ramos LR, et al. Human longevity is associated with regular sleep patterns, maintenance of slow wave sleep, and favorable lipid profile. Front Aging Neurosci. 2014;6:134. https://doi.org/10.3389/fnagi.2014.00134.
12. Castro-Costa E, Dewey ME, Ferri CP, Uchôa E, Firmo JO, Rocha FL, et al. Association between sleep duration and all-cause mortality in old age: 9-year follow-up of the Bambuí Cohort Study. Brazil J Sleep Res. 2011;20(2):303–10. https://doi.org/10.1111/j.1365-2869.2010.00884.x.
13. Ohara T, Honda T, Hata J, Yoshida D, Mukai N, Hirakawa Y, et al. Association between daily sleep duration and risk of dementia and mortality in a Japanese community. J Am Geriatr Soc. 2018;66(10):1911–8. https://doi.org/10.1111/jgs.15446.
14. da Silva AA, de Mello RG, Schaan CW, Fuchs FD, Redline S, Fuchs SC. Sleep duration and mortality in the elderly: a systematic review with meta-analysis. BMJ Open. 2016;6(2):e008119. https://doi.org/10.1136/bmjopen-2015-008119.
15. Foley D, Ancoli-Israel S, Britz P, Walsh J. Sleep disturbances and chronic disease in older adults: results of the 2003 National Sleep Foundation Sleep in America Survey. J Psychosom Res. 2004;56(5):497–502. https://doi.org/10.1016/j.jpsychores.2004.02.010.
16. Casale G, de Nicola P. Circadian rhythms in the aged: a review. Arch Gerontol Geriatr. 1984;3(3):267–84. https://doi.org/10.1016/0167-4943(84)90028-1.
17. Lucchesi L, Lucchesi M, Tufik S. Alterações do ciclo sono-vigília na depressão. In: Lacerda A, Quarantini L, Miranda-Scippa A, Del Porto J, editors. Depressão: do neurônio ao funcionamento social. Porto Alegre: Artmed; 2009. p. 360.
18. Campbell SS, Murphy PJ, Stauble TN. Effects of a nap on nighttime sleep and waking function in older subjects. J Am Geriatr Soc. 2005;53(1):48–53. https://doi.org/10.1111/j.1532-5415.2005.53009.x.
19. Bloom HG, Ahmed I, Alessi CA, Ancoli-Israel S, Buysse DJ, Kryger MH, et al. Evidence-based recommendations for the assessment and management of sleep disorders in older persons. J Am Geriatr Soc. 2009;57(5):761–89. https://doi.org/10.1111/j.1532-5415.2009.02220.x.
20. Patel D, Steinberg J, Patel P. Insomnia in the elderly: a review. J Clin Sleep Med. 2018;14(6):1017–24. https://doi.org/10.5664/jcsm.7172.
21. Lucchesi LM, Pradella-Hallinan M, Lucchesi M, Moraes WA. Sleep in psychiatric disorders. Braz J Psychiatry. 2005;27 Suppl 1:27–32. https://doi.org/10.1590/s1516-44462005000500006.
22. Tufik S, Santos-Silva R, Taddei JA, Bittencourt LR. Obstructive sleep apnea syndrome in the Sao Paulo Epidemiologic Sleep Study. Sleep Med. 2010;11(5):441–6. https://doi.org/10.1016/j.sleep.2009.10.005.
23. Hachul H, Brandão LC, D'Almeida V, Bittencourt LR, Baracat EC, Tufik S. Isoflavones decrease insomnia in postmenopause. Menopause. 2011;18(2):178–84. https://doi.org/10.1097/gme.0b013e3181ecf9b9.
24. Moraes WAS, Poyares D. Sono e envelhecimento. In: Tufik S, editor. Medicina e Biologia do Sono. Barueri: Editora Manole; 2008. p. 429–39. ISBN 978-85-204-1485-9.
25. Morin CM, Colecchi C, Stone J, Sood R, Brink D. Behavioral and pharmacological therapies for late-life insomnia: a randomized controlled trial. JAMA. 1999;281(11):991–9. https://doi.org/10.1001/jama.281.11.991.

26. Vitiello MV, Rybarczyk B, Von Korff M, Stepanski EJ. Cognitive behavioral therapy for insomnia improves sleep and decreases pain in older adults with co-morbid insomnia and osteoarthritis. J Clin Sleep Med. 2009;5(4):355–62.
27. Benjafield AV, Ayas NT, Eastwood PR, Heinzer R, Ip MSM, Morrell MJ, et al. Estimation of the global prevalence and burden of obstructive sleep apnoea: a literature-based analysis. Lancet Respir Med. 2019;7(8):687–98. https://doi.org/10.1016/S2213-2600(19)30198-5.
28. Stone KL, Redline S. Sleep-related breathing disorder in the elderly. In: Ancoli-Israel S, editor. Sleep in older adult. Sleep Medicine Clinics. Philadelphia: W.B. Saunders-Elsevier; 2006;1(2):247–62. ISBN 1-4160-3565-6.
29. Verse T, Pirsig W. Impact of impaired nasal breathing on sleep-disordered breathing. Sleep Breath. 2003;7(2):63–76. https://doi.org/10.1007/s11325-003-0063-2.
30. Nery L, Moura S, Bittencourt L, Bagnato M, Gregório L, Tufik S. Síndrome da Apnéia do Sono Obstrutiva. In: Cukier A, Nakatani J, Morrone N, editors. Pneumologia - Atualização e Reciclagem. São Paulo: Atheneu; 1998. p. 104–11.
31. Bassiri A, Guilleminault C. Clinical features and evaluation of obstructive sleep apnea-hypopnea syndrome. In: Dement W, editor. Principles and practice of sleep medicine. 3rd ed. Philadelphia: WB Saunders; 2000. p. 869–78.
32. Larbi A, Franceschi C, Mazzatti D, Solana R, Wikby A, Pawelec G. Aging of the immune system as a prognostic factor for human longevity. Physiology (Bethesda). 2008;23:64–74. https://doi.org/10.1152/physiol.00040.2007.
33. Young T, Palta M, Dempsey J, Skatrud J, Weber S, Badr S. The occurrence of sleep-disordered breathing among middle-aged adults. N Engl J Med. 1993;328(17):1230–5. https://doi.org/10.1056/NEJM199304293281704.
34. Redline S, Tishler PV. The genetics of sleep apnea. Sleep Med Rev. 2000;4(6):583–602. https://doi.org/10.1053/smrv.2000.0120.
35. Bixler EO, Vgontzas AN, Lin HM, Ten Have T, Rein J, Vela-Bueno A, et al. Prevalence of sleep-disordered breathing in women: effects of gender. Am J Respir Crit Care Med. 2001;163(3 Pt 1):608–13. https://doi.org/10.1164/ajrccm.163.3.9911064.
36. Piovezan RD, Hirotsu C, Moizinho R, de Sá SH, D'Almeida V, Tufik S, et al. Associations between sleep conditions and body composition states: results of the EPISONO study. J Cachexia Sarcopenia Muscle. 2019;10(5):962–73. https://doi.org/10.1002/jcsm.12445.
37. Ancoli-Israel S. Sleep apnea in older adults--is it real and should age be the determining factor in the treatment decision matrix? Sleep Med Rev. 2007;11(2):83–5. https://doi.org/10.1016/j.smrv.2006.11.002.
38. Diaféria G, Santos-Silva R, Truksinas E, Haddad FLM, Santos R, Bommarito S, et al. Myofunctional therapy improves adherence to continuous positive airway pressure treatment. Sleep Breath. 2017;21(2):387–95. https://doi.org/10.1007/s11325-016-1429-6.
39. Allen RP, Picchietti D, Hening WA, Trenkwalder C, Walters AS, Montplaisi J, et al. Restless legs syndrome: diagnostic criteria, special considerations, and epidemiology. A report from the restless legs syndrome diagnosis and epidemiology workshop at the National Institutes of Health. Sleep Med. 2003;4(2):101–19. https://doi.org/10.1016/s1389-9457(03)00010-8.
40. Hublin C, Kaprio J, Partinen M, Koskenvuo M. Insufficient sleep--a population-based study in adults. Sleep. 2001;24(4):392–400. https://doi.org/10.1093/sleep/24.4.392.
41. Rizzo G, Manners D, Testa C, Tonon C, Vetrugno R, Marconi S, et al. Low brain iron content in idiopathic restless legs syndrome patients detected by phase imaging. Mov Disord. 2013;28(13):1886–90. https://doi.org/10.1002/mds.25576.
42. Eckeli AL, Gitaí LL, Dach F, Ceretta H, Sander HH, Passos AD, et al. Prevalence of restless legs syndrome in the rural town of Cassia dos Coqueiros in Brazil. Sleep Med. 2011;12(8):762–7. https://doi.org/10.1016/j.sleep.2011.01.018.
43. Karroum EG, Leu-Semenescu S, Arnulf I. Topography of the sensations in primary restless legs syndrome. J Neurol Sci. 2012;320(1–2):26–31. https://doi.org/10.1016/j.jns.2012.05.051.
44. Ohayon MM, O'Hara R, Vitiello MV. Epidemiology of restless legs syndrome: a synthesis of the literature. Sleep Med Rev. 2012;16(4):283–95. https://doi.org/10.1016/j.smrv.2011.05.002.

1 Defining Concepts

The term *sex* refers to the dichotomy between individuals such as male and female, related to glands or gonads, sex hormones, body anatomy, and genitals. Chromosomal sex refers to XX or XY at the time of fertilization (genotype); biological sex (phenotype) refers to secondary female or male sex characters from androgen hormones; gender identity refers to that inner feeling of belonging to the female or male universe and the ability to relate to both; gender role or social role refers to the way of being of each person, how it behaves before society as a whole (Table 1). This role already begins to be defined before birth (the sex of the fetus is known previously through ultrasonography), and after it, children should follow the set of values corresponding to what society establishes as to how they should be, feel, dress, and behave as a feminine or masculine person.

The term *gender* refers to how sexual characteristics and biological differences between women and men are understood and translated into social practice and relationships between people. It is how each culture identifies what is feminine and masculine; what are the obligations, rights, and standards to be followed by women and men [10, 11]. Women tend to multi-task (many activities at once), and so some research presents that women use more their brain than men do, needing more sleep.

Sex and gender are factors that significantly influence the health of women and men [12], as well as modulating women's and men's health standards and the level of disease of the general population. In this chapter, the sexual and gender differences of both normal sleep and sleep disorders will be addressed to assist in the clinical evaluation of physical therapists.

2 Normal Sleep in Women and Men

Girls have an increased sleep duration and sleep with more quality from childhood to early adolescence. From this moment on, there is a decrease in slow wave sleep (SWS) and a circadian delay that, if accentuated, may already predispose to insomnia symptoms in adolescents [13]. However, it is considered that the early pubertal maturation of young women (compared to boys) cannot be directly associated with the decline of the SWS, since even among boys, pubertal and electrophysiological time relationships were statistically independent of the sex difference [14].

Mallampalli and Carter presented a comprehensive report on differences in normal sleep of women and men: (i) sleep onset latency is longer in women; (ii) above

Table 1 Differences in the classification between sex and gender

Chromosomal sex or genotype	Biological sex or phenotype	Gender identity	Gender role or social role
XX	Female	Woman	Feminine
XY	Male	Man	Masculine

the age of 55, women report more drowsiness than men; (iii) as the age progresses, women have less sleep time than men; (iv) men have more N1 and N2 stages than women, who have more N3 stage [15].

3 Disturbed Sleep Between Gender

Understanding the difference between women's and men's sleep disorders has so far focused on the biological dimension [4, 13, 16] and in studies with men [4]. Advanced age is a risk factor for sleep difficulties in both sexes. However, hormonal and anatomical factors influence and alter women's sleep, especially from menarche to postmenopause, requiring specialized knowledge in the conduction of their problems.

There is little scientific evidence about how psychological and socio-cultural factors intensify the differences in the sleep-wake cycle between women and men. After a night of sleep deprivation, the performance of cognitive functions in women was more impaired than men [17]. These findings can be explained by the several commitments assumed by the female role, such as double working hours between work and family, impacting on the health of workers with children [18]. Women work 7.5 hours more per week than men, and 90% of them reported doing domestic work in addition to paid work [19], thus being more disposed to sleep deprivation. This lifestyle may be related to increased surveillance [20, 21] and may also be associated with mood disorders such as anxiety and depression [22], which in turn, influence and impair sleep.

Women have an increased risk of insomnia of 40% compared to men [10], which justifies greater attention from health professionals. Insomnia in women seems to be associated with mood disorders, and insomnia in men seems to be associated with clinical comorbidities. Insomnia is also more prevalent in separated, widowed, or single women [23].

Obstructive sleep apnea (OSA) is more prevalent in men, and obesity is a relevant risk factor [24]. However, the quality of life of women with OSA is more affected than that of men [25]. The symptoms of OSA presented in women at a less severe level when compared to men, with mild snoring, minor Apnea-hypopnea index (AHI), shorter obstruction events [26] and usually report difficulties in initiating and maintaining sleep, nightmares, fatigue, and depression [2, 27]. This clinical condition may lead to the diagnosis of OSA in women. Men with OSA usually have more pronounced AHI and symptoms such as loud and strong snoring witnessed apnea, and daytime drowsiness. The consequences of OSA are also distinct: hypertension and depression are more common in women and diabetes and heart disease in men [28]. Women with OSA severity like those of men usually present impairments in quality of life and attend health services more intensively [29]. In the treatment of OSA with Continuous Positive Airway Pressure (CPAP), women tend to be less adherent to therapy, using alternative treatments [30]. In clinical practice, women report that they do not want to be seen by their spouse using the equipment during sleep.

Other sleep disorders present prevalence between genders and can be found in Table 2.

Table 2 Prevalence and relevance of sleep disorders between genders

Sleep disorder	Prevalence	Relevance
Circadian rhythm	♀	♀ are more prone to morning-type and increased wakefulness
Insomnia	♀	♀ are more prone to morning-type and increased wakefulness Risk of up to 40% more than ♂ Cognitive impairment is greater in women with sleep deprivation ♀ report unsatisfactory sleep during different stages of life Peri- and post-menopause accentuate risk factors ♀ double workday affects the quantity and quality of sleep
Obstructive sleep apnea	♂	Increased waist circumference is a risk factor for OSA severity in ♂ ♂ have more pronounced AHI ♀ are underdiagnosed, have nonspecific symptoms Depression is associated with OSA in ♀
Restless legs syndrome	♀	Associated with anemia, pregnancy, iron deficiency
Central sleep apnea	♂	Lower BMI and age above 65 years
REM behavioral sleep disorder	♂	♂ tend to have dreams of more violent content and with more explicit physical manifestations than ♀ Ratio ♂ /♀ of 1.62/1
Sleep-related eating disorders	♀	Associated with eating problems in childhood
Narcolepsy	♂	With or without cataplexy, ratio about ♂ /♀ of 1.4 / 1.8

AHI apnea-hypopnea index, *OSA* obstructive sleep apnea, *BMI* body mass index, ♂ man, ♀ woman

3.1 Sleep in Different Phases Across Women's Life

The sleep pattern is experienced in a unique way between women in different stages of life, either by physiological, cultural, or behavioral factors. There are changes that occur in the cycles of female life that influence and are influenced by sleep: menarche (which indicates the beginning of the reproductive phase) and monthly periods (also called pre-menopause); pregnancy (a fluctuation of hormones throughout 3 trimesters); peri-menopause (the phase that marks the end of a woman's reproductive life, with an approach to the last period, around the age of 50, which happens by the decrease in estrogen production and precedes menopause); menopause itself (the last first day of a period); and post-menopause (clinically recognized when there is amenorrhea (absence of menstruation) in the last 12 months, ruled out pathological causes) [31]. All these hormone-controlled phases physiologically impact the sleep pattern (Fig. 1) [16].

Menarche and the new infradian rhythm of the menstrual cycle tend to promote changes in the young woman's quality of life. From this time on, girls are prone to the development of mood disorders, twice as much as boys [16]. Symptoms of the perimenstrual syndrome, dysmenorrhea, and night bleeding are early associated with a compromised sleep pattern. In PSG examination there is an increase in EEG

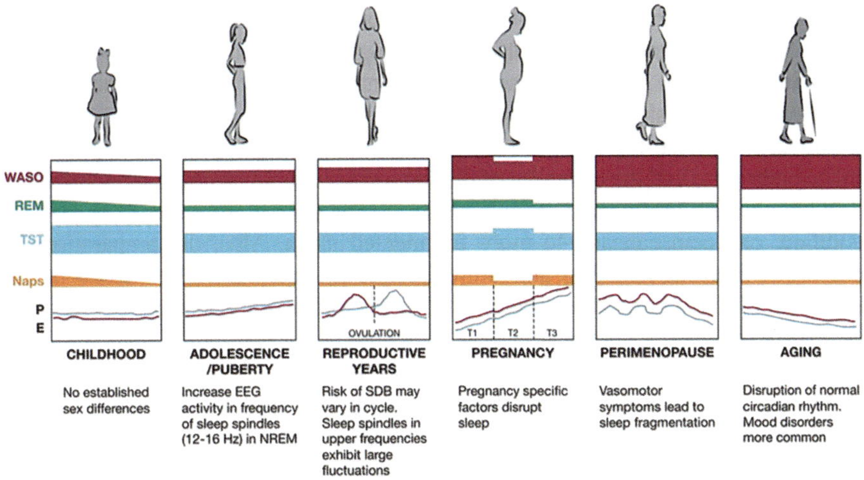

Fig. 1 Sleep in women across the life span. E estrogen, NREM non-rapid eye movement, P progesterone, REM rapid eye movement, SDB sleep-disordered breathing, T trimester, TST total sleep time, WASO wake after sleep onset. (Reprinted with permission from Pengo et al. [16])

activity, and N2 stage sleep spindles in the post-ovulatory luteal phase [32] already indicating a change in the sleep architecture. The menstrual cycle is divided into the pre-ovulatory follicular phase and post-ovulatory luteal phase, in which the onset of the period marks the beginning of a new cycle. Sleep complaints appear at the end of the luteal phase (pre-menstrual) and at the beginning of the follicular phase, as worsening in the quality of sleep and insomnia symptoms [33]. Additionally, women with irregular menstrual cycles had twice the chance of having sleep problems, compared to women with regular menstrual cycle patterns [34]. Premenstrual syndrome can be accompanied by complaints of insomnia, unpleasant dreams, poor sleep quality, daytime sleepiness, and fatigue [35]. Dysmenorrhea and lower sleep efficiency are negatively interlaced [36]. Instructing the patients to keep a three-month diary is a good opportunity to working out whether the sleep problems are related to the menstrual cycle and therefore seek help.

Pregnancy is a period of physical and psychological changes that modify the quality of life and contribute negatively to the duration and consolidation of sleep. Sleeping during pregnancy (for two or more!) is a challenge. As many as 97% of pregnant women say that their sleep is disturbed, especially in the third semester. Pregnant women have typical sleep disorders when compared to non-pregnant ones [37], and a poor quality sleep in the first months was associated with the development of gestational diabetes mellitus [38]. During pregnancy, the narrowing of the upper airway is a risk factor for the presence of rhinitis, nasal congestion, snoring, and even OSA. There is an even higher prevalence of restless leg syndrome due to iron deficiency and hormonal influences. In the first trimester, high levels of progesterone increase daytime and sleepiness and the need for sleep. Progesterone also increases urine production and can disturb sleep as the enlarged uterus presses on

References

1. Ferrara M, De Gennaro L. How much sleep do we need? Sleep Med Rev. 2001;5(2):155–79.
2. Collop NA, Adkins D, Phillips BA. Gender differences in sleep and sleep-disordered breathing. Clin Chest Med. 2004;25(2):257–68.
3. Zhang B, Wing YK. Sex differences in insomnia: a meta-analysis. Sleep. 2006;29(1):85–93.
4. Mong JA, et al. Sleep, rhythms, and the endocrine brain: influence of sex and gonadal hormones. J Neurosci. 2011;31(45):16107–16.
5. Goel N, Kim H, Lao RP. Gender differences in polysomnographic sleep in young healthy sleepers. Chronobiol Int. 2005;22(5):905–15.
6. Lee KA, Kryger MH. Women and sleep. J Womens Health (Larchmt). 2008;17(7):1189–90.
7. Hirotsu C, et al. Sleep complaints in the Brazilian population: impact of socioeconomic factors. Sleep Sci. 2014;7(3):135–42.
8. Berger K, et al. Sex and the risk of restless legs syndrome in the general population. Arch Intern Med. 2004;164(2):196–202.
9. Money J. Gender: history, theory and usage of the term in sexology and its relationship to nature/nurture. J Sex Marital Ther. 1985;11(2):71–9.
10. Van Reeth O, et al. Nocturnal exercise phase delays circadian rhythms of melatonin and thyrotropin secretion in normal men. Am J Physiol. 1994;266(6 Pt 1):E964–74.
11. da Costa RP. The eleven sexes: the multiple faces of human sexuality. Vol. 4th ed; 2005. São Paulo: Kondo Editora.
12. Barsky AJ, Peekna HM, Borus JF. Somatic symptom reporting in women and men. J Gen Intern Med. 2001;16(4):266–75.
13. Franco P, et al. Sleep during development: sex and gender differences. Sleep Med Rev. 2020;51:101276.
14. Campbell IG, et al. Sex, puberty, and the timing of sleep EEG measured adolescent brain maturation. Proc Natl Acad Sci U S A. 2012;109(15):5740–3.
15. Mallampalli MP, Carter CL. Exploring sex and gender differences in sleep health: a Society for Women's Health Research report. J Womens Health (Larchmt). 2014;23(7):553–62.
16. Pengo MF, Won CH, Bourjeily G. Sleep in women across the life span. Chest. 2018;154(1):196–206.
17. Santhi N, et al. Sex differences in the circadian regulation of sleep and waking cognition in humans. Proc Natl Acad Sci U S A. 2016;113(19):E2730–9.
18. Rotenberg L, Portela LF, Duarte RA. Gender and sleep in nightworkers: a quantitative analysis of sleep in days off. J Hum Ergol (Tokyo). 2001;30(1–2):333–8.
19. IPEA., I.o.A.E.R. Study shows gender and race inequality in 20 years. December 12th, 2020. Available from: Available at: http://www.ipea.gov.br/portal/index.php?option=com_content&id=29526.
20. Verbrugge LM. Gender and health: an update on hypotheses and evidence. J Health Soc Behav. 1985;26(3):156–82.
21. Lieban RW. Gender and symptom sensitivity: report on a Philippine study. Am J Orthopsychiatry. 1985;55(3):446–50.
22. Walker WH 2nd, et al. Circadian rhythm disruption and mental health. Transl Psychiatry. 2020;10(1):28.
23. Ohayon M. Epidemiological study on insomnia in the general population. Sleep. 1996;19(3 Suppl):S7–15.
24. Tufik S, et al. Obstructive sleep apnea syndrome in the Sao Paulo Epidemiologic Sleep Study. Sleep Med. 2010;11(5):441–6.
25. Schiza SE, Bouloukaki I. Does gender matter: sex-specific aspects of symptoms, outcome, and therapy of obstructive sleep apnea. Curr Opin Pulm Med. 2020;26(6):642–9.
26. Wimms A, et al. Obstructive sleep apnea in women: specific issues and interventions. Biomed Res Int. 2016;2016:1764837.
27. Shaib F, Attarian H. Sex and gender differences in sleep disorders: an overview. In: Principles of gender-specific medicine: gender in the genomic era; 2017. USA: Elsevier. p. 585–601.

28. Bostan OC, et al. Impact of gender on symptoms and comorbidities in obstructive sleep apnea. Eurasian J Med. 2021;53(1):34–9.
29. Greenberg-Dotan S, et al. Gender differences in morbidity and health care utilization among adult obstructive sleep apnea patients. Sleep. 2007;30(9):1173–80.
30. Jayaraman G, et al. Influence of gender on continuous positive airway pressure requirements in patients with obstructive sleep apnea syndrome. Sleep Breath. 2011;15(4):781–4.
31. Research on the menopause in the 1990s. Report of a WHO Scientific Group. World Health Organ Tech Rep Ser. 1996;866:1–107.
32. Baker FC, et al. Sleep quality and the sleep electroencephalogram in women with severe premenstrual syndrome. Sleep. 2007;30(10):1283–91.
33. Baker FC, Driver HS. Self-reported sleep across the menstrual cycle in young, healthy women. J Psychosom Res. 2004;56(2):239–43.
34. Hachul H, et al. Does the reproductive cycle influence sleep patterns in women with sleep complaints? Climacteric. 2010;13(6):594–603.
35. Nowakowski S, Meers J, Heimbach E. Sleep and women's health. Sleep Med Res. 2013;4(1):1–22.
36. Woosley JA, Lichstein KL. Dysmenorrhea, the menstrual cycle, and sleep. Behav Med. 2014;40(1):14–21.
37. Christian LM, et al. Associations of postpartum sleep, stress, and depressive symptoms with LPS-stimulated cytokine production among African American and White women. J Neuroimmunol. 2018;316:98–106.
38. Xu YH, et al. Association between sleep duration during pregnancy and gestational diabetes mellitus: a meta-analysis. Sleep Med. 2018;52:67–74.
39. Rychnovsky J, Hunter LP. The relationship between sleep characteristics and fatigue in healthy postpartum women. Womens Health Issues. 2009;19(1):38–44.
40. Davis SR, et al. Menopause. Nat Rev Dis Primers. 2015;1:15004.
41. Frange C, et al. Impact of insomnia on pain in postmenopausal women. Climacteric. 2017;20(3):262–7.
42. Frange C, et al. Insomnia with musculoskeletal pain in postmenopause: associations with symptoms, mood, and quality of life. J Menopausal Med. 2018;24(1):17–28.
43. Frange C, et al. Temporal analysis of chronic musculoskeletal pain and sleep in postmenopausal women. J Clin Sleep Med. 2019;15(2):223–34.
44. Harlow SD, et al. Executive summary of the Stages of Reproductive Aging Workshop + 10: addressing the unfinished agenda of staging reproductive aging. Menopause. 2012;19(4):387–95.
45. Hachul H, et al. The effect of menopause on objective sleep parameters: data from an epidemiologic study in Sao Paulo, Brazil. Maturitas. 2015;80(2):170–8.
46. Dell PF. Beyond homeostasis: toward a concept of coherence. Fam Process. 1982;21(1):21–41.
47. Hasler BP, Troxel WM. Couples' nighttime sleep efficiency and concordance: evidence for bidirectional associations with daytime relationship functioning. Psychosom Med. 2010;72(8):794–801.
48. A, D.H.a.D. Couple relationships are associated with increased rem sleep - a proof-of-concept analysis of a large dataset using ambulatory polysomnography. Front Psych. 2021;12:641102.
49. Gunn HE, et al. Sleep concordance in couples is associated with relationship characteristics. Sleep. 2015;38(6):933–9.
50. Drews HJ, et al. Bed-sharing in couples is associated with increased and stabilized REM sleep and sleep-stage synchronization. Front Psych. 2020;11:583.
51. March 20, 2020. Available from: https://www.sleepreviewmag.com/sleep-health/parameters/quality/philips-releases-global-satisfaction-trends.
52. Luyster FS, et al. Patient and partner experiences with obstructive sleep apnea and CPAP treatment: a qualitative analysis. Behav Sleep Med. 2016;14(1):67–84.
53. Tramonti F, et al. Relationship quality of persons with obstructive sleep apnoea syndrome. Psychol Health Med. 2017;22(8):896–901.

Sleep in Neurologic Diseases

Lúcio Huebra Pimentel Filho, Marcos Manoel Honorato, and Fernando Morgadinho Santos Coelho

Systemic diseases have a complex relationship with circadian rhythm, sleep, and sleep disorders. Many neurological diseases present intensification of their symptoms at a certain time of the day, right after waking up, close to bedtime, or even during sleep. Several conditions, especially neurological diseases, can present themselves as precipitating or perpetuating factors of sleep disorders. Also, sleep disorders can be aggravating factors of the symptoms of several diseases. The proper approach to sleep disorders in patients affected by neurologic diseases becomes important. It is necessary to know the main sleep symptoms related to the underlying neurological diseases, how to investigate them to enable treatment with consequent improvement in the quality of life. In this chapter, we will stick to the following neurological diseases, due to their higher prevalence and their association with sleep: stroke, epilepsy, Parkinson's disease, Alzheimer's disease, neuromuscular diseases, and headache.

L. H. P. Filho (✉)
Neurology and Neurosurgery Department, Escola Paulista de Medicina, Universidade Federal de São Paulo, São Paulo, SP, Brazil

M. M. Honorato
Neurology and Neurosurgery Department, Escola Paulista de Medicina, Universidade Federal de São Paulo, São Paulo, SP, Brazil

Universidade do Estado do Pará, Santarém, Pará, Brazil

F. M. S. Coelho
Neurology and Neurosurgery Department; Department of Psychobiology, Escola Paulista de Medicina, Universidade Federal de São Paulo, São Paulo, SP, Brazil

C. Frange, F. M. S. Coelho (eds.), *Sleep Medicine and Physical Therapy*,
https://doi.org/10.1007/978-3-030-85074-6_27

Another epilepsy that has an intimate relationship with sleep is encephalopathy with an epileptic status of slow-wave sleep (ESES). It may also have a genetic etiology. Persistent discharges are activated by slow-wave sleep [25].

Authors reported that epilepsy alone already changes the architecture of sleep, with low sleep efficiency and changes in the distribution of REM and non-REM stages being frequent [26].

Although the electroencephalogram (EEG) is the routine complementary exam in the evaluation of people with epilepsy, eventually epileptiform discharges may be observed during the recording of polysomnography [Fig. 1].

People with epilepsy are usually treated with anti-crisis medications. The mechanism of action is to block the sodium channels, which prevents the depolarization of hyperexcited neural networks. A common side effect of this class of drugs is excessive drowsiness, with emphasis on carbamazepine, oxcarbazepine, and pregabalin. Sleepiness also occurs after the use of GABAergic drugs such as phenobarbital and valproic acid [27]. Modern anti-crisis drugs such as lamotrigine also act on ion channels, but with a less sedative effect. Levetiracetam, an inhibitor of the release of synaptic vesicles, has a different profile and does not usually influence sleep [20, 27].

The ketogenic diet is an alternative treatment used for medication-refractory epilepsies in children and adolescents. It is rich in fats, suitable for proteins, and low in

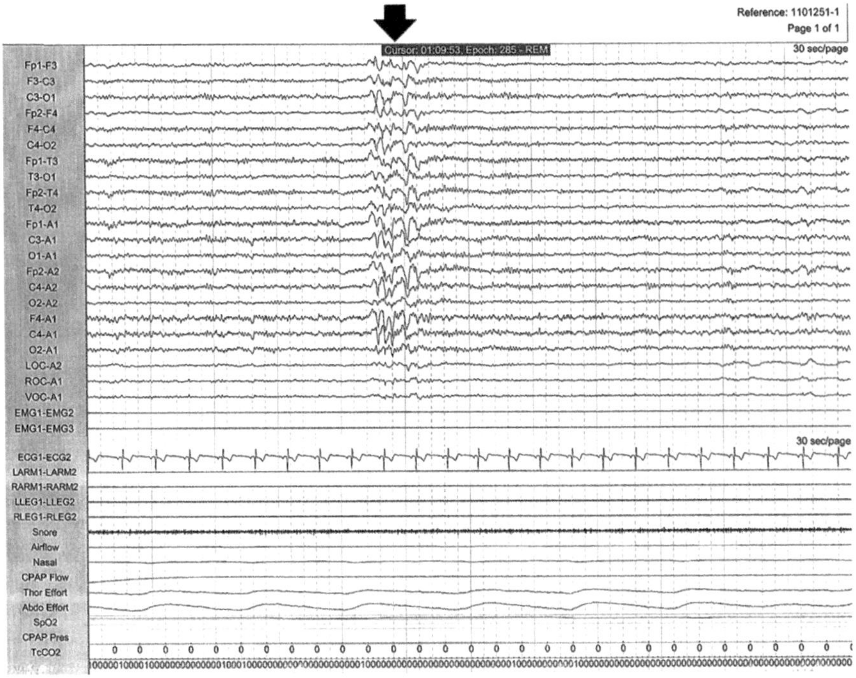

Fig. 1 Black arrow showing the epileptiform activity on the electroencephalogram, consisting of generalized high-voltage slow spike-wave patterns in this 30-second epoch of neurologic polysomnography. (Image courtesy from Dr. Fernando Morgadinho Santos Coelho)

carbohydrates [28]. Its effect on sleep was reported by some authors, who observed an increase in total sleep time and a reduction in non-REM sleep [28, 29].

Likewise, vagus nerve stimulation is useful in many cases of difficult-to-control epilepsy and can reduce excessive daytime sleepiness, minimizing the summative toxic effect of multiple drugs, but there are reports of increased occurrence and severity of sleep apnea in these patients [30, 31].

It is thought that some medications used for sleep disorders may have an anti-crisis effect, such as melatonin, used for disturbance of circadian rhythm. It was effective in reducing seizures in mice, but a meta-analysis was not effective in confirming these findings [32–34]. Modafinil, used to treat narcolepsy, also reduced epileptic seizures in experimental rat models. Pitolisant, which acts on the histamine H3 receptor, was effective in reducing the photo paroxysmal response in patients with photosensitive epilepsy, but the studied sample was small [35].

Understanding the biological basis of this relationship between epilepsy and sleep requires a brief review of the sleep-wake cycle regulation mechanism.

The ascending activator reticular system (ARDS) is a set of structures that regulates the sleep-wake cycle and consists of nuclei of the median raphe located in the brain stem that project into the cerebral cortex, with an activating effect. It is believed that this system is partly responsible for the fundamental rhythms observed in the normal electroencephalogram during surveillance [20].

Experimental models obtain synchronous neuronal activity and sleep induction after electrical stimulation of the thalamus, which suggests its participation as a primordial element in the synchronization of brain rhythms. In contrast, stimulation of ARDS causes sleep disruption and desynchronization of brain electrical activity, causing wakefulness [20].

These projection circuits to the cortex responsible for the wakefulness rhythm are largely excitatory, and the neurotransmitters most involved are acetylcholine and glutamate, which are also the neurotransmitters involved in epileptogenesis [20].

The inhibitory circuits are responsible for the synchronization and the sleep rhythm of slow waves and are mostly modulated by GABA (GABA-amino-butyric acid). The same structures seem to be responsible for the generation of generalized spike-slow-wave discharges [36].

As this circuit is involved in the control of cortical excitability, its dysfunction would be responsible in part for the hyper synchronization that would originate generalized epileptiform discharges [20]. Functional magnetic resonance and tractography studies reveal that thalamocortical connections are possibly involved in this process [37].

The suprachiasmatic nucleus functions as a relay that adjusts the sleep-wake cycle to the circadian rhythm. The routes related to it could explain the occurrence of crises in certain periods of the day. There is evidence that CLOCK gene expression may be reduced in patients with refractory epilepsy [38].

3 Parkinson's Disease and Sleep

Parkinson's disease is a neurodegenerative disease characterized primarily by bradykinesia associated with resting tremor, stiffness, and/or loss of postural reflexes. According to its pathophysiological characteristics, it is included in the group of neurodegenerative diseases known as synucleinopathies, which have similarities in their clinical presentation due to the presence of the motor symptoms already mentioned and the occurrence of non-motor symptoms, currently an important target of studies, such as changes in smell, loss of visual sensitivity to distinguish colors, constipation, and REM sleep behavior disorder.

Sleep disorders are seen in 50–60% of patients with Parkinson's disease and have an important impact on the quality of life. The disorders presented can be diverse, and the complaints presented vary from insomnia, excessive daytime sleepiness, non-restorative sleep, night fragmentation of sleep, or restless sleep [39].

Insomnia in patients with Parkinson's disease can occur for several reasons, from general conditions regardless of the underlying disease, such as poor sleep hygiene, inadequate environment, as well as the use of specific medications and disorders in this population. Selegiline (monoamine oxide B inhibitor) is metabolized to amphetamines and can generate alertness, causing difficulty in starting sleep according to the time of medication use [40]. The use of levodopa, amantadine, and trihexyphenidyl can also impair sleep quality. Patients with Parkinson's disease and insomnia should always be submitted to non-pharmacological treatment with guidance on sleep hygiene, specific cognitive-behavioral therapy for insomnia, the regularity of schedules, and the establishment of a routine of active activities during the day. Pharmacological treatment, when indicated, can be performed through non-benzodiazepine hypnotics such as zolpidem, zopiclone, zaleplon, or even the use of low doses of quetiapine [40].

In patients with difficulty falling asleep, symptoms of restless legs syndrome should always be actively questioned, since even when severely symptomatic patients may not directly complain about this condition. RLS has an increased prevalence among Parkinson's disease patients, affecting 10–20% of these patients. The first-line treatment is the use of dopaminergic agonists such as pramipexole and rotigotine. Gabapentin, opioids, and clonazepam can be used as a second-line or in case of augmentation syndrome with the use of the dopaminergic agonist [41].

Agitation at night can have an important social impact, generating fear and apprehension in family members and caregivers. Parkinson's disease patients commonly experience vivid dreams and nightmares arising from the use of dopaminergic therapy. The excessive rhythmic movement of the lower limbs can arise in the context of periodic limb movements of sleep (PLMS). If there is vocalization and complex movements suggestive of dream enhactment, REM sleep behavior disorder (RBD) should be remembered. RBD affects about 15–30% of Parkinson's disease patients and can precede the onset of motor symptoms of the disease and the moment of clinical diagnosis by decades [39]. During episodes of this parasomnia, patients show significant improvement in parkinsonian symptoms with increased voice volume, greater agility of movement, and absence of tremor. The episodes tend to be aggressive and can generate trauma for the patient or partner, even with serious injuries. In the clinical suspicion of RBD, it should be investigated by performing basal polysomnography with 4-limb electromyography and video monitoring, looking for episodes of loss of atony during REM sleep and behavioral changes in dreams experience. Symptoms generally respond well to treatment with the use of low doses of clonazepam or melatonin [39].

Excessive daytime sleepiness is another important complaint of patients with Parkinson's disease, being most of the time multifactorial. The frequent and generally undervalued reason is night fragmentation of sleep due to parkinsonian symptoms during sleep. The presence of significant stiffness with difficulty in moving during the night or the presence of tremors can generate multiple awakenings.

Obstructive sleep apnea does not seem particularly characteristic of Parkinson's disease, but the literature remains conflicting. The majority of studies reveal that the prevalence of OSA in Parkinson's disease is similar to the general population or matched control subjects [42]. But OSA should be investigated whenever there are other suggestive signs and symptoms such as snoring, dry mouth, morning headache, nocturia, overweight, and non-restorative sleep.

Sleep attacks, characterized as sudden drowsiness, can occur in 5.3% of patients on monotherapy with dopaminergic agonists and 7.3% of patients on the combined use of levodopa and dopaminergic agonists [39].

Clinical studies show that circadian disturbances are frequent in patients with Parkinson's disease, probably related to blunted circadian melatonin secretion and reduced amplitude of melatonin rhythm. These alterations may also be related to both insufficient exposures to bright light and phase advances related to treatment with dopaminergic drugs [43].

Exercise rehabilitation influences positively objective sleep patterns, changing sleep structure and acting as a promising supportive treatment for Parkinson's disease patients [44]. Fatigue and sleepiness are frequent complaints; a short nap after each rehabilitation session may improve tiredness [45].

4 Alzheimer's Disease and Sleep

Alzheimer's disease is a neurodegenerative disorder characterized by progressive cognitive decline with impaired memory, language, temporospatial orientation, executive functions, and other domains. It is considered the main irreversible cause of dementia in the elderly.

Sleep changes are part of the normal aging process, with an increase in nocturnal sleep fragmentation, nocturnal awakenings, and a greater tendency to sleep during the day. The prevalence of sleep disorders in Alzheimer's disease is estimated at 25% in mild cases and up to 50% in moderate to severe cases. Sleep disorders can take different forms such as excessive sleepiness during the day, difficulty sleeping in the night, fragmentation of night sleep, and early awakening. Sleep disorders can

Cluster headache attacks follow a striking circadian rhythm with an intriguing influence on sleep. Sleep quality is reduced in both types of episodic and chronic cluster headache [53].

Regular physical activity, in addition to its benefit in the quality of sleep, has a beneficial prophylactic effect in the control of headaches and should be encouraged, especially in patients with sleep disorders and migraines [54].

Sleep quality should always be questioned during the follow-up of patients with neurological diseases. It is only through questioning about sleep-related symptoms such as difficulty in initiating or maintaining sleep, early awakening, snoring, breathing pauses, daytime sleepiness, restlessness during the night, and non-restorative sleep that we can hypothesize that there is an associated sleep disorder and from there search the diagnosis and further start treatment. The treatment of sleep disorders comorbid to chronic neurological disorders is important for better control of the symptoms of the underlying pathology, greater adherence to treatment, and even for an overall improvement in the quality of life.

References

1. Kim AS, Cahill E, Cheng NT. Global stroke belt: geographic variation in stroke burden worldwide. Stroke. 2015;46:3564–70.
2. van Almenkerk S, Smalbrugge M, Depla MF, Eefsting JA, Hertogh CM. What predicts a poor outcome in older stroke survivors? A systematic review of the literature. Disabil Rehabil. 2013;35:1774–82.
3. Katzan IL, Thompson NR, Walia HK, Moul DE, Foldvary-Schaefer N. Sleep-related symptoms in patients with mild stroke. J Clin Sleep Med. 2020;16:55–64.
4. Kim KT, Moon H-J, Yang J-G, Sohn S-I, Hong J-H, Cho YW. The prevalence and clinical significance of sleep disorders in acute ischemic stroke patients—a questionnaire study. Sleep Breath. 2017;21:759–65.
5. Mello-Fujita L, Kim LJ, de Oliveira PL, et al. Treatment of obstructive sleep apnea syndrome associated with stroke. Sleep Med. 2015;16:691–6.
6. Culebras A. Sleep apnea and stroke. Curr Neurol Neurosci Rep. 2015;15:503.
7. Ramos AR, Seixas A, Dib SI. Obstructive sleep apnea and stroke: links to health disparities. Sleep Health. 2015;1:244–8.
8. Koo DL, Nam H, Thomas RJ, Yun C-H. Sleep disturbances as a risk factor for stroke. J Stroke. 2018;20:12.
9. Poryazova R, Huber R, Khatami R, et al. Topographic sleep EEG changes in the acute and chronic stage of hemispheric stroke. J Sleep Res. 2015;24:54–65.
10. Bollu C, Pandey A, Pesala S, Nalleballe K. Sleepiness after stroke: case report and review of literature on hypersomnia as a result of stroke. Madridge J Neurosci. 2017;1:4–6.
11. Jovanovic A, Stolic RV, Rasic DV, Markovic-Jovanovic SR, Peric VM. Stroke and diabetic ketoacidosis–some diagnostic and therapeutic considerations. Vasc Health Risk Manag. 2014;10:201.
12. Sarfo FS, Jenkins C, Mensah NA, et al. Prevalence and predictors of sleep apnea risk among Ghanaian stroke survivors. J Stroke Cerebrovasc Dis. 2017;26:1602–8.
13. Lyons OD, Ryan CM. Sleep apnea and stroke. Can J Cardiol. 2015;31:918–27.
14. Ito E, Inoue Y. The international classification of sleep disorders, American Academy of Sleep Medicine. Includes bibliographies and index. Nihon rinsho Jpn J Clin Med. 2015;73:916–23.

15. Mansukhani MP, Bellolio MF, Kolla BP, Enduri S, Somers VK, Stead LG. Worse outcome after stroke in patients with obstructive sleep apnea: an observational cohort study. J Stroke Cerebrovasc Dis. 2011;20:401–5.
16. Lau HL, Rundek T, Ramos AR. Sleep and stroke: new updates on epidemiology, pathophysiology, assessment, and treatment. Curr Sleep Med Rep. 2019;5:71–82.
17. Koretsi V, Eliades T, Papageorgiou SN. Oral interventions for obstructive sleep apnea: an umbrella review of the effectiveness of intraoral appliances, maxillary expansion, and maxillomandibular advancement. Dtsch Arztebl Int. 2018;115:200.
18. Parasram M, Segal AZ. Sleep disorders and stroke: does treatment of obstructive sleep apnea decrease risk of ischemic stroke? Curr Treat Options Neurol. 2019;21:29.
19. Coelho FMS, Georgsson H, Narayansingh M, Swartz RH, Murray BJ. Higher prevalence of periodic limb movements of sleep in patients with history of stroke. J Clin Sleep Med. 2010;6:428–30.
20. Wang Y-Q, Zhang M-Q, Li R, Qu W-M, Huang Z-L. The mutual interaction between sleep and epilepsy on the neurobiological basis and therapy. Curr Neuropharmacol. 2018;16:5–16.
21. Jain SV, Kothare SV. Sleep and epilepsy. Semin Pediatr Neurol. 2015;22(2):86–92.
22. Díaz-Negrillo A. Influence of sleep and sleep deprivation on ictal and interictal epileptiform activity. Epilepsy Res Treat. 2013;2013:492524.
23. Xu L, Guo D, Y-y L, Qiao D-D, Ye J-Y, Xue R. Juvenile myoclonic epilepsy and sleep. Epilepsy Behav. 2018;80:326–30.
24. Watanabe K, Negoro T, Aso K, Matsumoto A. Reappraisal of interictal electroencephalograms in infantile spasms. Epilepsia. 1993;34:679–85.
25. RamachandranNair R. Encephalopathy associated with electrical status epilepticus of sleep (ESES): a practical approach. Indian J Pediatr. 2020;87(12):1057–61.
26. Lanigar S, Bandyopadhyay S. Sleep and epilepsy: a complex interplay. Mo Med. 2017;114:453.
27. Jain SV, Glauser TA. Effects of epilepsy treatments on sleep architecture and daytime sleepiness: an evidence-based review of objective sleep metrics. Epilepsia. 2014;55:26–37.
28. Hallböök T, Lundgren J, Rosén I. Ketogenic diet improves sleep quality in children with therapy-resistant epilepsy. Epilepsia. 2007;48:59–65.
29. Iacovides S, Meiring RM. The effect of a ketogenic diet versus a high-carbohydrate, low-fat diet on sleep, cognition, thyroid function, and cardiovascular health independent of weight loss: study protocol for a randomized controlled trial. Trials. 2018;19:62.
30. Marzec M, Edwards J, Sagher O, Fromes G, Malow BA. Effects of vagus nerve stimulation on sleep-related breathing in epilepsy patients. Epilepsia. 2003;44:930–5.
31. Hallböök T, Lundgren J, Köhler S, Blennow G, Strömblad L-G, Rosén I. Beneficial effects on sleep of vagus nerve stimulation in children with therapy resistant epilepsy. Eur J Paediatr Neurol. 2005;9:399–407.
32. Jain SV, Horn PS, Simakajornboon N, et al. Melatonin improves sleep in children with epilepsy: a randomized, double-blind, crossover study. Sleep Med. 2015;16:637–44.
33. Banach M, Gurdziel E, Jędrych M, Borowicz KK. Melatonin in experimental seizures and epilepsy. Pharmacol Rep. 2011;63:1–11.
34. Khan S, Khurana M, Vyas P, Vohora D. The role of melatonin and its analogues in epilepsy. Rev Neurosci. 2021;32(1):49–67.
35. Trenité DK-N, Parain D, Genton P, Masnou P, Schwartz J-C, Hirsch E. Efficacy of the histamine 3 receptor (H3R) antagonist pitolisant (formerly known as tiprolisant; BF2. 649) in epilepsy: dose-dependent effects in the human photosensitivity model. Epilepsy Behav. 2013;28:66–70.
36. Sherin J, Shiromani P, McCarley R, Saper C. Activation of ventrolateral preoptic neurons during sleep. Science. 1996;271:216–9.
37. Mhuircheartaigh RN, Rosenorn-Lanng D, Wise R, Jbabdi S, Rogers R, Tracey I. Cortical and subcortical connectivity changes during decreasing levels of consciousness in humans: a functional magnetic resonance imaging study using propofol. J Neurosci. 2010;30:9095–102.

38. Daley JT, DeWolfe JL. Sleep, circadian rhythms, and epilepsy. Curr Treat Options Neurol. 2018;20:47.
39. Riquer IA, Bergareche A, Campos V. Sleep disorders in Parkinson disease. Neurologist. 2011;17(6 Suppl 1):S38–42.
40. Thenganatt MA, Frucht SJ. Treatment option for sleep dysfunction in Parkinson's disease. Curr Treat Options Neurol. 2011;13:473–87.
41. Rye DB. Parkinson's disease and RLS: the dopaminergic bridge. Sleep Med. 2004;5:317–28.
42. Mantovani S, Smith SS, Gordon R, O'Sullivan JD. An overview of sleep and circadian dysfunction in Parkinson's disease. J Sleep Res. 2018;27(3):e12673.
43. Stefani A, Högl B. Sleep in Parkinson's disease. Neuropsychopharmacology. 2019:1–8.
44. Amara AW, Wood KH, Joop A, et al. Randomized, controlled trial of exercise on objective and subjective sleep in Parkinson's disease. Mov Disord. 2020;35(6):947–58.
45. Frange C, Filho LHP, Aguilar AC, Coelho FMS. Exercise for "sleep rehabilitation" in Parkinson's disease. Mov Disord. 2020;35(7):1285.
46. Bliwise DL. Review: sleep in normal aging and dementia. Sleep. 1993;16:40–81.
47. Peter-Derex L, Yammine P, Bastuji H, Croisile B. Sleep and Alzheimer's disease. Sleep Med Rev. 2015;19:29–38.
48. Rasmussen MK, Mestre H, Nedergaard M. The glymphatic pathway in neurological disorders. Lancet Neurol. 2018;17(11):1016–24.
49. Arens R, Muzumdar H. Sleep, sleep disordered breathing, and nocturnal hypoventilation in children with neuromuscular diseases. Paediatr Respir Rev. 2010;11(1):24.
50. Benjamin SE. Sleep in patients with neurologic disease. Continuum. 2020;26(4):1016–33.
51. Vgontzas A, Pavlović JM. Sleep disorders and migraine: review of literature and potential pathophysiology mechanisms. Headache. 2018;58(7):1030–9.
52. Ferini-Strambi L, Galbiati A, Combi R. Sleep disorder-related headaches. Neurol Sci. 2019;40(Suppl 1):107–13.
53. Coo IF, Oosterhout WPJ, Willbrink LA, Zwet EW, Ferrari MD, Fronczek R. Chronobiology and sleep in cluster headache. Headache. 2019;59(7):1032–41.
54. Amin FM, Aristeidou S, Baraldi C, Czapinska-Ciepiela EK, et al. The association between migraine and physical exercise. J Headache Pain. 2019;19(1):83.

Sleep and Chronic Pain Interlaced Influences: Guidance to Physiotherapy Practice

Cristina Frange, Alberto Herrero Babiloni, Jacqueline Tu Anh Thu Lam, and Gilles J. Lavigne

1 What Is Pain

Pain was recently redefined by the International Association for Study of Pain (IASP) with more precision since the 1979 definition [1]. Pain is an unpleasant, sensory, and emotional experience in which a difference is clearly made between pain, nociception, and the person who experienced it (Table 1).

The recent joint effort of the IASP and the World Health Organization (WHO) resulted in a classification system for chronic pain syndromes. Nowadays, chronic pain is recognized as a disease, namely "chronic primary pain." Thus, pain can be

C. Frange (✉)
Department of Neurology and Neurosurgery, Escola Paulista de Medicina, Universidade Federal de São Paulo, Sao Paulo, SP, Brazil

Certified in Sleep Physiotherapy by the Brazilian Sleep Society (ABS), and The Brazilian Association of Cardiorespiratory Physiotherapy and Physiotherapy in Intensive Care (ASSOBRAFIR), Sao Paulo, SP, Brazil

World Physiotherapy Network for Health Promotion in Life and Work, Sao Paulo, SP, Brazil

A. H. Babiloni
Division of Experimental Medicine and Faculty of Dentistry, McGill University, Montreal, QC, Canada

Research Center of CIUSSS Nord Ile de Montréal, Sleep and Trauma Unit, Montréal, Montreal, QC, Canada

J. T. A. T. Lam
School of Rehabilitation, Faculty of Medicine, Université de Montréal, Montreal, QC, Canada

G. J. Lavigne
Faculties of Dental Medicine and Medicine, Université de Montréal; Research Center of CIUSSS Nord Ile de Montréal, Sleep and Trauma Unit and CHUM, Stomatology Department, Montreal, QC, Canada

C. Frange, F. M. S. Coelho (eds.), *Sleep Medicine and Physical Therapy*, https://doi.org/10.1007/978-3-030-85074-6_28

legs syndrome, and also 32% with obstructive sleep apnea (32%) [17]. Furthermore, patients with chronic pain experienced greater sleep fragmentation, more awakenings, and movement-related disruptions to sleep (apnea/hypopnea, PLMS) compared to pain-free individuals [17]. In this same investigation, sleep architecture seemed to be less affected by chronic pain, with only NREM 1 duration being longer. Remarkably, NREM 3 sleep, which has a restorative function [18], was not significantly shorter in chronic pain patients, though it did approach statistical significance, and might have been a finding with no statistical relevance but with clinical relevance. Reduction in NREM 3 sleep of chronic pain patients is presented in the literature with mixed results, with fibromyalgia reportedly being associated with reduced NREM 3 sleep [19], and rheumatoid arthritis associated with increased amounts, perhaps as a reparative response to inflammation [18].

2.1 Temporal Associations

On one hand, experimental models indicated that poor sleep, sleep disruption or deprivation, and sleep disturbances could contribute to an altered pain perception by triggering a hyperalgesic state/behaviors, with possible gender-specific effects [20]. On the other hand, it has been shown that besides delaying the onset of sleep and/or interrupting its stages [21], pain is able of causing frequent awakenings, thus disturbing the continuity of sleep [22]. However, the finding of pain disturbing sleep has been more inconsistent over the years [23, 24].

Regarding clinical populations, there are reports on changes of sleep architecture in patients with chronic musculoskeletal pain such as lower sleep efficiency, increased sleep onset, the lower density of slow-wave EEG activity, fewer sleep spindles in EEG activity, more frequent sleep stage shift and unstable deep sleep, and presence of more microarousals related to cyclic alternating patterns (changes in heart rate increase and increase in muscle tone) [25, 26]. In patients with fibromyalgia, for example, the intensity of chronic pain led to a sympathetic over-activity in both states, awake and asleep, due to possible autonomic nervous system dysfunction yet to be confirmed [26]. In longitudinal population studies (the ones that follow the subjects for many years to see if they develop any disease, symptoms, if they improve or not from a specific disease or condition), the severity of pain was related to the incidence or persistence of insomnia [27].

A representative study of the population of the United Kingdom with 4,236 participants over 50 years of age investigated the development of musculoskeletal pain over 10 years. After 10 years, 18.5% of the participants developed generalized chronic pain. Among these, 7.7% had no pain and 24.6% had “some pain” at baseline [28]. In the analysis, the authors found that anxiety and non-restorative sleep were predictors for the development of generalized chronic pain, the latter being the strongest predictor. An investigation of 12,350 women without musculoskeletal pain or physical disabilities demonstrated that after 10 years, almost 3% developed fibromyalgia [29]. The interesting fact lies in the dose-dependent association found in this study between poor sleep quality and the risk for fibromyalgia. This same investigation followed by 18-year found an increased chance of developing chronic pain conditions between 1.5 and 2.2-fold [30]. Interestingly, non-disturbed sleep had a significant effect, reducing in almost fourfold the resolution of multi-site pain (to no pain) [31], indicating the relevance of sleep on predicting the onset and resolution of pain. A large population-based survey with a 17-year follow-up showed that disrupted sleep along with non-specific health complaints were risk factors for the onset of chronic pain and predictive factor for an unfavorable course of chronic pain in the female population [32]. Specifically, disrupted sleep was an independent risk factor (2-fold chance) for the development of chronic pain in initially pain-free women [32].

3 Sleep Disorders and Pain

A recent comprehensive review listed the most likely sleep disorders associated with chronic pain [15]. This included insomnia, sleep apnea, up to sleep bruxism, and rarely, narcolepsy.

Insomnia is another sleep disturbance considered a risk factor for the development of chronic painful conditions. Complaints of insomnia predicted 93% of the risk of new cases of chronic widespread pain in pain-free participants [33] and were considered a risk factor, increasing by 1.4-fold the chance of developing back pain, with no inverse association [34]. In addition, the treatment of insomnia complaints (symptoms) in participants with osteoarthritis and insomnia leads to improvements in pain severity and osteoarthritis symptoms [35]. Taken together this data points out to a uni-directionality of insomnia as a plausible risk factor for the development of chronic pain.

Obstructive sleep apnea (see chapter "Obstructive Sleep Apnea: An Overview" in this volume for more information) is also associated with chronic pain, both in increased prevalence and pain intensity, such as orofacial pain [36], psoriasis, an immune-mediated chronic inflammatory painful disease [37], or fibromyalgia (almost 50%) [38]. Indeed, clinical symptoms are increased, and prognosis and physical function is decreased when patients present both chronic pain and OSA, which may interfere in the rehabilitation of musculoskeletal diseases [39, 40].

Another sleep disorder that has been associated with chronic pain in the orofacial area is sleep bruxism (see chapter "Sleep Bruxism: An Overview" in this volume for more information). The association of awake and sleep bruxism to chronic pain is largely debated, and causality remains to be proven [41]. Indeed, sleep bruxism has been categorized as a risk or contributory factor to dental pain and/or temporomandibular disorders (TMD), although these reports are very variable depending on the subjective or objective nature of the bruxism reports [42]. Indeed, large polysomnographic studies have shown that the distribution of TMD between bruxers and non-bruxers is similar [43], and the occurrence of TMD pain is not associated with the intensity of sleep bruxism [44, 45]. Nevertheless, different subgroups of individuals might present different characteristics that can make them more vulnerable to develop pain or any other comorbidity. For instance, a very recent study using recent machine learning in the general population of Sao Paulo showed that the association between insomnia and sleep bruxism was more prevalent among middle-aged females when compared to other sex and age groups [46]. Although the investigation of the association between sleep bruxism and sleep continuity and disturbances across different phenotypes is active and progressing [43, 47], given the important link between sleep and chronic pain, more studies accounting for chronic pain as well are needed.

Patients with narcolepsy types 1 and 2 (with and without cataplexy, respectively) had a high prevalence of chronic pain and fatigue, increased symptoms of comorbid depression and anxiety, and negatively impacted quality of life. Both types presented a higher frequency of chronic pain: 84.8% for type 1 and 75.7% for type 2; 42.4% of all patients presented daily pain compared to controls regardless of its type; and surprisingly increased risk factor for pain, such as almost 21-fold in type 1, and 12-fold in type 2, compared with controls [48].

In longitudinal investigations, poor sleep has also been found as a predictor for next-day pain. A sequential relationship between sleep and pain was found in an analysis of 30-day self-reported ratings of pain and sleep in participants with fibromyalgia: a night of poor sleep was followed by a painful day, and a more painful day preceded a night of poorer sleep [49]. In postmenopausal women, the co-existence of insomnia and chronic musculoskeletal pain resulted in greater pain intensity and alterations in sleep homeostasis [50]. In this sense, sleep disorders should be considered as possible risk factors for the onset and/or worsening of musculoskeletal pain and treated when treating a patient with pain.

In summary, individuals suffering from sleep disturbances are at elevated risk for the development of pain over time frames from 1 year to 28 years [51–53]. Together, all these investigations from different groups and countries suggest that sleep impairments contribute exponentially to the development of somatic symptoms such as chronic pain in some time-point.

4 Mechanisms Involved in Sleep and Pain Relation

There are many hypotheses on the mechanisms of sleep and pain interaction. One hypothesis is that brain structures involved in the generation and maintenance of sleep are also involved in pain modulation, thus providing a neurobiological substrate for this relationship. For example, animal studies have shown that the periaqueductal gray matter of the midbrain is responsible for the modulation of both sleeps [54] and pain [55, 56]. In humans, sleep and pain processing often share afferent circuits such as the parabrachial-amygdala and parabrachial hypothalamic pathways [57]. Likewise, the thalamus is associated with excitation and the processing of nociceptive stimuli sent to the cerebral cortex in animals [58].

Another hypothesis, derived from animal research, is the pain-on and pain-off neurons' concept. These neurons, which are situated in the *nucleus raphe Magnus*, respectively, facilitate and inhibit nociceptive impulses to thalamocortical pathways and are influenced by the wake-sleep cycle: inhibitory pain-off neurons are activated during NREM N3 sleep, while excitatory pain-on neurons are activated during wakefulness [22].

Moreover, recent human neuroimaging studies have shown that acute sleep deprivation amplifies pain reactivity in the primary somatosensory cortex and that the degree of this amplification predicts the expansion of experienced pain across individuals. However, sleep deprivation seems to blunt pain reactivity in higher-order valuation and decision-making regions of the striatum and insular cortex, which are brain areas also involved in pain modulation [59]. In addition, sleep disruption increased reward-related connectivity between the *nucleus accumbens* and the anterior midcingulate cortex at pain onset [60], suggesting among others that sleep disruption could affect pain via attention and reward mechanisms.

Other possible underpinnings of the interaction formed between sleep and pain problems are the increase in distinct inflammatory markers potentially leading to a generalized inflammatory state, the influence and mediation of mood disorders (e.g., anxiety, depression) and affect issues, and the alteration of endogenous substances apparently related with both sleep and pain processes such as dopamine, or perhaps melatonin, vitamin D, or orexin/hypocretin as recently summarized in a comprehensive review [7].

Other hypothesized mechanisms involved in sleep and pain relation described neuronal and non-neuronal components such as (i) the opioid system (inadequate sleep deteriorates the function of the opioid antinociceptive system); (ii) the monoaminergic system (serotonin is known to promote wakefulness and to inhibit REM sleep [61] and is involved in both sleep-wake and pain control); (iii) the orexinergic system (also known as hypocretin, orexin neurons are active during wake and nearly silent during sleep, and orexin deficiency is associated with narcolepsy, and are also involved in nociception, specifically pain transmission and modulation, found in spinal dorsal horn); (iv) the immune system (an upregulation of inflammatory mediators such as cytokines and prostaglandins is observed both in pain conditions and in sleep impairments); (v) the pineal melatonin system (having innumerable functions, including sleep promoting effect [62], anti-inflammatory and analgesic, improving endogenous pain inhibition); (vi) the endocannabinoid system (modulation of pain and sleep and a possible treatment which still needs more research); (vii) the hypothalamus-pituitary-adrenal axis (HPA, dysregulations of HPA axis responses can be a marker for comorbid pain and sleep deficiency); (viii) the adenosine signaling (which has sleep-regulatory and sleep-promoting properties, and its increased activity is related to increased pain); (ix) the nitric oxide signaling (contributes in the homeostatic regulation of sleep and wakefulness, as nitric oxide is increased during sleep deprivation (and followed by an increase in adenosine), and together, nitric oxide and adenosine regulate sleep pressure and also are an important mediator of pain in periaqueductal gray matter area), among others [24].

is essential to understand that their management should be conducted by the sleep physician.

Therefore, after adequate indications, the PT will proceed to individualized treatment of the pain condition. One important point to remember is that the first-line choice for chronic pain and sleep treatment is the *active* involvement of the patient, as a partner. To reach such, a variety of complementary approaches and techniques are available, including education and self-management (e.g., neuroscience pain education or cognitive behavior therapy for pain (CBT-P)); therapeutic exercise including strengthening-coordination-function, activities of daily living, use of proper body mechanics (motor control), physical activity, and exercise (choose type, duration, frequency, and intensity), knowing the effects of exercise on both sleep and pain to induce hypoalgesia (e.g., aerobic training, resistance exercise, stretching, isometric exercises, and mind-based exercises); passive techniques (manual therapy such as mobilizations, manipulations, soft tissue massage, muscle energy, traditional massage, and Rolfing; movement therapies such as Feldenkrais, proprioceptive neuromuscular facilitation, and global postural reeducation; *watsu* (a form of hydrotherapy which encompasses stretches, massages, and acupressure in warm water used for deep relaxation and passive exercises; and relaxation); and electrotherapeutic and dry needling modalities (Table 2). Note that all chronic pain conditions cited have sleep impairments such as non-refreshing sleep, fragmented sleep, or disturbances.

In addition, sleep hygiene tips and cognitive behavior therapy for insomnia and other sleep disturbances (please have a look at chapter "Optimizing Behavior Strategies for Sleep" of this book) can be added, in order to improve sleep and to make the patient have knowledge and action in the treatment. Sleep hygiene is always a subject that should be discussed in PTs treatment. Furthermore, sleep positioning should be addressed for any sort of musculoskeletal pain; the positioning can always be improved (see chapter "Sleep Ergonomics" of this book).

The restoration of adequate sleep is essential to avoid the exacerbation of painful symptoms. In this sense, we encourage PTs to look at sleep habits/routine and symptoms in patients who seek assistance.

This is complex work to be done and may take a longer time. In order to maximize efficiency and manage more comprehensively the patient with sleep disturbance and chronic pain, an interdisciplinary approach where PT collaborates with other health professionals such as psychologists, dentists, pharmacists, and physicians is essential [7, 72].

Of importance, we need to reiterate that adequate acute pain treatment can prevent the development of chronic pain, and poor sleep to insomnia and/or exacerbation of concomitant sleep disorders. Improving patient quality of life and satisfaction with care, as well as enhancing clinical resource management and reducing long-term costs, remains one of the major health decision-makers' objectives.

Table 2 Summary of physical therapy techniques in the management of chronic primary and secondary pain, including examples of pain condition, qualitative level of evidence and references. (Note that level of evidence is low to modest for most)

PT techniques		Chronic pain condition	Level of evidence	References
Education and self-management	Neuroscience pain education	Musculoskeletal pain	Strong	Watson et al. [73]
	Biopsychosocial approach	Chronic pain	Strong (short- and medium-term) Low (long-term)	Gianola et al. [74]
		Subacute low back pain	Very low–low	Marin et al. [75]
Physical activity and exercise	Aerobic training	Knee osteoarthritis	Strong	Loew et al. [76]
		Rheumatoid arthritis	Strong	Scarvel and Elkins [77]; Hurkmans et al. [78]
	Resistance exercise/ strengthening	Fibromyalgia	Strong	Busch et al. [79]
		Mechanical neck disorders	Low	Gross et al. [80]
		Nonspecific neck pain	Strong	Sihawong et al. [106]
		Nonspecific shoulder pain	Strong	van den Dolder et al. [90]
		Patelofemoral pain syndrome	Strong (short-term), low (long-term)	Searle et al. [109]
	Stabilization exercises	Nonspecific low back pain	Strong	Smith et al. [107]
	Isometric exercises	Mechanical neck disorders	Moderate	Gross et al. [80]
	Pilates	Nonspecific back pain	Strong	Patti et al. [81]
		Nonspecific low back pain	Very low–moderate	Yamato et al. [82]
	Meditative movement-based exercises (Yoga, Tai Chi, Qigong)	Fibromyalgia (yoga)	Strong	Langhorst et al. [83]
		Fibromyalgia (qigong)	Low	Lauche et al. [84]
		Nonspecific low back pain	Very low–moderate	Nascimento et al. [85]
	Aquatic exercises	Musculoskeletal conditions	Strong, but moderate effects	Barker et al. [86]
		Fibromyalgia	Low–moderate	Bidonde et al. [87]
		Knee and hip osteoarthritis	Strong	Bartels et al. [88]
	Motor control exercises	Nonspecific low back pain	Very low–moderate	Saragiotto et al. [89]

(continued)

Table 2 (continued)

PT techniques		Chronic pain condition	Level of evidence	References
Manual therapy	Soft tissue massage	Nonspecific shoulder pain	Strong	van den Dolder et al. [90]
		Post-operative cardiopulmonary surgery	Very low–moderate	Nerbass et al. [91]
	Manipulation or mobilization	Nonspecific low back pain	Very low–moderate	Nascimento et al. [85]
	Trigger point	Chronic non-cancer pain	Very low	Denneny et al. [92]
	McKenzie Method	Low back pain	Moderate–strong	Lam et al. [93]
Electrotherapeutic modalities	Ultrasound	Musculoskeletal pain conditions	Insufficient evidence	Wu et al. [94]
		Knee osteoarthritis	Strong	Wu et al. [94]
		Shoulder calcific tendinosis	Strong	Ebenbichler et al. [108]
	Phonophoresis	Musculoskeletal pain conditions	Low	Watson [97]
		Knee osteoarthritis	Low (not more effective than ultrasound alone)	Wu et al. (94)
	Photobiomodulation (Laser)	Joint pain	Strong	Bjordal et al. [95]
		Knee osteoarthritis	Strong	Bjordal et al. [96]
		Myofascial trigger points	Strong	Law et al. [98]
	Interferential current		Effective for a temporary decrease of pain	Fernando [99]
	Transcutaneous electrical nerve stimulation (TENS)	Low back pain	Inconclusive	Resende et al. [100]
		Central pain in multiple sclerosis	Moderate	Sawant et al. [101]
		Painful diabetic neuropathy	Strong	Stein et al. [102]
		Neuropathic pain	Very low–moderate	Jin et al. [103]
Needling modalities	Dry needling	Myofascial pain syndrome	Very low–moderate	Fogelman et al. [104]
	Acupuncture	Nonspecific low back pain	Very low–moderate	Nascimento et al. [85]
		Musculoskeletal pain	Very low–moderate	Kelly et al. [105]

References

1. International Association for the Study of Pain, P.t. [cited December, 12th 2020]. Available from: https://www.iasp-pain.org/Education/Content.aspx?ItemNumber=1698#Pain.
2. Treede RD, et al. Chronic pain as a symptom or a disease: the IASP Classification of Chronic Pain for the International Classification of Diseases (ICD-11). Pain. 2019;160(1):19–27.
3. Flor H, Turk D. Chronic pain: an integrated biobehavioral approach. Seattle: IASP Press; 2011.
4. Moldofsky H, et al. Musculosketal symptoms and non-REM sleep disturbance in patients with "fibrositis syndrome" and healthy subjects. Psychosom Med. 1975;37(4):341–51.
5. Wolfe F, et al. Fibromyalgia criteria and severity scales for clinical and epidemiological studies: a modification of the ACR Preliminary Diagnostic Criteria for Fibromyalgia. J Rheumatol. 2011;38(6):1113–22.
6. Roizenblatt M, et al. Pain-related diseases and sleep disorders. Braz J Med Biol Res. 2012;45(9):792–8.
7. Herrero Babiloni A, et al. Sleep and pain: recent insights, mechanisms, and future directions in the investigation of this relationship. J Neural Transm (Vienna). 2020;127(4):647–60.
8. Creed F. A review of the incidence and risk factors for fibromyalgia and chronic widespread pain in population-based studies. Pain. 2020;161(6):1169–76.
9. de Rooij A, et al. Factors associated with sleep quality in patients with chronic widespread pain attending multidisciplinary treatment. Pain Pract. 2020;20(5):471–9.
10. Knutson K. Sleep and pain: summary of the 2015 Sleep in America Poll. Sleep Health. 2015;1(2):85.
11. Hirshkowitz M, et al. National Sleep Foundation's sleep time duration recommendations: methodology and results summary. Sleep Health. 2015;1(1):40–3.
12. Edwards RR, et al. Duration of sleep contributes to next-day pain report in the general population. Pain. 2008;137(1):202–7.
13. Morin CM, Gibson D, Wade J. Self-reported sleep and mood disturbance in chronic pain patients. Clin J Pain. 1998;14(4):311–4.
14. Sivertsen B, et al. The epidemiology of insomnia: associations with physical and mental health. The HUNT-2 study. J Psychosom Res. 2009;67(2):109–16.
15. Andersen ML, et al. Sleep disturbance and pain: a tale of two common problems. Chest. 2018;154(5):1249–59.
16. Ohayon MM. Relationship between chronic painful physical condition and insomnia. J Psychiatr Res. 2005;39(2):151–9.
17. Mathias JL, Cant ML, Burke ALJ. Sleep disturbances and sleep disorders in adults living with chronic pain: a meta-analysis. Sleep Med. 2018;52:198–210.
18. Drewes AM, et al. A longitudinal study of clinical symptoms and sleep parameters in rheumatoid arthritis. Rheumatology (Oxford). 2000;39(11):1287–9.
19. Wu YL, et al. Sleep disturbances in fibromyalgia: a meta-analysis of case-control studies. J Psychosom Res. 2017;96:89–97.
20. Smith BH, et al. The IASP classification of chronic pain for ICD-11: applicability in primary care. Pain. 2019;160(1):83–7.
21. Finan PH, Goodin BR, Smith MT. The association of sleep and pain: an update and a path forward. J Pain. 2013;14(12):1539–52.
22. Foo H, Mason P. Brainstem modulation of pain during sleep and waking. Sleep Med Rev. 2003;7(2):145–54.
23. Herrero Babiloni A, et al. Towards the endotyping of the sleep-pain interaction: a topical review on multitarget strategies based on phenotypic vulnerabilities and putative pathways. Pain. 2021;162(5):1281–8.
24. Haack M, et al. Sleep deficiency and chronic pain: potential underlying mechanisms and clinical implications. Neuropsychopharmacology. 2020;45(1):205–16.
25. Lavigne G, Smith M, Denis R, Zucconi M. Pain and sleep. In: Kryger HM, Roth T, Dement WC, editors. Principles and practice of sleep medicine. St. Louis: Elsevier Saunders; 2017. p. 1442–51.

74. Gianola S, Andreano A, Castellini G, Moja L, Valsecchi MG. Multidisciplinary biopsychosocial rehabilitation for chronic low back pain: the need to present minimal important differences units in meta-analyses. Health Qual Life Outcomes. 2018;16(1):91.
75. Marin TJ, Van Eerd D, Irvin E, et al. Multidisciplinary biopsychosocial rehabilitation for subacute low back pain. Cochrane Database Syst Rev. 2017;6(6):CD002193.
76. Loew L, Brosseau L, Wells GA, et al. Ottawa panel evidence-based clinical practice guidelines for aerobic walking programs in the management of osteoarthritis. Arch Phys Med Rehabil. 2012;93(7):1269–85.
77. Scarvell J, Elkins MR. Aerobic exercise is beneficial for people with rheumatoid arthritis. Br J Sports Med. 2011;45(12):1008–9.
78. Hurkmans E, van der Giesen FJ, Vliet Vlieland TP, Schoones J, Van den Ende EC. Dynamic exercise programs (aerobic capacity and/or muscle strength training) in patients with rheumatoid arthritis. Cochrane Database Syst Rev. 2009;2009(4):CD006853.
79. Busch AJ, Barber KA, Overend TJ, Peloso PM, Schachter CL. Exercise for treating fibromyalgia syndrome. Cochrane Database Syst Rev. 2007;(4):CD003786. Published 2007.
80. Gross A, Kay TM, Paquin JP, et al. Exercises for mechanical neck disorders. Cochrane Database Syst Rev. 2015;1:CD004250.
81. Patti A, Bianco A, Paoli A, et al. Effects of Pilates exercise programs in people with chronic low back pain: a systematic review. Medicine (Baltimore). 2015;94(4):e383.
82. Yamato TP, Maher CG, Saragiotto BT, et al. Pilates for low back pain. Cochrane Database Syst Rev. 2015;(7):CD010265.
83. Langhorst J, Klose P, Dobos GJ, Bernardy K, Hauser W. Efficacy and safety of meditative movement therapies in fibromyalgia syndrome: a systematic review and meta-analysis of randomized controlled trials. Rheumatol Int. 2013;33:193–207.
84. Lauche R, Cramer H, Dobos G, Langhorst J, Schmidt S. A systematic review and meta-analysis of mindfulness-based stress reduction for the fibromyalgia syndrome. J Psychosom Res. 2013;75(6):500–10.
85. Nascimento PRCD, Costa LOP, Araujo AC, Poitras S, Bilodeau M. Effectiveness of interventions for non-specific low back pain in older adults. A systematic review and meta-analysis. Physiotherapy. 2019;105(2):147–62.
86. Barker AL, Talevski J, Morello RT, Brand CA, Rahmann AE, Urquhart DM. Effectiveness of aquatic exercise for musculoskeletal conditions: a meta-analysis. Arch Phys Med Rehabil. 2014;95(9):1776–86.
87. Bidonde J, Busch AJ, Webber SC, et al. Aquatic exercise training for fibromyalgia. Cochrane Database Syst Rev. 2014;(10):CD011336.
88. Bartels EM, Lund H, Hagen KB, Dagfinrud H, Christensen R, Danneskiold-Samsøe B. Aquatic exercise for the treatment of knee and hip osteoarthritis. Cochrane Database Syst Rev. 2007;(4):CD005523.
89. Saragiotto BT, Maher CG, Yamato TP, et al. Motor control exercise for chronic non-specific low-back pain. Cochrane Database Syst Rev. 2016;(1):CD012004.
90. van den Dolder PA, Ferreira PH, Refshauge KM. Effectiveness of soft tissue massage and exercise for the treatment of non-specific shoulder pain: a systematic review with meta-analysis. Br J Sports Med. 2014;48(16):1216–26.
91. Nerbass FB, Feltrim MIZ, Souza SA, Ykeda DS, Lorenzi-Filho G. Effects of massage therapy on sleep quality after coronary artery bypass graft surgery. Clinics. 2010;65(11):1105–10.
92. Denneny D, Frawley HC, Petersen K, et al. Trigger Point Manual Therapy for the Treatment of Chronic Noncancer Pain in Adults: A Systematic Review and Meta-analysis. Arch Phys Med Rehabil. 2019;100(3):562–77.
93. Lam OT, Strenger DM, Chan-Fee M, Pham PT, Preuss RA, Robbins SM. Effectiveness of the McKenzie Method of Mechanical Diagnosis and Therapy for Treating Low Back Pain: Literature Review With Meta-analysis. J Orthop Sports Phys Ther. 2018;48(6):476–90. https://doi.org/10.2519/jospt.2018.7562.

94. Wu Y, Zhu S, Lv Z, et al. Effects of therapeutic ultrasound for knee osteoarthritis: a systematic review and meta-analysis. Clin Rehabil. 2019;33(12):1863–75.
95. Bjordal JM, Couppé C, Chow RT, Tunér J, Ljunggren EA. A systematic review of low level laser therapy with locationspecific doses for pain from chronic joint disorders. Aust J Physiother. 2003;49(2):107–16.
96. Bjordal JM, Johnson MI, Lopes-Martins RA, Bogen B, Chow R, Ljunggren AE. Short-term efficacy of physical interventions in osteoarthritic knee pain. A systematic review and meta-analysis of randomised placebo-controlled trials. BMC Musculoskelet Disord. 2007;8:51.
97. Watson T. Physiology of pain. Orthopaedic Physical Therapy Clinics of North America. Pain Management. 1995;4:423–42.
98. Law D, McDonough S, Bleakley C, Baxter GD, Tumilty S. Laser acupuncture for treating musculoskeletal pain: a systematic review with meta-analysis. J Acupunct Meridian Stud. 2015;8(1):2–16.
99. Fernando C. Physical therapy and pain management. In Weiner, RS (Ed.), Pain management: A practical guide for clinicians. 6th ed., Boca Raton, FL:CRC Press; pp. 739–46, 2002.
100. Resende L, Merriwether E, Rampazo ÉP, et al. Meta-analysis of transcutaneous electrical nerve stimulation for relief of spinal pain. Eur J Pain. 2018;22(4):663–78.
101. Sawant A, Dadurka K, Overend T, Kremenchutzky M. Systematic review of efficacy of TENS for management of central pain in people with multiple sclerosis. Mult Scler Relat Disord. 2015;4(3):219–27.
102. Stein C, Eibel B, Sbruzzi G, Lago PD, Plentz RD. Electrical stimulation and electromagnetic field use in patients with diabetic neuropathy: systematic review and meta-analysis. Braz J Phys Ther. 2013;17(2):93–104.
103. Jin Y, Xing G, Li G, et al. High Frequency Repetitive Transcranial Magnetic Stimulation Therapy For Chronic Neuropathic Pain: A Meta-analysis. Pain Physician. 2015;18(6):E1029–E1046.
104. Fogelman Y, Kent J. Efficacy of dry needling for treatment of myofascial pain syndrome. J Back Musculoskelet Rehabil. 2015;28(1):173–79.
105. Kelly RB, Willis J. Acupuncture for Pain. Am Fam Physician. 2019;100(2):89–96.
106. Sihawong R, Janwantanakul P, Sitthipornvorakul E, Pensri P. Exercise therapy for office workers with nonspecific neck pain: a systematic review. J Manipulative Physiol Ther. 2011;34(1):62–71.
107. Smith BE, Littlewood C, May S. An update of stabilisation exercises for low back pain: a systematic review with meta-analysis. BMC Musculoskelet Disord. 2014;15:416.
108. Ebenbichler GR, Erdogmus CB, Resch KL, et al. Ultrasound therapy for calcific tendinitis of the shoulder. N Engl J Med. 1999;340(20):1533–38.
109. Searle A, Spink M, Ho A, Chuter V. Exercise interventions for the treatment of chronic low back pain: a systematic review and meta-analysis of randomised controlled trials. Clin Rehabil. 2015;29(12):1155–67.

Part V
Physiotherapeutic Resources to Improve Sleep

requiring vasodilation of the distal extremities and increasing peripheral blood flow [1, 2]. Thus, an exercised-induced increase in body temperature could promote sleep onset through the heat dissipation mechanism [3].

Research on the effect of aerobic exercise on body temperature has shown divergent results such as positive changes in slow-wave sleep or lack of changes, highlighting the time of day and the intensity of aerobic exercise as important factors that may lead to different effects on body temperature and, consequently, on sleep [4–6].

1.2 Repair and Restoration

Two theories regarding the purpose of sleep, the energy conservation and repair and restoration theories, postulate that sleep is a way to conserve or restore the metabolically active tissues that are impacted by exercise. Both of these theories assume that increases in energy expenditure would be related to increases in the duration of sleep and slow-wave sleep; therefore, the exercise would represent a stimulus for the depletion of energy reserves, playing a significant role in sleep [7]. These theories are based on homeostatic mechanisms of sleep regulation with adenosine being strongly related to sleep drive [8]. Studies [9, 10] with protocols of moderate- to high-intensity aerobic exercise have observed increases of 2.9% in slow-wave sleep duration in humans after high-intensity exercise and in adenosine concentrations measured after high-intensity exercise in animal models [9, 11].

1.3 Anxiolytic and Antidepressant Role of Exercise

Sleep disorders are closely associated with mental health conditions [12–14]. Anxiety and depression are commonly observed in patients with sleep problems and are risk factors for the development of insomnia; relatedly, insomnia is a risk factor for the development of anxiety and depression, highlighting the bidirectionality between insomnia and anxiety and depression [15]. Thus, considering the beneficial effect of exercise on anxiety and depression [16], the antidepressant and anxiolytic role of exercise may serve as a potential mechanism to reduce sleep disorder severity and improve sleep quality.

1.4 Changes in the Circadian System

Exercise performed at different times of day may influence the timing of the circadian system, advancing or delaying the sleep/wake cycle. Considering that several sleep disorders are related to circadian function, in this hypothesis, exercise could modulate the timing of the circadian system, advancing when performed during the day or delaying when performed in the evening [17]. Thus, exercise could be an external facilitator of circadian adaptation in people who need to alter the timing of the sleep-wake cycle, such as travelers and night workers [18].

1.5 Impact of Exercise on Sleep Quality

Although sleep quality is an indicator widely used by the general population to assess sleep in clinical practice and in laboratory settings, its concept is quite broad and involves several parameters. There is still no consensus on what constitutes good sleep quality with its assessments generally occurring in a self-reported manner [19]. Some variables (e.g., latency, number of arousals, arousals after sleep onset, efficiency) can be considered indicators of sleep quality [20]. Although research reports that exercise improves sleep quality [21–23], there is a paucity of studies evaluating the isolated effect of interventions, with sleep quality often being assessed in conjunction with other sleep parameters in a variety of populations and conditions.

For example, a meta-analysis [24] with 6 studies and 305 adults examined the effect of interventions between 10 and 16 weeks with moderate-intensity aerobic exercise and/or strength training on sleep quality assessed with the Pittsburgh Sleep Quality Index (PSQI). In addition to an improvement in overall sleep quality, they observed decreases in sleep latency and sleeping pill usage.

Another systematic review [25] evaluated the acute and chronic effects of strength training alone and combined with aerobic training on the sleep quality of adults. The authors observed that combined training (aerobic training plus strength training) promoted better results in the subjective parameters of sleep quality, primarily assessed using the PSQI. Despite the interesting results, the methodological differences between studies included in this review do not allow us to indicate how combined training was superior in improving sleep quality when compared to aerobic or strength training performed alone.

The results of clinical trials similarly have demonstrated heterogeneity in findings according to the population studied. For example, in a sample of adolescents, 12 weeks of moderate-intensity aerobic and strength training improved sleep quality by 67%, sleep efficiency by 7.6%, and sleep duration by 64 minutes [23].

In a sample of inactive older adults, Jurado-Fasoli et al. [21] evaluated the effect of 12 weeks of exercise training on PSQI-assessed sleep quality. They observed sleep quality improvements in the group that practiced physical activity according to the recommendations of the World Health Organization (34% reduction in PSQI score), in the group that performed high-intensity interval training (34% reduction), and in the group that performed high-intensity interval training plus whole-body electrostimulation (40% reduction) [21]. In another study, strength training performed for 12 weeks significantly improved the sleep quality of patients with breast cancer [26]. On the other hand, in a sample of middle-aged women, improvements in PSQI after

4 months of practicing yoga and walking exercise were not observed [27]. Finally, in a robust review recently published by Kline and colleagues, it was observed that longer bouts of exercise training resulted in better sleep quality outcomes [28].

Thus, considering the findings presented, exercise training can be recommended as a tool for improving sleep quality. Despite this recommendation, due to the methodological limitations, it remains challenging to establish which type (e.g., aerobic or strength training), intensity (e.g., moderate, or high), or duration (e.g., 2, 6, or 12 weeks) would promote better responses in the sleep quality in various populations. Thus, the available evidence does not support the prerogative that evening exercise leads to poor sleep quality.

2 Exercise Timing

Although exercise performed in the evening is sometimes discouraged due to concerns that it may disrupt sleep, little evidence corroborates this assumption [29, 30]. Experimental studies have not found negative effects of exercising in the evening [10, 31]. Based on data from the National Sleep Foundation's "Sleep in America" poll, Buman et al. evaluated respondents' sleep according to the time of day of exercise; they found that most participants believed that their sleep was of equal or better quality (97%) and longer duration (98%) on the days they exercised in the evening (i.e., <4 h before bedtime) compared to the days they did not exercise [32]. The paucity of negative effects of evening exercise on sleep was also evidenced in a recent meta-analysis by Stutz et al. [33]; across 23 studies, exercise in the evening (i.e., <4 h before bedtime) promoted an increase of 7.7 minutes in rapid eye movement latency, an increase of 1.3% in slow-wave sleep, and a decrease of 1.0% in stage 1 sleep.

3 Effect of Exercise Training on Sleep Disorders

The most evident literature on the effect of exercise on sleep disorders has been observed among people with sleep-related breathing disorders, insomnia, or daytime sleepiness resulting from these conditions. Although the small evidence base does not provide an indication of the best type of exercise for each situation, current data suggest that there is an important role of exercise in the management of these disorders.

3.1 Obstructive Sleep Apnea

Among sleep-related breathing disorders, obstructive sleep apnea (OSA) is an important public health problem associated with hypersomnia, increased cardiovascular mortality, and metabolic dysfunction [34]. Characterized by recurrent episodes of total or partial upper airway obstruction and influenced by genetic and environmental factors [35], the prevalence of OSA in Brazil is estimated at 33% of the adult population, with men showing higher prevalence than women (40.6% against 26.1%, respectively) [36].

In epidemiological research, the literature indicates that exercise has been associated with a lower risk of developing both mild and moderate to severe OSA [35, 37]. For example, in a study with more than 14,000 participants, Murillo et al. [38] observed in a cross-sectional study that 150 minutes per week of moderate- to vigorous-intensity physical activity was associated with 24% lower odds of having mild or moderate to severe OSA [38]. Corroborating these data, da Silva and colleagues [39] studied 5453 men and women and observed that adults who practiced structured exercise had 23% and 34% lower odds of having moderate or severe forms of OSA, respectively, while those who performed occupational activities (based on the employee's reported significant engagement in standing, walking, sitting, lifting, carrying, pushing, and pulling at work) did not show any reduction in the odds of having OSA [37]. Despite these suggestive findings, the methodological designs of these investigations did not allow the establishment of cause-and-effect relationships on the role of exercise training in the treatment of OSA.

Although no study has focused on the effect of an acute bout of exercise on OSA, several studies have investigated the effect of long-term exercise training [40–45]. Some systematic reviews [22, 46, 47] observed that exercise intervention lasting between 4 and 16 weeks with a frequency between 3 and 6 days a week and between 25 and 60 minutes per training session resulted in a reduction of approximately 30% in OSA severity despite no effect on total body weight. In addition, exercise training promoted a positive effect in aspects associated with daily functioning, such as a 13% improvement in quality of life and a 16.5% reduction in daytime sleepiness [22].

Aerobic exercise training [42, 44, 48–50] and combined training (i.e., aerobic exercise plus strength exercise) [40, 43, 45, 50] have been the most investigated types of exercise. For example, in a seminal work [48] of 6 months duration with moderate-intensity aerobic training, a 50% reduction in OSA severity was observed. Similar results were found in a study by Servantes et al. [50], in which an OSA severity reduction of 40% was observed with a 12-week aerobic training plus strength training intervention. On the other hand, increased exercise intensity does not seem to have additional effects in the improvement of OSA, as modest OSA severity reduction in the order of 24% was observed in adults with severe OSA after 12 weeks of high-intensity interval training [44].

On the other hand, combined training (i.e., when the intervention is composed of aerobic exercise plus strength exercise) has also had a positive impact on reducing OSA severity. For example, a 12-week trial that featured 150 minutes per week of moderate-intensity aerobic training and 2 days per week of moderate-intensity strength training [40] promoted a reduction in OSA severity of approximately 25% in adults with moderate OSA.

Although the results point to a clear benefit of exercise for reducing OSA severity, the underlying mechanisms of the relationship between OSA and exercise

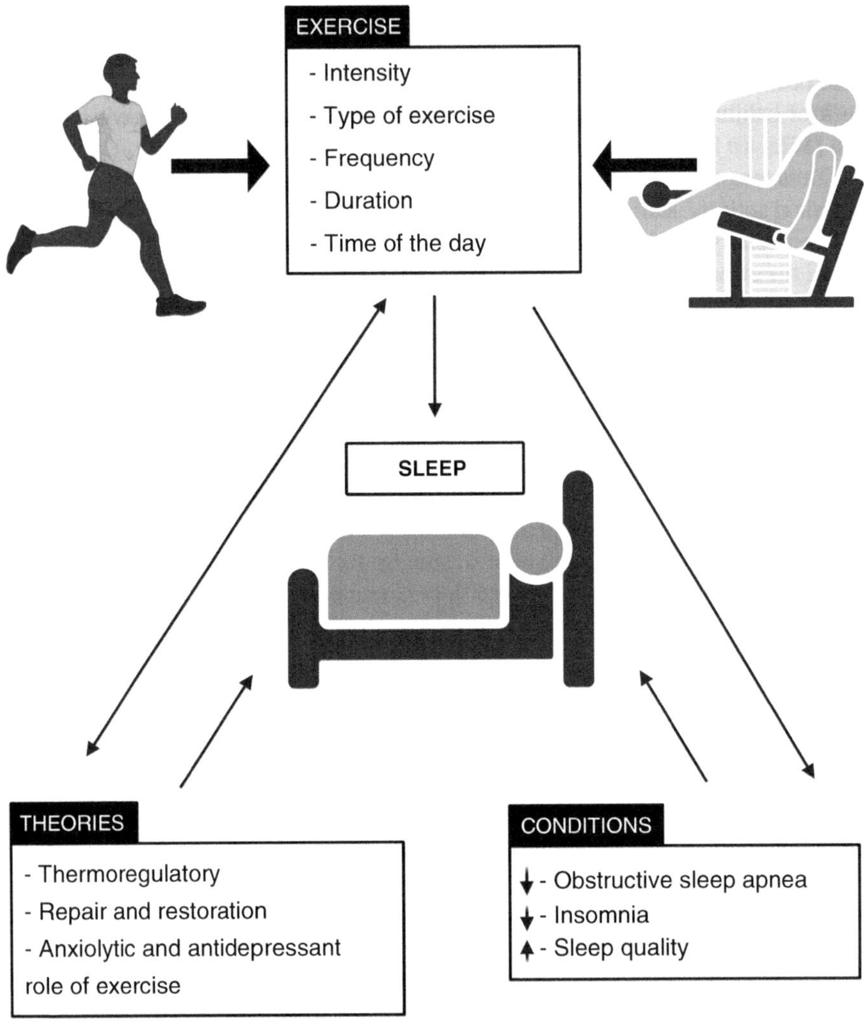

Fig. 1 Exercise training impacts sleep in those with and without sleep problems. In addition, it is known that conditions such as obstructive sleep apnea, insomnia, and poor sleep quality can be improved by exercise. Many different mechanisms could potentially explain how exercise promotes sleep. However, considering that there are several factors involved in the prescription of exercise (e.g., intensity, duration, frequency, mode, timing), it remains unclear how these various factors influence the effect of exercise on sleep

References

1. Horne JA, Staff LH. Exercise and sleep: body-heating effects. Sleep. 1983;6(1):36–46. https://doi.org/10.1093/sleep/6.1.36.
2. Rogers NL, Bowes J, Lushington K, Dawson D. Thermoregulatory changes around the time of sleep onset. Physiol Behav. 2007;90(4):643–7. https://doi.org/10.1016/j.physbeh.2006.11.018.
3. Raymann RJ, Swaab DF, Van Someren EJ. Skin temperature and sleep-onset latency: changes with age and insomnia. Physiol Behav. 2007;90(2–3):257–66. https://doi.org/10.1016/j.physbeh.2006.09.008.
4. Miller DJ, Sargent C, Roach GD, Scanlan AT, Vincent GE, Lastella M. Moderate-intensity exercise performed in the evening does not impair sleep in healthy males. Eur J Sport Sci. 2020;20(1):80–9. https://doi.org/10.1080/17461391.2019.1611934.
5. O'Connor PJ, Breus MJ, Youngstedt SD. Exercise-induced increase in core temperature does not disrupt a behavioral measure of sleep. Physiol Behav. 1998;64(3):213–7. https://doi.org/10.1016/s0031-9384(98)00049-3.
6. Thomas C, Jones H, Whitworth-Turner C, Louis J. High-intensity exercise in the evening does not disrupt sleep in endurance runners. Eur J Appl Physiol. 2020;120(2):359–68. https://doi.org/10.1007/s00421-019-04280-w.
7. Driver HS, Taylor SR. Exercise and sleep. Sleep Med Rev. 2000;4(4):387–402. https://doi.org/10.1053/smrv.2000.0110.
8. Landolt HP. Sleep homeostasis: a role for adenosine in humans? Biochem Pharmacol. 2008;75(11):2070–9. https://doi.org/10.1016/j.bcp.2008.02.024.
9. Dworak M, Diel P, Voss S, Hollmann W, Struder HK. Intense exercise increases adenosine concentrations in rat brain: implications for a homeostatic sleep drive. Neuroscience. 2007;150(4):789–95. https://doi.org/10.1016/j.neuroscience.2007.09.062.
10. Dworak M, Wiater A, Alfer D, Stephan E, Hollmann W, Struder HK. Increased slow wave sleep and reduced stage 2 sleep in children depending on exercise intensity. Sleep Med. 2008;9(3):266–72. https://doi.org/10.1016/j.sleep.2007.04.017.
11. Youngstedt SD, O'Connor PJ, Crabbe JB, Dishman RK. The influence of acute exercise on sleep following high caffeine intake. Physiol Behav. 2000;68(4):563–70. https://doi.org/10.1016/s0031-9384(99)00213-9.
12. Arenas DJ, Thomas A, Wang J, DeLisser HM. A systematic review and meta-analysis of depression, anxiety, and sleep disorders in US adults with food insecurity. J Gen Intern Med. 2019;34(12):2874–82. https://doi.org/10.1007/s11606-019-05202-4.
13. Kalmbach DA, Anderson JR, Drake CL. The impact of stress on sleep: pathogenic sleep reactivity as a vulnerability to insomnia and circadian disorders. J Sleep Res. 2018;27(6):e12710. https://doi.org/10.1111/jsr.12710.
14. Riemann D, Baglioni C, Bassetti C, Bjorvatn B, Dolenc Groselj L, Ellis JG, et al. European guideline for the diagnosis and treatment of insomnia. J Sleep Res. 2017;26(6):675–700. https://doi.org/10.1111/jsr.12594.
15. Alvaro PK, Roberts RM, Harris JK. A systematic review assessing bidirectionality between sleep disturbances, anxiety, and depression. Sleep. 2013;36(7):1059–68. https://doi.org/10.5665/sleep.2810.
16. Hallgren M, Herring MP, Owen N, Dunstan D, Ekblom O, Helgadottir B, et al. Exercise, physical activity, and sedentary behavior in the treatment of depression: broadening the scientific perspectives and clinical opportunities. Front Psych. 2016;7:36. https://doi.org/10.3389/fpsyt.2016.00036.
17. Youngstedt SD, Elliott JA, Kripke DF. Human circadian phase-response curves for exercise. J Physiol. 2019;597(8):2253–68. https://doi.org/10.1113/JP276943.
18. Richardson CE, Gradisar M, Short MA, Lang C. Can exercise regulate the circadian system of adolescents? Novel implications for the treatment of delayed sleep-wake phase disorder. Sleep Med Rev. 2017;34:122–9. https://doi.org/10.1016/j.smrv.2016.06.010.

19. Kline C. Sleep quality. In: Gellman M, editor. Encyclopedia of behavioral medicine. New York: Springer; 2020.
20. Ohayon M, Wickwire EM, Hirshkowitz M, Albert SM, Avidan A, Daly FJ, et al. National Sleep Foundation's sleep quality recommendations: first report. Sleep Health. 2017;3(1):6–19. https://doi.org/10.1016/j.sleh.2016.11.006.
21. Jurado-Fasoli L, De-la OA, Molina-Hidalgo C, Migueles JH, Castillo MJ, Amaro-Gahete FJ. Exercise training improves sleep quality: a randomized controlled trial. Eur J Clin Invest. 2020;50(3):e13202. https://doi.org/10.1111/eci.13202.
22. Lins-Filho OL, Pedrosa RP, Gomes JML, Dantas Moraes SL, Vasconcelos BCE, Lemos CAA, et al. Effect of exercise training on subjective parameters in patients with obstructive sleep apnea: a systematic review and meta-analysis. Sleep Med. 2020;69:1–7. https://doi.org/10.1016/j.sleep.2019.12.022.
23. Mendelson M, Borowik A, Michallet AS, Perrin C, Monneret D, Faure P, et al. Sleep quality, sleep duration and physical activity in obese adolescents: effects of exercise training. Pediatr Obes. 2016;11(1):26–32. https://doi.org/10.1111/ijpo.12015.
24. Yang PY, Ho KH, Chen HC, Chien MY. Exercise training improves sleep quality in middle-aged and older adults with sleep problems: a systematic review. J Physiother. 2012;58(3):157–63. https://doi.org/10.1016/S1836-9553(12)70106-6.
25. Kovacevic A, Mavros Y, Heisz JJ, Fiatarone Singh MA. The effect of resistance exercise on sleep: a systematic review of randomized controlled trials. Sleep Med Rev. 2018;39:52–68. https://doi.org/10.1016/j.smrv.2017.07.002.
26. Steindorf K, Wiskemann J, Ulrich CM, Schmidt ME. Effects of exercise on sleep problems in breast cancer patients receiving radiotherapy: a randomized clinical trial. Breast Cancer Res Treat. 2017;162(3):489–99. https://doi.org/10.1007/s10549-017-4141-8.
27. Elavsky S, McAuley E. Lack of perceived sleep improvement after 4-month structured exercise programs. Menopause. 2007;14(3 Pt 1):535–40. https://doi.org/10.1097/01.gme.0000243568.70946.d4.
28. Kline CE, Hillman CH, Bloodgood Sheppard B, Tennant B, Conroy DE, Macko RF, et al. Physical activity and sleep: an updated umbrella review of the 2018 Physical Activity Guidelines Advisory Committee report. Sleep Med Rev. 2021;58:101489. https://doi.org/10.1016/j.smrv.2021.101489.
29. Morin CM, Hauri PJ, Espie CA, Spielman AJ, Buysse DJ, Bootzin RR. Nonpharmacologic treatment of chronic insomnia. An American Academy of Sleep Medicine review. Sleep. 1999;22(8):1134–56. https://doi.org/10.1093/sleep/22.8.1134.
30. Santiago LDCS, Lyra MJ, Cunha Filho M, Cruz PWDS, Santos MAMD, Falcão APST. Efeito de uma sessão de treinamento de força sobre a qualidade do sono de adolescentes. Rev Bras Med Esporte. 2015;21:148–52.
31. Flausino NH, Da Silva Prado JM, de Queiroz SS, Tufik S, de Mello MT. Physical exercise performed before bedtime improves the sleep pattern of healthy young good sleepers. Psychophysiology. 2012;49(2):186–92. https://doi.org/10.1111/j.1469-8986.2011.01300.x.
32. Buman MP, Phillips BA, Youngstedt SD, Kline CE, Hirshkowitz M. Does nighttime exercise really disturb sleep? Results from the 2013 National Sleep Foundation Sleep in America Poll. Sleep Med. 2014;15(7):755–61. https://doi.org/10.1016/j.sleep.2014.01.008.
33. Stutz J, Eiholzer R, Spengler CM. Effects of evening exercise on sleep in healthy participants: a systematic review and meta-analysis. Sports Med. 2019;49(2):269–87. https://doi.org/10.1007/s40279-018-1015-0.
34. Javaheri S, Barbe F, Campos-Rodriguez F, Dempsey JA, Khayat R, Javaheri S, et al. Sleep apnea: types, mechanisms, and clinical cardiovascular consequences. J Am Coll Cardiol. 2017;69(7):841–58. https://doi.org/10.1016/j.jacc.2016.11.069.
35. Quan SF, O'Connor GT, Quan JS, Redline S, Resnick HE, Shahar E, et al. Association of physical activity with sleep-disordered breathing. Sleep Breath. 2007;11(3):149–57. https://doi.org/10.1007/s11325-006-0095-5.

36. Tufik S, Santos-Silva R, Taddei JA, Bittencourt LR. Obstructive sleep apnea syndrome in the Sao Paulo Epidemiologic Sleep Study. Sleep Med. 2010;11(5):441–6. https://doi.org/10.1016/j.sleep.2009.10.005.
37. Simpson L, McArdle N, Eastwood PR, Ward KL, Cooper MN, Wilson AC, et al. Physical inactivity is associated with moderate-severe obstructive sleep apnea. J Clin Sleep Med. 2015;11(10):1091–9. https://doi.org/10.5664/jcsm.5078.
38. Murillo R, Reid KJ, Arredondo EM, Cai J, Gellman MD, Gotman NM, et al. Association of self-reported physical activity with obstructive sleep apnea: results from the Hispanic Community Health Study/Study of Latinos (HCHS/SOL). Prev Med. 2016;93:183–8. https://doi.org/10.1016/j.ypmed.2016.10.009.
39. da Silva RP, Martinez D, Pedroso MM, Righi CG, Martins EF, Silva LM, et al. Exercise, occupational activity, and risk of sleep apnea: a cross-sectional study. J Clin Sleep Med. 2017;13(2):197–204. https://doi.org/10.5664/jcsm.6446.
40. Kline CE, Crowley EP, Ewing GB, Burch JB, Blair SN, Durstine JL, et al. The effect of exercise training on obstructive sleep apnea and sleep quality: a randomized controlled trial. Sleep. 2011;34(12):1631–40. https://doi.org/10.5665/sleep.1422.
41. Kline CE, Ewing GB, Burch JB, Blair SN, Durstine JL, Davis JM, et al. Exercise training improves selected aspects of daytime functioning in adults with obstructive sleep apnea. J Clin Sleep Med. 2012;8(4):357–65. https://doi.org/10.5664/jcsm.2022.
42. Ueno LM, Drager LF, Rodrigues AC, Rondon MU, Braga AM, Mathias W Jr, et al. Effects of exercise training in patients with chronic heart failure and sleep apnea. Sleep. 2009;32(5):637–47. https://doi.org/10.1093/sleep/32.5.637.
43. Desplan M, Mercier J, Sabate M, Ninot G, Prefaut C, Dauvilliers Y. A comprehensive rehabilitation program improves disease severity in patients with obstructive sleep apnea syndrome: a pilot randomized controlled study. Sleep Med. 2014;15(8):906–12. https://doi.org/10.1016/j.sleep.2013.09.023.
44. Karlsen T, Nes BM, Tjonna AE, Engstrom M, Stoylen A, Steinshamn S. High-intensity interval training improves obstructive sleep apnoea. BMJ Open Sport Exerc Med. 2016;2(1). https://doi.org/10.1136/bmjsem-2016-000155.
45. Servantes DM, Javaheri S, Kravchychyn ACP, Storti LJ, Almeida DR, de Mello MT, et al. Effects of exercise training and CPAP in patients with heart failure and OSA: a preliminary study. Chest. 2018;154(4):808–17. https://doi.org/10.1016/j.chest.2018.05.011.
46. Iftikhar IH, Kline CE, Youngstedt SD. Effects of exercise training on sleep apnea: a meta-analysis. Lung. 2014;192(1):175–84. https://doi.org/10.1007/s00408-013-9511-3.
47. Andrade FMDD, Pedrosa RP. The role of physical exercise in obstructive sleep apnea. J Bras Pneumol. 2016;42:457–64.
48. Norman JF, Von Essen SG, Fuchs RH, McElligott M. Exercise training effect on obstructive sleep apnea syndrome. Sleep Res Online. 2000;3(3):121–9.
49. Sengul YS, Ozalevli S, Oztura I, Itil O, Baklan B. The effect of exercise on obstructive sleep apnea: a randomized and controlled trial. Sleep Breath. 2011;15(1):49–56. https://doi.org/10.1007/s11325-009-0311-1.
50. Servantes DM, Pelcerman A, Salvetti XM, Salles AF, de Albuquerque PF, de Salles FC, et al. Effects of home-based exercise training for patients with chronic heart failure and sleep apnoea: a randomized comparison of two different programmes. Clin Rehabil. 2012;26(1):45–57. https://doi.org/10.1177/0269215511403941.
51. Gottlieb DJ, Punjabi NM. Diagnosis and management of obstructive sleep apnea: a review. JAMA. 2020;323(14):1389–400. https://doi.org/10.1001/jama.2020.3514.
52. Peppard PE, Young T, Palta M, Dempsey J, Skatrud J. Longitudinal study of moderate weight change and sleep-disordered breathing. JAMA. 2000;284(23):3015–21. https://doi.org/10.1001/jama.284.23.3015.
53. Newman AB, Foster G, Givelber R, Nieto FJ, Redline S, Young T. Progression and regression of sleep-disordered breathing with changes in weight: the Sleep Heart Health Study. Arch Intern Med. 2005;165(20):2408–13. https://doi.org/10.1001/archinte.165.20.2408.

be in between 33 °C and 35 °C to produce therapeutic effects without cooling or overheating, being more pleasant and inducing to more relaxed muscles and joints [3].

The use of heated water, as a bath, near bedtime and having total or partial immersion of the body, has been proven to promote muscle relaxation with a consequent decrease of muscle tone, and increase of peripheral blood flow and heat dissipation through peripheral vasodilation [13]. These events result in a decrease in the activation of the sympathetic autonomic nervous system [13], thus facilitating quietness behavior with consequent decrease of sleep onset latency, and also ensuring the restorative sleep [1, 3, 12, 14–16].

The control of central body temperature is performed by the diencephalic structure (i.e., hypothalamus), in association with the suprachiasmatic nucleus [17]. Except for a fever, the central body temperature remains virtually constant varying around 0.6 °C. Thus, the average central body temperature usually ranges from 36.5 °C to 37 °C [18]. The circadian rhythm of thermoregulation is influenced by the balance between heat loss and production throughout the day, closely related to the waking and sleep phases, and to the change of behavior from higher to lower physical and mental activity [14, 19]. The temperature of the skin, also called peripheral temperature, has a wider range ranging from 24 °C to 33 °C, being 29 °C considered a thermoneutral temperature. However, the temperature of the skin surface varies between the regions of the body and does not have, therefore, a fixed value, as it depends on individual vasomotor variability, ambient temperature, and blood flow redistribution [19–22]. With that information in mind, it is possible to think about the effects that immersion in water can cause in the body: relaxation, decrease of the sympathetic nervous system tonus, change of body temperature, and muscle fatigue. These effects induce sleep [1], in addition to all the effects, on sleep, related to the practice of physical exercise (see chapter "Exercise and Sleep").

Chronic pain, which usually is related to muscle tension and insomnia, is a clinical condition that commonly alters the autonomic nervous system, as it keeps its sympathetic division predominantly activated at the expense of the activation of the parasympathetic division. This scenario affects, negatively, the onset and maintenance of sleep [23]. Body and mental relaxation are attainable goals with hydrotherapy. However, it is noteworthy that these conditions often require multidisciplinary intervention and, when necessary, a combination of non-pharmacological and pharmacological treatment modalities [24–26].

It should be noted that healthy people also present difficulty to initiate sleep sometimes and that some strategies, as the use of heated water in the feet, are able to favor the beginning of sleep by promoting the dilation of peripheral blood vessels. This dilation increases the temperature and heat loss in the body ends, favoring the loss of central body heat. This mechanism figures as the best physiological predictor for the quick onset of sleep [15].

A structured and appropriate hydrotherapeutic program requires the identification of the biological and social rhythm of the patient, in order to establish the best time for the practice, the water temperature that is pleasant and capable of promoting peripheral vasodilation, and whether the immersion will be partial or total, in addition to establishing the aquatic activity and the duration of the intervention [3].

Horne, one of the pioneers in considering the effects of passive body heating on sleep, conducted a pilot study back in 1987 to verify whether passive body heating would influence the amount of slow-wave sleep (SWS, N3 stage). Six healthy men with no sleep complaints underwent immersion in a bath heated at 41 °C for 30 minutes, 3 times a week for 2 weeks. Immersion occurred at 2 scheduled hours: 17 h and 21 h. Each intervention happened with a 3-day range. The polysomnography exam (PSG) and the Stanford Sleepiness Scale were the instruments used, each day of the intervention, to evaluate the objective sleep pattern and sleepiness. The researchers found that in the days of immersion at 21 h there was an increase of 15.4 minutes in SWS [27]. This finding demystifies the statement that taking a warm bath around bedtime can be harmful to sleep. It is worth noting that 21 h, except for night workers or shift workers, is a favorable time to decrease body temperature, as it is also the average time when the individual is more prone to quietness. With passive body heating, by means of peripheral vasodilation, there will be an exchange of heat with the environment (water), which will induce the decrease of the core body temperature, in addition to greater muscle relaxation – being these two crucial factors for a good night's sleep.

An investigation with older women, with an average age between 60 and 72 years old and with insomnia diagnosis, addressed the sleep changes caused by passive body heating (immersion in hot water in a bathtub). The participants underwent two baths with different controlled water temperatures: first, ranging between 40 °C and 40.5 °C, and second ranging from 37.5 °C to 38.5 °C, during 2 consecutive nights, for 30 minutes immersed until the level of the chest [28]. The baths took place 90 minutes before the usual time of sleeping. The sleep period was then monitored by PSG, and the participants also answered specific questionnaires on sleep quality. After bathing with water temperature between 40 °C and 40.5 °C, there was a significant decrease in the number of awakenings after the sleep onset (WASO), and an increase in the amount of SWS [28]. In both temperature ranges, the participants reported an improvement in the perception of sleep quality. Correspondingly, when they answered the post-sleep questionnaire, they considered that the sleep was deeper and restorative and felt more willing to wake up in the morning [28]. Regardless of the specific mechanism that explains the effects of passive body heating, this can be considered an effective non-pharmacological method, which improved the sleep of older women with insomnia, further suggesting that a passive body heating routine is beneficial for both the sleep and waking phases, for deep and restorative sleep favoring better performance of activities in the waking phase.

Using a milder temperature of 36.1 °C, postmenopausal women diagnosed with fibromyalgia were submitted to 15 sessions (5×/week for 3 weeks) of passive immersion in a temperature-controlled bathtub. The participants were comfortably positioned in dorsal decubitus with water up to the level of the sternal manubrium and stayed there for 30 minutes. This protocol was performed between 18 h and 20 h for 15 days. The PSG was performed in the following moments: 1st PSG, adaptation aiming at familiarization with team and equipment; 2nd PSG, baseline, in order to determine the sleep pattern; 3rd PSG, acute, after the 1st intervention; 4th PSG, chronic, performed on the 15th day; and the follow-up PSG, performed after 15 days of the 4th PSG. As a result, the chronic and follow-up evaluations showed a decrease in WASO, sleep latency, and REM sleep, as well as an increase in sleep efficiency. The increase of SWS was observed only at the chronic assessment [29]. This finding demonstrates that the establishment of a heated bath routine prior to bedtime may be beneficial for a restorative sleep night with consequent relief of pain and improvement in quality of sleep and, therefore, quality of life.

In addition to the proposals of passive body heating without the direct intervention of the physiotherapist, there is a well-known technique in the literature, called Watsu, in which the physiotherapist takes the patient in his arms and leads him, passively, by the heated pool combining muscle and mental relaxation, stretching, joint mobilization, and Shiatsu. The Watsu method is recommended for people of any age with acute or chronic pain complaints, and is also indicated for people with sleep complaints [30].

Sleep and wakefulness regulation is well synchronized by two processes called circadian and homeostatic [31]. The sleep pressure imposed by the homeostatic process depends on the energy expenditure throughout the day, and, most often, people who cannot enjoy restorative sleep cannot have enough energy to perform regular physical activity, becoming increasingly sedentary and susceptible to increased body weight and other unfavorable clinical conditions that will negatively impact their sleep quality. The incentive to exercise in the aquatic environment is generally well accepted because it is more pleasant to perform intense exercises than in the ground, whether focused on muscle strength gain, cardiovascular, individual, or group fitness. Thus, with greater energy expenditure, there will certainly be greater pressure on sleep. It is important to emphasize that group activities promote the socialization of people with a tendency to social isolation, impacting positively on anxiety and depression symptoms. Aquatic exercise supports body weight and reduces stress in the musculoskeletal, aspects that are very important for the elderly because it decreases the risk of falls, which is commonly a barrier to perform ground exercises [32–34].

A hydrotherapeutic method used to gain muscle strength and improve body perception is named Bad Ragaz ring method [35]. A recent study, while not directly investigating the sleep variable, found that by proposing and performing hydrotherapeutic intervention via Bad Ragaz and Ai Chi aquatic methods for participants with low back pain, pain complaints decreased after 4 weeks of treatment using these methods [36].

1 Final Words

Although there are several hydrotherapeutic techniques, it is worth noting that the most important is to have knowledge about the physical properties of water, selecting the appropriate and pleasant temperature for the patients in an individualized way, and proposing an intervention that meets the specific needs and objectives of the patient. This can be through hydro kinesiotherapy [37], referring to specific approaches aimed at mitigating the consequences of clinical conditions (e.g., fibromyalgia, fatigue, anxiety, stress, sleep disorders). In this way, physiotherapists will be assertive in promoting a good night's sleep, with consequent positive effects in the waking period.

Although in clinical practice we realize that hydrotherapy presents promising results mainly for sleep disorders that require prior relaxation (e.g., insomnia), there are no consensus and guidelines, or research into the theme that calls for 100% of this practice. Thus, further scientific research is needed using population-representative samples, disease-specific, focusing on the use of water resources specifically related to the improvement of sleep.

References

1. Mooventhan A, Nivethitha L. Scientific evidence-based effects of hydrotherapy on various systems of the body. N Am J Med Sci. 2014;6(5):199–209.
2. Fleming SA, Gutknecht NC. Naturopathy and the primary care practice. Prim Care. 2010;37(1):119–36.
3. Becker BE. Aquatic therapy: scientific foundations and clinical rehabilitation applications. PM R. 2009;1(9):859–72.
4. Burns SB, Burns JL. Hydrotherapy. J Altern Complement Med. 1997;3(2):105–7.
5. Vitorino DF, Carvalho LB, Prado GF. Hydrotherapy and conventional physiotherapy improve total sleep time and quality of life of fibromyalgia patients: randomized clinical trial. Sleep Med. 2006;7(**3**):293–6.
6. Vignochi CM, Teixeira PP, Nader SS. Effect of aquatic physical therapy on pain and state of sleep and wakefulness among stable preterm newborns in neonatal intensive care units. Rev Bras Fisioter. 2010;14(3):214–20.
7. Latorre-Roman PA, et al. Effect of a 12-day balneotherapy programme on pain, mood, sleep, and depression in healthy elderly people. Psychogeriatrics. 2015;15(1):14–9.
8. An J, Lee I, Yi Y. The thermal effects of water immersion on health outcomes: an integrative review. Int J Environ Res Public Health. 2019;16(7):1280.
9. Rapoliene L, et al. Balneotherapy for musculoskeletal pain: does the mineral content matter? Int J Biometeorol. 2020;64(6):965–79.
10. Macfarlane GJ, et al. EULAR revised recommendations for the management of fibromyalgia. Ann Rheum Dis. 2017;76(2):318–28.
11. Edlich RF, et al. Bioengineering principles of hydrotherapy. J Burn Care Rehabil. 1987;8(6):580–4.
12. Szymusiak R. Body temperature and sleep. Handb Clin Neurol. 2018;156:341–51.
13. Sato D, et al. Water immersion decreases sympathetic skin response during color-word Stroop test. PLoS One. 2017;12(7):e0180765.
14. Krauchi K. The thermophysiological cascade leading to sleep initiation in relation to phase of entrainment. Sleep Med Rev. 2007;11(6):439–51.
15. Krauchi K, et al. Warm feet promote the rapid onset of sleep. Nature. 1999;401(6748):36–7.
16. Harding EC, Franks NP, Wisden W. The temperature dependence of sleep. Front Neurosci. 2019;13:336.
17. Saper CB, Scammell TE, Lu J. Hypothalamic regulation of sleep and circadian rhythms. Nature. 2005;437(7063):1257–63.
18. Guyton AC, Hall JE. Textbook of medical physiology. 11th ed. Philadelphia: WB Sounders Company; 2006. p. 1152.
19. Van Someren EJ. Mechanisms and functions of coupling between sleep and temperature rhythms. Prog Brain Res. 2006;153:309–24.

1 Sleep Hygiene

One of these single-component therapies is sleep hygiene. Sleep hygiene is a set of rules, a guide, to adopt behaviors that are hindering sleep. Sleep hygiene was described as:

> (...) education is intended to provide information about lifestyle (diet, exercise, substance use) and environmental factors (light, noise, temperature) that may interfere with or promote better sleep. Sleep hygiene also may include general sleep-facilitating recommendations, such as allowing enough time to relax before bedtime and information about benefits of maintaining a regular sleep schedule. [4]

Sleep hygiene aims to eliminate anxiety generated by the anticipated fear of not sleeping, negative thoughts related to sleep, or that bedtime will be stressful [5–7]. Sleeping and waking up at the same time every day, including weekends and holidays, helps the rhythm required for melatonin production and other factors that depend on circadian rhythm. In normal circumstances, daytime naps are unnecessary and hinder nighttime sleep. Unless you need a scheduled nap for a specific reason (i.e., narcolepsy) and they are part of the routine, following time and duration. The regularity of meals is also important, as its regularity during the day and the choice of food at dinner and dinner time are all related to sleep, as they are external cues for entrainment of the circadian system. The room environment should be quite suitable and comfortable for the promotion of sleep: good support from the mattress and the pillow, room temperature (slightly cooler is optimal), no noises, blackout curtains, or light control should be suitable. Attention to stimulating screens, such as television, tablets, smartphones, computer, games, etc., as they emit a blue light that can interrupt the melatonin release and therefore disrupt sleep. The balance between work and leisure should also be observed. Many activities accumulate tiredness (increase sleep pressure) and delay bedtime. The routine for sleeping well includes a period for rest and shutdown of thoughts, especially problems, worries, and work for the next day.

Sleep hygiene is used to teach the individual healthy habits and behaviors that can disrupt sleep (Table 1). There are no contraindications, as sleep hygiene is a benign intervention.

Sleep hygiene is one of the multicomponent approaches of the CBT, and not CBT solely. There is a need for the physical therapist to explain the rationale and the relevance for each of the instructions, emphasizing that they are not casual and scientific-based and that they may also contribute to the development of insomnia. Also, the individual's willingness to change habits is fundamental to the success of CBT. Other problems that affect behavior change include the place where the individual lives (if there is noise, light, danger, or neighbors that disturb), the help of the family (if there are sick, alcoholic, aggressive individuals), the type of work/study (time, distance, stressful activities), and if there is a possibility of leisure (children, relaxing activities, physical activity), among others.

Using a sleep diary can help the patient to be aware of his sleeping habits, and the PT to understand the routine or lack of it, and to what extent, to change and

Table 1 Sleep hygiene education for patients and rationale. (Adapted with permission from: Siengsukon et al. [8])

Sleep hygiene rule		Rationale
Routine	Go to sleep and wake up at the same time every day. This will help set your natural biological clock. Exposure to bright natural light when you first wake up is also helpful to set your natural biological clock	This regularity and the exposure to sunlight will allow the biological clock to be synchronized, indicating to the brain that it's time to wake up. On the other hand, avoiding exposure to light in the early evening will be key to favoring the release of melatonin which is a sleep-inducing hormone
Bed = sleep	Use your bed for only sleep and sexual activity to help train your brain that if you are in your bed, you should be sleeping. Do not eat, work, or watch TV in bed. Do these activities outside of the bedroom. Leave bed if unable to fall asleep within 20 minutes and return when sleepy. If unable to leave the bed due to limited mobility or safety concerns, do something relaxing (i.e., relaxation techniques) until sleepy and able to fall to sleep	To promote better circadian cycling, set an alarm to go to sleep and to wake up every day at the same time
Relaxing routine prior to sleep	Develop a relaxing bedtime routine. This may include taking a warm bath, reading a book, meditation, or stretching. Avoid stimulating activities right before bedtime, including watching TV or discussing a stressful topic	The heating promoted by the bath, for example, can cause a downregulation of the central temperature and facilitate the onset of sleep and the deepen of sleep
Physical exercises	Avoid moderate to vigorous exercise at least 2–3 hours before bedtime. Exercising immediately before bedtime stimulates your body and brain making it hard to fall asleep. There is evidence however that doing regular (preferably moderate to vigorous) exercise improves your sleep at night. Talk to your physical therapist about an appropriate exercise program	Doing intense physical exercises close to bedtime can stimulate the body and brain making it difficult to lower body temperature, necessary for the onset of sleep. On the other hand, there is evidence that regular physical exercise helps reduce pre-sleep anxiety, facilitating the onset of sleep and helps synchronize the wakefulness cycle-sleep. In addition, regular practice of physical exercises has antidepressant and anxiolytic effect, associating the improvement of sleep quality. Aerobic exercise can deepen sleep. Deeper sleep is more restorative and protect against noise, pain, and hot flashes. Unclear whether exercise can help sleep a greater amount and more quickly

(continued)

Table 1 (continued)

Sleep hygiene rule		Rationale
Caffeine	Avoid caffeinated foods and drinks at least 4 hours before bedtime (includes most tea, coffee, chocolate, and soft drinks). Check the presence of caffeine in your drink or food by reading the label. Caffeine can cause difficulty falling asleep and increase the number of times you wake up during the night	Scientific evidence indicates that caffeine is antagonistic to adenosine receptors, in addition to delaying the rhythm of melatonin, and thus hinders the onset of sleep and dysregulate our biological clock
Alcohol and cigarettes	Refrain from drinking alcohol or smoking at least 3–4 hours before bedtime. Although people may think drinking alcohol causes relaxation before bedtime, it can increase the number of times you wake up during the night and can cause you to wake up early. Nicotine in cigarettes can cause difficulty falling asleep	Alcohol consumption can cause relaxation before bedtime; however, alcohol directly interferes with sleep, especially in REM sleep, decreasing its amount, and increases the nocturnal awakenings and wake earlier in the morning. Nicotine in turn is a stimulant that impairs asleep
Sleeping pills	Do not take un-prescribed or over-the-counter sleeping pills	
Naps	Avoid daytime napping so that you are tired at night and can fall asleep easily. If you feel you need to take a nap, limit the nap to 30 minutes and avoid napping in the evening	If you choose this habit, take this nap preferably after lunch (when we have a slight fall in body temperature). Avoid napping at other times and for an extended time. This will impair night sleep in quantity and quality
Sleep environment	Make your sleeping environment comfortable and relaxing. This includes avoiding too much light and disturbing noises. Stop using light-emitting electronics (i.e., television, computer, smartphone) at least 30 minutes before bedtime, as the blue light that is emitted can disrupt sleep by suppressing melatonin production. Use ear plugs, light-blocking curtains, or an eye mask if needed. Also, keep the temperature comfortable. Being too warm or cold may disturb your sleep. Also, use a comfortable and supportive pillow and mattress	The wavelength of blue light emitted by these devices impairs sleep induction by suppressing melatonin production and informing the brain that it is daytime. Another fundamental point is to seek a comfortable and preferably well-aligned posture. Choose the mattress and pillows well – not only the one that will support the head, but others of support that can assist in the optimal adjustment of posture
Food and liquids	Avoid eating a large meal or spicy food 2–3 hours before going to bed. Your digestive system slows down while you are sleeping which can stimulate acid secretions that cause heart burn. A light snack may be helpful if you are hungry. Avoid excessive liquid 2–3 hours before bedtime. Remember: it's not only *what* you eat, but also *when* you eat	The digestion of large or very caloric meals impairs so much sleep, as the digestive system slows down at night and can stimulate the secretion of acids that cause heartburn and reflux Avoid liquids before going to sleep so you don't have to wake up at night to go to the bathroom
Help	Talk to your doctor or health professional if you still have trouble sleeping	

improve sleep [9]. The sleep diary is explained in chapter "Subjective Assessment of Sleep" of this book. Sleep diary provides information about sleep duration, the number of awakenings during the night, sleep efficiency, sleep latency period, whether there is regularity in bedtime and waking up during the week and on weekends, naps during the day.

In the 1980s, the first CBT protocols for insomnia emerged, combining cognitive and behavioral techniques for changes in sleep habits. CBT has been indicated in clinical guidelines as an evidence-based treatment of choice for chronic insomnia, but can be used for sleep disorders, aiming to increase sleep time and improve sleep efficiency [10–15]. When used alone, cognitive, and behavioral techniques have a clinical effect, proved to be more efficient and lasting, together with other treatments. As a single treatment, it does not present scientific evidence in all sleep disorders, except for insomnia, but within subjective parameters, not objective ones [1].

2 Cognitive Behavioral Therapy

CBT aims to reduce sleep-related negative behavioral symptoms and reduce anxiety-related cognitive symptoms related to sleep. CBT requires customized forms of application [10] (internet, group, individual, self-application, etc.); a different number of sessions (from 4 to 8); duration of the sessions (60–120 minutes); and techniques applied according to the needs of each individual [16].

The CBT applied in person or at a distance can count on the aid of ready texts or pamphlets, and its effectiveness has proven both individually and in groups [10, 16]. In many countries, it can be applied by any health professional qualified in CBT, such as a psychologist, physician, nurse, occupational therapist, speech therapist, and/or social worker, and by the physiotherapist [10].

CBT uses a commonly employed multi-component package that combines sleep restriction therapy, stimulus control therapy, relaxation, paradoxical stimulation, and cognitive therapy [3].

3 Sleep Restriction Therapy

Sleep restriction (or time-in-bed restriction, a more accurate name) aims to increase sleep efficiency, which is the relationship between how much time is spent sleeping in the time that the individual set out to sleep (sleep time/time in bed × 100%) [10, 12]. Many individuals stay in bed too long trying to sleep or waiting for sleep to come, thus causing an increase in anxiety, usually leading to irritability in the absence of sleep, spending much more energy trying to sleep than effectively sleeping. Sleep restriction therapy consists of reducing the time in bed which can result in consolidation of sleep without interruptions and reduction of anticipatory sleep anxiety. This therapy is indicated for those who have sleep difficulties, in which sleep efficiency is less than 85%, indicated by a 1- or 2-week (preferably with is to help patients to learn how to control physiological parameters such as muscle tension and finger temperature, for example, to reduce somatic arousal [18]. In other words, biofeedback actively involves the patient in the therapeutic process and provides the awareness of the patient's own sensations and response to stressors. The individual is trained to use his own body signals to relax. Monitoring physiological reactions, especially those related to anxiety and stress, helps the person to perceive the changes that occur in his body during relaxation. Biofeedback is also used as a form of cognitive restructuring, in pain control, in the elimination of organic symptoms, and in the rehabilitation of muscle functions.

6 Paradoxical Intention Therapy

Paradoxical intention aims to eliminate the anxiety that inhibits falling asleep [10, 12] and the maladaptive relationship between effort to sleep and ability to sleep. This technique has shed light on investigations that participants with insomnia had more success falling asleep when they tried to remain awake when they had to try to fall asleep [19]. The individual should be prepared to spend the whole night awake performing an activity compatible with your sleep routine (e.g., watching a movie), without going to sleep. It is about taking a different perspective of sleep and sleep habits, beliefs, and fears. The instruction for the patient to stay awake as long as possible after getting into bed, to persistently involve in the feared action (staying awake) to reduce anxiety and conscious intent to sleep that misperceives associated goal-directed performance (falling asleep). This method eases the patient's disproportionate focus on sleep and anxiety over not sleeping; as a result, sleep becomes less difficult to initiate. There are elements of paradoxical intention incorporated into CBT techniques (Table 2).

7 Cognitive Therapy for Dysfunctional Beliefs About Sleep

Cognitive Therapy aims to identify beliefs (dysfunctional thoughts), attitudes, and knowledge of the individual in relation to sleep, in order to replace them with more appropriate/adapted thoughts and behaviors [10, 12]. Cognitive restructuring should help the individual understand what normal sleep is, how many hours of sleep are needed, what hours one should sleep, what are the bodily signs of sleep, how to distract unwanted thoughts, causes the individual to be aware, to recognize and review his expectations about sleep. For the AASM, cognitive therapy is "[…] a set of strategies including structured psychoeducation, Socratic questioning, use of thought records, and behavioral experiments designed to identify and modify unhelpful beliefs about sleep that may support sleep-disruptive habits and/or raise performance anxiety about sleeping" [3].

Table 2 Paradoxical aspects of other Cognitive Behavioral Therapy methods. (Reprinted with permission from Espie [20])

CBT method	Patient concern	Therapeutic response
Sleep restriction therapy	*I have got insomnia. I feel I am not getting enough sleep.*	*What are going to do is to reduce the time you spend in bed, so you need to stay awake for longer...*
Stimulus control	*I keep awakening up during the night and can't get back to sleep.*	*Get up out of your bed, and get out of your bedroom, and go and read a book instead.*
Progressive muscle relaxation	*I feel wound up and unable to let go.*	*Tense up muscles in your fingers and your hands to make a fist, keep the tension going at a steady rate, ...*
Cognitive therapy	*I feel that if I don't sleep soon, then I am going to be completely useless tomorrow.*	*So what's the worst that could happen if you don't sleep? You could try that as an experiment.*
Keeping a sleep diary	*I just can't stop thinking about my sleep. How I sleep and how I feel the next day is constantly in my mind.*	*I would like you to start keeping a detailed and careful note of your sleep pattern and sleep quality in a diary. Now every day you need to fill this in accurately...*

Education about sleep, circadian rhythm (internal clock, effect of hormones), on the influence of age and gender, and the effects of sleep deprivation promote decreased anxiety and reformulation of sleep. The control of concerns can be done through guidance to put on paper everything that is thought, as well as the tasks that were performed that day and the planning of the next day, in the late afternoon or early evening, in a different place from the bedroom. Listing problems and possible solutions have proven to be an efficient resource to reduce sleep time concerns. Relaxation techniques and mental training also help to avoid this schedule.

The repetition of new habits turns them into routines in 4 weeks. As the problems of everyday life do not end and life is a succession of them, some nights of insomnia may reappear. But using the trained techniques, the patient can sleep the next night and recreate the good sleeping conditions and beliefs. This is the educational character of cognitive therapy.

8 Final Words

Sleep education considers appropriate habits and personal needs to make up a good sleep routine. Proper eating, physical activity, sleeping environment, regularity of bedtime, and waking up influence good sleep habits. Having positive experiences with sleep too. Resting and turning off thoughts are important behaviors in preparing for sleep. The presented techniques aim to reduce sleep-related behavioral symptoms that make the patient sleep poorly and reduce anxiety-related cognitive symptoms to fall asleep.

Acknowledgment Our acknowledgment to Dr. Catherine Siengsukon, PT, Ph.D. for her inputs on this chapter.

References

1. Mitchell LJ, et al. The impact of cognitive behavioural therapy for insomnia on objective sleep parameters: a meta-analysis and systematic review. Sleep Med Rev. 2019;47:90–102.
2. Ong JC, Arnedt JT, Gerhman PR. Insomnia diagnosis, assessment, and evaluation. In: Kryger MH, Roth T, Dement WC, editors. Principles and practice of sleep medicine. Philadelphia: WB Saunders; 2017. p. 785–93.
3. Edinger JD, et al. Behavioral and psychological treatments for chronic insomnia disorder in adults: an American Academy of Sleep Medicine systematic review, meta-analysis, and GRADE assessment. J Clin Sleep Med. 2021;17(2):263–98.
4. Hauri PJ. Sleep disorder. Kalamazoo: Upjohn; 2004.
5. Morgan K. Daytime activity and risk factors for late-life insomnia. J Sleep Res. 2003;12(3):231–8.
6. Ohayon MM, et al. How age and daytime activities are related to insomnia in the general population: consequences for older people. J Am Geriatr Soc. 2001;49(4):360–6.
7. Sivertsen B, et al. Sleep problems in general practice: a national survey of assessment and treatment routines of general practitioners in Norway. J Sleep Res. 2010;19(1 Pt 1):36–41.
8. Siengsukon CF, Al-Dughmi M, Stevens S. Sleep health promotion: practical information for physical therapists. Phys Ther. 2017;97(8):826–36.
9. Prado GF, Carvalho L, Prado LBF. Insônia: guia prático sobre diagnóstico e tratamento. São Paulo: Eventos Omnifarma; 2011.
10. Teixeira CM, Teixeira L, Prado LBF, Prado GF, Carvalho LBC. Terapia Cognitiva Comportamental para Insônia: revisão sistemática. Rev Neurocienc. 2016;240:1–33.
11. Qaseem A, et al. Management of chronic insomnia disorder in adults: a clinical practice guideline from the American College of Physicians. Ann Intern Med. 2016;165(2):125–33.
12. Schutte-Rodin S, et al. Clinical guideline for the evaluation and management of chronic insomnia in adults. J Clin Sleep Med. 2008;4(5):487–504.
13. van Straten A, et al. Cognitive and behavioral therapies in the treatment of insomnia: a meta-analysis. Sleep Med Rev. 2018;38:3–16.
14. Wu JQ, et al. Cognitive behavioral therapy for insomnia comorbid with psychiatric and medical conditions: a meta-analysis. JAMA Intern Med. 2015;175(9):1461–72.
15. van der Zweerde T, et al. Cognitive behavioral therapy for insomnia: a meta-analysis of long-term effects in controlled studies. Sleep Med Rev. 2019;48:101208.
16. Seyffert M, et al. Internet-delivered cognitive behavioral therapy to treat insomnia: a systematic review and meta-analysis. PLoS One. 2016;11(2):e0149139.
17. Jacobsen E. Progressive relaxation: a psychological and clinical investigation of muscular states and their significance in psychology and medical practice. Chicago: University of Chicago Press; 1929.
18. Morgenthaler T, et al. Practice parameters for the psychological and behavioral treatment of insomnia: an update. An American Academy of Sleep Medicine report. Sleep. 2006;29(11):1415–9.
19. Ascher LM, Efran JS. Use of paradoxical intention in a behavioral program for sleep onset insomnia. J Consult Clin Psychol. 1978;46(3):547–50.
20. Espie CA. Chapter 6: Paradoxical intention therapy. In: Perlis M, Aloia M, Kuhn B, editors. Behavioral treatments for sleep disorders; a comprehensive primer of behavior sleep medicine intervention. 1st ed. Amsterdam: Academic Press/Elsevier; 2011. p. 69.

Sleep Ergonomics

Silmara Bueno and Cristina Frange

It is during sleep that the whole body recomposes and prepares itself for the next day. Being asleep is a state of physical and mental restoration, essential to the body, where the plasticity of the entire organism occurs. Thus, body supporting during sleep is of major importance. The human spine must be supported by the combination of a mattress, a bed base, and a pillow to adopt its natural position. The acquisition of a non-neutral position may influence painful processes, and in particular, musculoskeletal system pathologies.

Sleep quality and comfort are frequent questions of patients in the daily practice of physiotherapists, as the number of hours and the quality of sleep is well established to affect overall health – and to acquire that one must sleep on a proper surface. The posture adopted during sleep influences the physical health of the individual and may be correlated with musculoskeletal disorders in the shoulders, neck, lumbar region, as well as headaches, for example, that can, in turn, predispose to sleep fragmentation, poor quality, and quantity, leading to sleep disturbances.

A proper sleep system (i.e., mattress and support structure, and head pillow) can align the spine to some extent in its neutral posture which is the same as the spine alignment in the upright position [1]. A non-neutral posture can affect lateral bending and unbalanced loading on intervertebral disks and facet joints. For the intervertebral disks, growth and restoration depend on the amount of pressure and

S. Bueno
Personal do Sono Sleep Consulting, São Paulo, SP, Brazil

C. Frange (✉)
Department of Neurology and Neurosurgery, Escola Paulista de Medicina, Universidade Federal de São Paulo, Sao Paulo, SP, Brazil

Certified in Sleep Physiotherapy by the Brazilian Sleep Society (ABS), and The Brazilian Association of Cardiorespiratory Physiotherapy and Physiotherapy in Intensive Care (ASSOBRAFIR), Sao Paulo, SP, Brazil

World Physiotherapy Network for Health Promotion in Life and Work, Sao Paulo, SP, Brazil

C. Frange, F. M. S. Coelho (eds.), *Sleep Medicine and Physical Therapy*,
https://doi.org/10.1007/978-3-030-85074-6_32

resistance increases the risk of inflammatory or degenerative processes that affect the skeletal muscle system [14].

Postural assessment at bedtime makes it possible to assess imbalances to restructure posture through ideal support for the entire skeletal muscle system. The pelvic area of the human body is broader and heavier than other body parts. The thoracic area, because of the presence of the lungs is wider but not heavier. When lying in a lateral decubitus for sleep, on a very firm mattress, there is unsuitable spinal support, as only the broader areas of the body are supported (e.g. pelvis and shoulder). When these forces are not respected, ischemia may appear in body regions that are in contact with the surface. Ischemia generates metabolic substances (which will stimulate the nerve extremities and lead to discomfort and pain in lumbar and neck regions. The continuity of this factor can cause chronic muscular pain in the neck spine [15, 16]. Postural discomfort due to continuous muscle contraction can decrease blood supply, increase tension (stretching tight), or ligament compression, usually leading the individual to change the posture. Different studies have shown the association of microtrauma with pain and functional disability caused by poor posture during sleep [14, 17–19], highlighting the importance to have ideal support for the body and a correct and aligned posture.

The adopted posture for sleeping is something incredibly unique and particular. We move more than 10 times during sleep, this tends to decrease with age, and most of the time we are unable to remember the position in which we fall asleep or wake up. The body requires a position according to the degree of comfort and habit, so the body tends to adapt during a change in the musculoskeletal system.

2 Mattress: Alignment of the Body

In comparison about the mattress, custom-made surface, firm, and soft matters showed that the custom-made matters have maintained the natural alignment of the spine, arranged with different stiffness zones (Fig. 2a).

In the firm matters, the spine has bent down in the lumbar area, as only the shoulder and pelvis received good support on these surfaces (Fig. 2b). The softness of the soft mattress caused the pelvic area to sag more into the mattress, while the position of the vertebra C7 on soft surfaces is higher than that of the pelvis, due to the relatively lower mass of the upper part of the body (Fig. 2c) [20]. Therefore, the

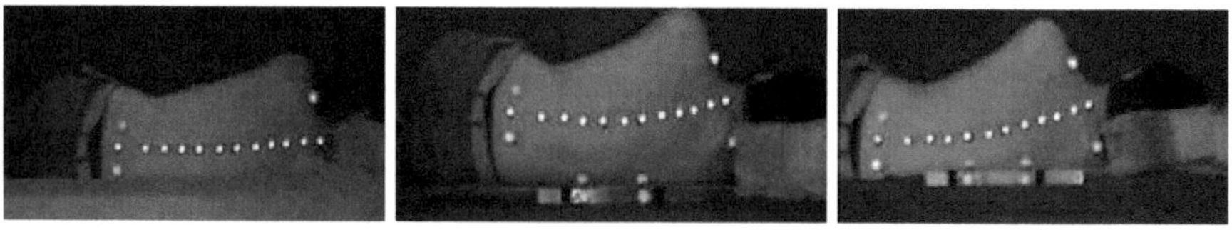

Fig. 2 Alignment of the spine on custom-made (**a**), firm (**b**), and soft (**c**), surfaces. (Reprinted with permission from Leilnahari et al. [20])

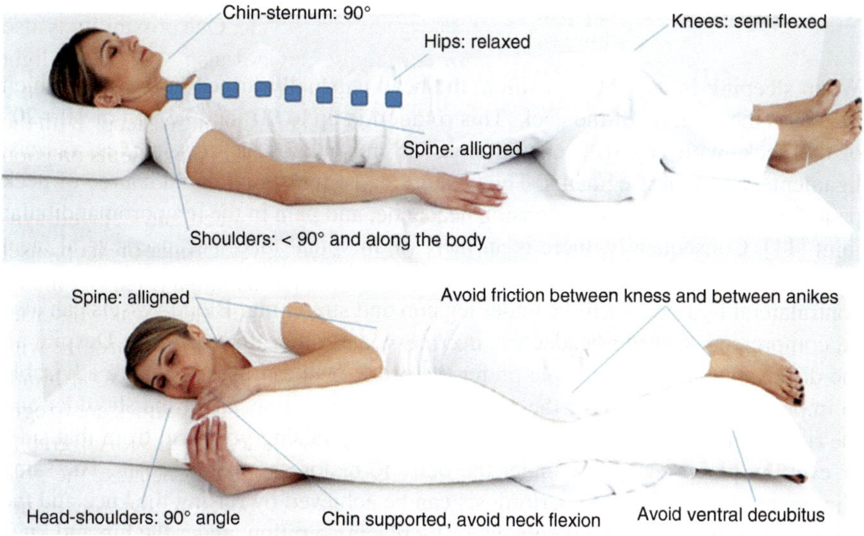

Fig. 3 Supine position with roll under the knees to protect the lumbar region, hips, and knees; and lateral decubitus with supported contour-shaped body pillow. (Image courtesy from Dr. Silmara Bueno.)

custom-made mattress allowed the neutral alignment of the spine, close to the natural standing position.

In the supine position, the center of gravity is a result of all segmental centers of gravity in relation to weight, having as many centers of gravity as there are positions to be adopted. The individual is in stable balance in the supine position when the line drawn from their centers of gravity coincides with the base of support [21].

The most common sleeping position in adults is the lateral decubitus (57%) [22], most likely due to the increased support of the spinal structures [23], followed by the supine position (17%) and the prone position (11%), despite this last one not being indicated for sleep. The other postures are variations of the positions in which the individual lies down to sleep [24]. The supine and the lateral decubitus are the sleeping postures most indicated, as they allow greater comfort and efficiency [25]. Yet, both positions require the use of two pillows (or a bigger one): one supporting the head and the other, below or between the knees (Fig. 3). The supine position allows the alignment of the spine with the use of pillows, cushions, and supports. For this case, it is recommended to use a pillow for the head and another pillow under the knees to align the pelvis.

3 Pillows: Neck Support

When sleeping in the prone position, the head is usually turned to the side, which increases the rotation of the neck. This rotation is up to 90° and flexion of 10°–20° of the neck, with negative repercussions on muscular structures, nerves, vessels, ligaments, and other segments. This posture constitutes a potential source of neck pain, fatigue, muscle tension, tension headache, and pain in the temporomandibular joint [11]. Consequently, there is an increase in spinal load, because several facet joints of the most cranial vertebra are compressed on the ipsilateral side, while the contralateral ligaments will be under tension and stretching. Blood vessels can also be compressed, causing headaches, dizziness, and other disorders [1]. Despite all the disadvantages, many people prefer the prone position. It is therefore advisable to improve the alignment of the spine by placing a pillow, under the shoulder and the ribcage next to which the head is facing, or by raising your arm from that side, or even by placing a pillow under the belly to restore lumbar lordosis. The same alignment of an eventual hyperlordosis can be achieved by raising the knee and the hip next to which the head is rotated, or by placing a pillow under the hip and knee on this side. In fact, most of the aforementioned corrections implement a slight change of position to an almost lateral position [1].

Inadequate posture of the head when sleeping imposes a considerable consumption of muscle energy in the neck region. Poor neck posture during sleep, increase biomechanical stresses on neck spine structures, producing neck pain and stiffness, headache, and scapular or arm pain, resulting in low-quality sleep [26]. A suitable pillow is a proper support for neck lordosis [27]. Choosing an adequate pillow can

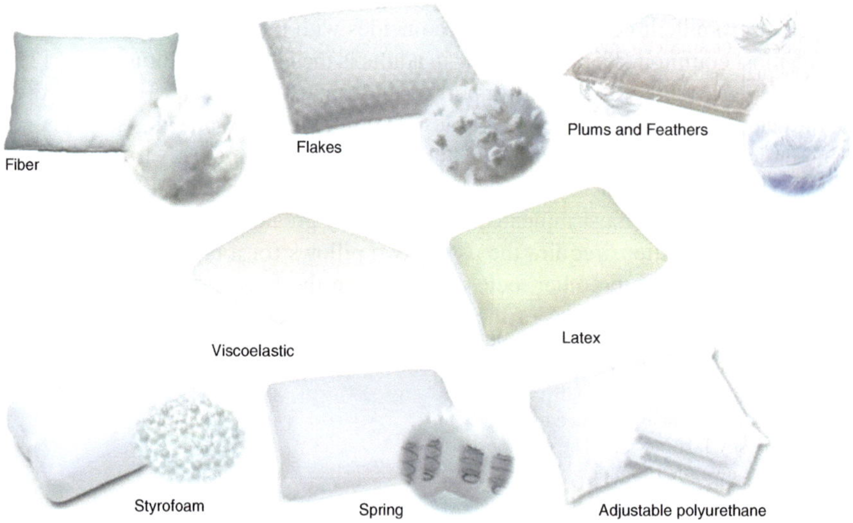

Fig. 4 Different materials with different supports for pillows. (Image courtesy from Dr. Silmara Bueno.)

reduce pain and improve sleep quality [28]. The big question is: "How is the suitable pillow? How do I chose one? Where do we have it on the market?" There is still no consensus regarding the best type of material for pillows, or their shapes and heights, which are still under debate in the literature (Fig. 4).

The main role of a pillow during sleep is to support the neck spine in a neutral position. A neutral position of the spine prevents loss of neck spine curvature and neck waking symptoms by minimizing end-range positioning of spinal segments [23, 29]. In addition, proper support can increase the contact area between the neck and the pillow so the pressure exerted upon the muscles can be evenly distributed [30]. Modifications of the neck inclination from 10 to 15 degrees alter muscle activity and blood supply in the region [31]. During the neck flexion, the horizontal distance between the center of gravity of the head and the axis joint at the atlanto-occipital joint increases considerably. The contraction of the scapular elevator muscles, with repercussions on the brachial plexus, is expressed by symptoms of pain, tingling, and decreased strength of the upper limbs [31]. Likewise, such manifestations can be observed when lying down, maintaining the prolonged positioning of the neck in semi-flexion.

Neck and spine pain as a whole has been described as one of the factors that can interfere with sleep quality. Pain and discomfort were related to higher and longer electromyographic (EMG) activities of trapezius in participants who have neck and shoulder pain. However, the relation of comfort and EMG activity of the neck and upper trunk during lateral sleeping position in different pillow heights is still a gap in the literature [32].

We already know that many people might not fall asleep when the neck was stiff and shoulder muscles were not relaxed. In addition, we should use props to relax the joints and loosen stiff muscles having proper support [33].

Pillow temperature must also be taken into consideration. A pillow that helps reduce core and head temperatures during nighttime sleep has been shown to be important for deep sleep (slow wave sleep) [34]. The reason individuals using a pillow made of a material that helps the pillow surface stay cool could fall asleep more easily and sleep well is strongly related to the lowered core and head temperatures and slowed heart rate [35]. Moreover, a pillow designed to reduce the temperature of the head can reduce sweating and whole-body temperature, and indirectly improve sleep quality [36].

An investigation on the effects of three types of pillows with different contents on neck lordosis, pillow temperature, and pillow comfort was conducted [37]. The three pillows were made of different materials: the orthopedic pillow (a roll-shaped pillow containing multiple polypropylene capsules), the memory foam pillow (contoured pillow consisting of polyurethane foam), and the feather pillow (regularly shaped pillow filled with 100% goose feathers). The Cobb angle from C2-C7 of the participants was measured from a radiograph, and when comparing the pre-Cobb angle in a standing position and the post-Cobb angle in a supine position with the use of the three different pillows, the researches found that the angle was significantly increased with the orthopedic pillow, from -3.83° at baseline to 7.70° (Fig. 5). The memory foam pillow increased the Cobb angle from -3.83° to -0.33°,

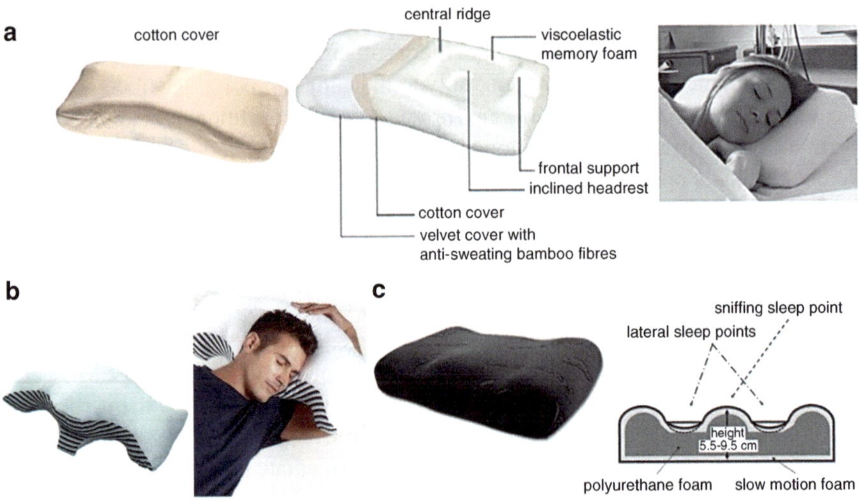

Fig. 6 Different types of sleep positioning pillows for obstructive sleep apnea. (**a**) Visual aspect of the pillow's external cotton cover; observable underlying foam structure beneath illustrated velvet cover; subject's head and neck placement in lateral position; (**b**) pillow that only adjusts the head and neck in lateral decubitus with an arm space; (**c**) polyurethane head positioning pillow. (Modified with permission from Newell et al. [43])

(Fig. 6c) in a sample of post-stroke patients showed a significant reduction of supine position and AHI, having an acceptable adherence following 3 months [45].

In addition, the head positioning pillow for 2 consecutive nights in mild to moderate positional OSA patients showed significant reductions of subjective and objective snoring severity in normal-weight patients, in contrast to overweight patients where only a reduction in subjective snoring was shown [46].

Positional therapy may therefore present as a valuable first-time intervention in positional OSA. Individualized care for positional OSA treatment by determining who will benefit from positional therapy alone or as an adjunct therapy is still needed, as well as guidelines on the theme.

5 Final Words

Material properties of a sleep system should be adjusted to personal needs in an objective way and preferences, for the reason that they are the underlying determinants of most physical ergonomic features (e.g., spine support). For example, obese patients need a firmer mattress in order to prevent the pelvic girdle from dropping too deep into the mattress. Materials therefore must be developed and combined to optimize general sleep system characteristics. Here, we point out a new avenue for research and increase the interest for the physical therapist to be evolved in positioning for better sleep.

References

1. Haex B. Back and bed. Ergonomic aspect of sleeping. 2nd ed. New York: CRC Press; 2004.
2. Huysmans T, et al. A 3D active shape model for the evaluation of the alignment of the spine during sleeping. Gait Posture. 2006;24(1):54–61.
3. Sakata RK, Issy AM, Vlainich R. Cervicobraquialgias. Rev Faces Dor. 2002;2:5–6.
4. Grandjean E, Manual de ergonomia: adaptando o trabalho ao homem. Stein, João Pedro 4a ed. 1998, Porto Alegre: Artes Médicas.
5. Gardiner MD. Manual de terapia por exercícios. São Paulo: Santos; 1995.
6. Kendall FP, McCreary EK, Provance PG. Músculos: provas e funções. 4th ed. Manole: São Paulo; 1995.
7. Smith LK, Weiss EL, Lehmkuhl LD. Cinesiologia clínica de Brunnstrom. 5th ed. São Paulo: Manole; 1997.
8. Iida I. Ergonomia: projeto e produção. São Paulo: Edgar Blucher; 1990.
9. Nachemson AL. The lumbar spine: an orthopedic challenge. Spine. 1976;1(1):59–71.
10. Almeida GCD. Efeitos de uma intervenção postural durante o sono na percepção da dor na coluna vertebral, na qualidade de vida e na qualidade do sono. In: Faculdade de Motricidade Humana. Lisboa: Universidade de Lisboa, FMH/FL; 2015. p. 244.
11. Kisner C, Colby LA. Exercícios terapêuticos: fundamentos e técnicas. 3rd ed. São Paulo: Manole; 1995.
12. Oliver J, Middleditch A. Anatomia funcional da coluna vertebral. Rio de Janeiro: Revinter; 1998.
13. Chaffin DB, Anderson GB, Martin BJ. Biomecânica ocupacional. Belo Horizonte: Ergo; 2001.
14. Grandjean E, Hunting W. Ergonomics of posture--review of various problems of standing and sitting posture. Appl Ergon. 1977;8(3):135–40.
15. Haex B. Back and bed: ergonomic aspects of sleeping. Reino Unido: CRC Press; 2005.
16. Yim JE. Optimal pillow conditions for high-quality sleep: a theoretical review. Indian J Sci Technol. 2015;8(5):135–9.
17. Bork BE, et al. Work-related musculoskeletal disorders among physical therapists. Phys Ther. 1996;76(8):827–35.
18. Cromie JE, Robertson VJ, Best MO. Work-related musculoskeletal disorders in physical therapists: prevalence, severity, risks, and responses. Phys Ther. 2000;80(4):336–51.
19. Mierzejewski M, Kumar S. Prevalence of low back pain among physical therapists in Edmonton. Canada Disabil Rehabil. 1997;19(8):309–17.
20. Leilnahari K, et al. Spine alignment in men during lateral sleep position: experimental study and modeling. Biomed Eng Online. 2011;10:103.
21. Bienfait M. Os desequilíbrios estáticos: fisiologia, patologia e tratamento fisioterápico. 2nd ed. São Paulo: Summus; 1995.
22. De Koninck J, Lorrain D, Gagnon P. Sleep positions and position shifts in five age groups: an ontogenetic picture. Sleep. 1992;15(2):143–9.
23. Gordon SJ, Grimmer-Somers KA, Trott PH. A randomized, comparative trial: does pillow type alter cervico-thoracic spinal posture when side lying? J Multidiscip Healthc. 2011;4:321–7.
24. Santiago R. Para uma noite bem dormida. Cited 2018 December 4th, 2018. http://ruisantiago.com/Docs/dormir.pdf.
25. Locks RT, Merino GSAD, Merino EAD. Levantamento e identificação dos aspectos básicos para a correta escolha do travesseiro de fibra. Blucher Design Proc. 2014;1(4):2331–43.
26. Gordon SJ, Grimmer-Somers KA, Trott PH. Pillow use: the behavior of cervical stiffness, headache and scapular/arm pain. J Pain Res. 2010;3:137–45.
27. Ambrogio N, et al. A comparison of three types of neck support in fibromyalgia patients. Arthritis Care Res. 1998;11(5):405–10.
28. Lavin RA, Pappagallo M, Kuhlemeier KV. Cervical pain: a comparison of three pillows. Arch Phys Med Rehabil. 1997;78(2):193–8.
29. Mc DJ. Sleep posture; its implications. Br J Phys Med. 1946;9:46–52.

30. Chen HL, Cai D. Body dimension measurements for pillow design for Taiwanese. Work. 2012;41 Suppl 1:1288–95.
31. Mercúrio R. Dor nas costas nunca mais. São Paulo: Manole; 1997.
32. Mork PJ, Westgaard RH. The association between nocturnal trapezius muscle activity and shoulder and neck pain. Eur J Appl Physiol. 2004;92(1–2):18–25.
33. Hannon JC. Pillow talk: the use of props to encourage repose. J Bodyw Mov Ther. 1999;3(1):55–64.
34. Liu SF, Lee YL, Liang JC. Shape design of an optimal comfortable pillow based on the analytic hierarchy process method. J Chiropr Med. 2011;10(4):229–39.
35. Kawabata A, Tokura H. Effects of two kinds of pillow on thermoregulatory responses during night sleep. Appl Human Sci. 1996;15(4):155–9.
36. Okamoto-Mizuno K, Tsuzuki K, Mizuno K. Effects of head cooling on human sleep stages and body temperature. Int J Biometeorol. 2003;48(2):98–102.
37. Jeon MY, et al. Improving the quality of sleep with an optimal pillow: a randomized, comparative study. Tohoku J Exp Med. 2014;233(3):183–8.
38. Persson L, Moritz U. Neck support pillows: a comparative study. J Manipulative Physiol Ther. 1998;21(4):237–40.
39. Her JG, et al. Development and comparative evaluation of new shapes of pillows. J Phys Ther Sci. 2014;26(3):377–80.
40. Verhaert V. Ergonomic analysis of integrated bed measurements: towards smart sleep systems. Lovaina: Universidade Católica de Leuven; 2011. p. 210.
41. Hage M. Dor nas costas: deixe de reclamar e resolve de uma vez. São Paulo: Gente Editora; 1997.
42. Sacco IC, et al. The effect of pillow height on muscle activity of the neck and mid-upper back and patient perception of comfort. J Manipulative Physiol Ther. 2015;38(6):375–81.
43. Newell J, Mairesse O, Neu D. Can positional therapy be simple, effective and well tolerated all together? A prospective study on treatment response and compliance in positional sleep apnea with a positioning pillow. Sleep Breath. 2018;22(4):1143–51.
44. Zuberi NA, Rekab K, Nguyen HV. Sleep apnea avoidance pillow effects on obstructive sleep apnea syndrome and snoring. Sleep Breath. 2004;8(4):201–7.
45. Svatikova A, et al. Positional therapy in ischemic stroke patients with obstructive sleep apnea. Sleep Med. 2011;12(3):262–6.
46. Chen WC, et al. Treatment of snoring with positional therapy in patients with positional obstructive sleep apnea syndrome. Sci Rep. 2015;5:18188.

Part VI
Evidence from Basic Science and Its Contribution to Physical Therapy in Sleep Medicine

constantly considered and updated; and of which scientists, health professionals, and the general population must be aware.

2 Animal Models for Sleep Research

Animals are used in sleep research as analogs for human sleep or sleep disorders. The use of animals in research presents practical and scientific advantages as they are easily manageable, which makes for better control of experimental conditions and helps avoid experimental biases. Further, the use of standardized species across experiments and in multiple laboratories ensures the replicability of results.

The use of animals, however, also presents obstacles, since there are no species that perfectly emulate the physiology of human sleep. For this reason, animal models are treated as mere approximations and do not fully replace the use of humans in sleep research. In practice, scientists choose very carefully which animal model to use depending on the phenomenon under investigation. In some cases, a species or strain is chosen for its biology, while in other settings scientists use clever experimental designs to mimic human sleep disorders that would otherwise not be present in animals.

Human sleep presents typical events that must be at least partially represented by a model for it to be useful in research. These events include the release of hormones, the occurrence of sleep phases, specific electroencephalographical (EEG) patterns, and other phenomena [5]. The animals most commonly used in sleep science are rats, mice, cats, and dogs [6, 7], all of which carry some level of similarity to human sleep.

A defining trait in human sleep is the intercalation of rapid eye movement (REM) sleep with non-REM (NREM) sleep, two different phases that can be detected by EEG. REM sleep presents desynchronized, low-amplitude EEG wave patterns that resemble those observed when an individual is awake, which also gives it the name "paradoxical sleep." Human NREM sleep presents synchronized, high-amplitude wave patterns and can be subdivided into stages 1, 2, and 3, each with progressively deeper sleep and slower waves.

In 1970, it was found that rats show sleep stages analogous to those found in humans [8], which eventually made them the most widely used animal model in sleep science. The most commonly used species of rat are *R. rattus* (the house rat) and *Rattus norvegicus albinus* (an albino variation of the brown rat bred specifically for scientific purposes). Unlike humans, rats sleep in a polyphasic manner, that is, they sleep multiple times a day in short sections of about 12 minutes each, averaging a total of 13 hours of sleep per day [6, 9]. Rats are nocturnal animals, meaning they explore, eat, interact, reproduce, and carry out other activities mostly during the dark phase of the 24-hour cycle.

As stated previously, the architecture of sleep in rats is remarkably similar to that of humans. Rats alternate between REM and NREM sleep, and their NREM sleep is subdivided into three stages, SS_I, SS_{II}, and SS_{III}, which, like humans, present increasingly slow and synchronous wave patterns as sleep gets deeper [8]. The order of sleep stages in rats is not constant, meaning that, after any given state, either the previous one may resume, or a new stage may begin.

Another valuable model species is the mouse (*M. musculus*). This species has a long history of use in science [6, 10], and there are currently over 11,000 strains being used in research [11]. Sleep varies between strains, but, on average, mice sleep for between 11 and 15 hours every day. Similar to rats, mice have polyphasic sleep, presenting sleep bouts of 2–4 minutes each. Characteristics such as the ratio between light and dark phase sleep, the percentage of R and NREM stages, the presence or absence of sleep disorders, and others vary between strains, which must be considered when choosing a strain for research.

Cats (*F. catus*) and dogs (*C. familiaris*) are also prominent models utilized in sleep research. Cats were used in the first study to ever describe REM sleep in a non-human animal [12] and have been used to this day to study neuroanatomy, physiology, and mechanisms of REM sleep. Dogs have been utilized since the nineteenth century in sleep research [13] and are currently used to model sleep disorders. Narcolepsy naturally occurs in many domestic animals, including cats, dogs, and mice, which led to the discovery of a mutation in the orexin/hypocretin receptor II gene as one of the main causes of the disease. Interestingly, this discovery was made independently by two different groups, one studying dogs and one studying mice, both of which published their results in August 1999 [14, 15].

Restless leg syndrome (RLS) studies point to two probable underlying causes in patients: abnormalities in the dopaminergic system and iron deficiency in the cerebrospinal fluid [7], and animals with these abnormalities are used as models for RLS. Rats with induced depletion of the diencephalic A11 dopaminergic nuclei showed improvements after treatment consistent with clinical results in humans, although subjective measures, such as the sensation of discomfort in the legs, cannot be evaluated [16]. Mice with iron deficiency showed increases in wake time prior to light-phase onset, which, since mice are nocturnal animals, corresponded to the time of day when RLS is most severe in humans, pointing to iron deficiency as a possible model for RLS in mice [17].

Obstructive sleep apnea (OSA) is the most common sleep disorder in humans, affecting nearly 1/3 of the adult population [18]. For this reason, many animal models have been developed in an attempt to study and combat it. English bulldogs are suitable for this due to their upper airway anatomy, which hinders airflow to the lungs during their sleep, mimicking many of the symptoms observed in humans [19]. A few other species naturally present OSA symptoms, including minipigs and a few strains of rats and mice [20].

3 Sleep Interventions

Sleep interventions provide means for the development of models for sleep disorders in animals that do not present them naturally. Interventions usually come in the form of mechanisms that interfere with sleep, or bioactive molecules that influence the molecular pathways of sleep. Sleep deprivation is a frequently used intervention that allows the measurement of the consequences of the lack of sleep in animals. Experimental designs usually mimic patterns of sleep deprivation present in humans, such as insomnia or chronic sleep restriction, and measure effects linked to the lack of sleep, including worsening of attention, reflexes, and pain [21, 22].

To induce sleep deprivation, a technique called "gentle handling" is often employed, in which a technician actively keeps an animal awake for a set period of time. When the animal shows signs of sleep onset, the researcher may introduce or remove objects from the cage, generate acoustic stimuli, or even touch the animal to keep it awake. This technique must be performed in such a way that avoids acoustic or physical pain while generating the minimum amount of stress possible, as it is known that stress hormones, such as corticosterone and adrenocorticotropic hormone, interfere with sleep patterns and may bias the experimental [23].

The correct performance of gentle handling depends heavily on the experience of each technician, which makes it difficult to standardize and replicate. To avoid this and to keep stress levels to a minimum, a number of devices have been developed that completely automate the process, thus eliminating the need for a technician. These mechanisms detect when an animal is falling asleep via computerized systems, and gently move the cage in order to wake them up [24, 25]. Alternatively, when the experimental design requires sleep fragmentation without complete sleep deprivation, a specialized cage coupled with an automated sweeping bar can be employed. The bar moves across the cage floor at a constant speed, touching the animals whenever they are asleep, thus waking them up for a brief period of time at regular intervals [26].

In some instances, the experimental design requires deprivation of the R stage exclusively, in which case the most popular strategy is the "platform method" [27]. In this method, the animals are placed in a tank containing small platforms (usually five) surrounded by water for a set period. When REM sleep initiates, the accompanying muscular atonia makes them fall into the water, thus waking them up. This method has been improved over the years to reduce the stress caused by REM sleep deprivation. A modern variation is the multiple platform method [28], which uses a greater number of platforms (usually ten), allowing the animals to swim between them during the experiment.

It is possible to mimic OSA symptoms in models that do not present them naturally by inducing an anesthetic state, leptin hormone deficiency, or obesity [20]. Another common strategy is to induce the symptoms mechanically. OSA patients suffer from collapses of the upper airway during sleep, which usually causes snoring and cessation of airflow into the lungs. This results in a periodic lack of oxygen in the blood and tissues in a process known as "intermittent hypoxia," which results in short and frequent awakenings during the night that is not perceived by the patient but induces sleep fragmentation [18].

It is possible to induce intermittent hypoxia in animals with the use of a "hypoxia chamber." This device consists of a sealed chamber that does not allow gas exchange with the exterior. Gas cylinders are attached to a computerized system that discharges pre-set concentrations of oxygen, carbon dioxide, and nitrogen at regular intervals. By alternating between atmospheric and infra-atmospheric saturation levels of oxygen, this system induces intermittent hypoxia in the animals placed inside the chamber. This condition simulates, and allows assessment of, the gas imbalances present in naturally occurring OSA, including oxygen desaturation and hypercapnia [7].

An important aspect of sleep interventions is the ability to influence the circadian rhythm. Sleep is mainly regulated by two mechanisms: the endogenous biological clock, which consists of a set of genes expressed at regular intervals throughout the light-dark cycle that synchronize most bodily functions, and by environmental cues captured by sensorial organs. Light plays an important role in modulating both the circadian clock and sleep [29]. In the laboratory, scientists use light to artificially influence sleep for experimental purposes. In this setting, lighting variables, such as spectral composition, intensity, and the duration of the photoperiod are carefully controlled to produce effects in the studied animals. The complete absence of light removes the environment as a modulator of the circadian rhythm, leaving only the biological clock as a regulator of physiological functions, a process known as "free-running."

4 Pharmaceutical Interventions

Drugs that modulate particular neurophysiological states can be employed to induce or alter sleep. Animal models have been widely used to study and discover these drugs, and, conversely, these drugs have been used to study the sleep process in animals and humans.

An important class of drugs consists of hypnotics, molecules capable of inducing sleep that is usually employed to treat insomnia. Benzodiazepines and Z-drugs are examples of hypnotics that target the GABAergic system of receptors, as GABA (gamma-aminobutyric acid) is a major inhibitory neurotransmitter in mammals [30], although other molecules may be used to modulate different receptor families. The use of hypnotics in sleep science and for treatment must be carefully considered, as each pharmaceutical may influence different stages of sleep, and many are involved with unrelated neuronal circuits [30].

Stimulant drugs have the opposite effect, inducing alertness and arousal, and delaying the onset of sleep. Examples include modafinil and dextroamphetamine, but the most common stimulant molecule consumed by humans is caffeine [31]. This drug acts by inhibiting the adenosine receptors associated with the accumulation of sleepiness after extended periods of the vigil, thus prolonging wakefulness. Stimulants are widely used to instill alertness and enhance attention, but they may have other uses, such as in the treatment for attention deficit and hyperactivity disorder [31].

There are classes of molecules capable of modulating the circadian rhythm, which is known as chronobiotics [32]. These molecules act by delaying or advancing the circadian clock, which, in turn, affects the onset of sleep. The most

Sleep and Musculoskeletal System

Helton de Sá Souza, Ana Claudia Pelissari Kravchychyn, and Sara Quaglia de Campos Giampá

What is the relationship between sleep and skeletal muscle? Before answering this question, it is important to note that understanding sleep alone is not an easy task. Sleep is a physiological phenomenon that remains a scientific enigma. However, it is recognized due to its importance and its impacts on health when it becomes inadequate [1]. Adequate sleep functions are attributed to health; on the other hand, the sleep debt generates significant negative organic changes, with emphasis on metabolic, hormonal, immunological, and cognitive functions. Collectively these changes can disrupt skeletal muscle homeostasis and compromise the normal functioning of this tissue.

There is a "popular knowledge" that skeletal muscle "grows" and recovers during sleep. Nevertheless, many questions remain without answers about the role of sleep in muscle recovery, as well as its influence on muscle physiology. In mid-2011, studies on the subject were published and gained notoriety by demonstrating the possible mechanisms underlying the sleep-skeletal muscle binomial [2]. However, there are still gaps to be filled. This chapter aims to discuss the complex and bidirectional relationship between sleep and skeletal muscle.

H. de Sá Souza (✉)
Department of Physical Education, Universidade Federal de Viçosa, Viçosa, MG, Brazil

A. C. P. Kravchychyn
Department of Physical Education and Department of Nutrition,
University Center of Volta Redonda, Unifoa, Volta Redonda, Rio de Janeiro, Brazil

S. Q. de Campos Giampá
Department of Cardiology, Faculdade de Medicina da Universidade de São Paulo,
São Paulo, SP, Brazil

C. Frange, F. M. S. Coelho (eds.), *Sleep Medicine and Physical Therapy*,
https://doi.org/10.1007/978-3-030-85074-6_34

1 Skeletal Muscle

Skeletal muscle is one of the most dynamic and plastic tissues of the human body; representing about 40% of the total body weight, they can store between 50 and 75% of all body proteins and are responsible for 30–50% of the whole body's protein "turnover" (balance *between* synthesis and degradation). Muscles are composed mainly of water (75%), protein (20%), and other substances (5%) (i.e., inorganic salts, minerals, fats, and carbohydrates) [3]. There are more than 600 muscles distributed throughout the human body, and these tissues have several functions, including mechanical, structural, metabolic, and endocrine [3, 4].

In this context, skeletal muscles have been seen as much more than effectors of muscle actions or structure for skeletal support. The literature is concise in showing that skeletal muscles are able to synthesize, store, and secrete substances (myokines) that can signal the muscle itself (autocrine function), neighboring tissues (paracrine function), or modulate the activity of various other body systems (endocrine function). In addition to these functions, it is known that skeletal muscles contribute to weight loss, together with the immune system activity and endocrine function, highlighted in recent years [5].

Therefore, understanding the factors that can influence skeletal muscle tissue, such as sleep or its damage, becomes essential to develop effective intervention strategies to promote and maintain population health.

2 Sleep and Skeletal Muscle: What Is the Relationship?

In 2005, Siegel proposed that sleep is a highly complex, active, and dynamic behavior that modulates cognitive activity, mood, and immune, endocrine, cardiovascular, and neuromuscular systems [6]. The main theories related to sleep functions are allocated into three categories: energy metabolism; related to modulation of the immune system and inflammatory processes, and, finally, the key role of sleep in the process of physical restoration [6, 7].

These categories of sleep functions are directly related to the physiology of skeletal muscle tissue, making it possible to establish the relationship between them. Furthermore, sleep seems to modulate factors related to memory and mood. Thus, while REM sleep is often associated with processes of maintaining cognitive aspects and mood, NREM sleep, especially slow-wave sleep (SWS or NREM N3), has been pointed out as one of the main responsible for modulating the immune system, energy conservation, and physical restoration [7].

Precisely to physical restoration, it is known that N3 stage plays an important role in the modulation of hormone secretion that has fundamental functions for skeletal muscle tissue, such as insulin and growth hormone (GH) [8, 9]. In contrast, global impairments in the sleep pattern of young adults were associated with a decrease in the secretion of testosterone, GH, insulin, and an increase in cortisol levels, which represents catabolic signals, [10, 11] as well as inflammatory markers, such as Interleukin 6 (IL-6), Interleukin 1 (IL-1), and tumor necrosis factor-alpha (TNF-α), which can also negatively influence the integrity of skeletal muscle tissue [10, 12–17].

The first study that proposed the pathway by which sleep (adequate or inadequate) could influence skeletal muscle was done in 2011 [2]. Later, the same group demonstrated in animal models that this hypothesis could, in fact, be true. Therefore, it was observed that rats deprived of sleep for 96 hours presented reduction of muscle volume with a concomitant increase in corticosterone concentrations and testosterone reduction [18]. These initial results stimulated the development of a series of other studies that proposed to investigate intervention strategies that could minimize the deleterious effects of sleep debt on skeletal muscle tissue and biochemical pathways by which this phenomenon could be explained. To understand these paths, it is necessary, first, to remember how the protein turnover occurs.

2.1 *Muscle Metabolism*

In general, regardless of the type of stimulus, skeletal muscle tissue morphological adaptations are pervaded by changes in protein turnover. Strictly speaking, when there are higher signals of synthesis than of protein degradation, there are an accumulation of muscle mass (hypertrophy/hyperplasia), while when there are higher rates of protein degradation there is a reduction in the amount of this tissue (muscular atrophy).

As previously mentioned, protein turnover is regulated by different factors, among which are anabolic hormones testosterone, GH, and insulin-like growth factor 1 (IGF-1) [19].

In this perspective, it is necessary to consider that skeletal muscle tissue integrity is associated with the nutritional status of the person, i.e., in situations where there is prolonged fasting or poor distribution of macronutrients, the reduction of muscle mass can occur. On the other hand, when the diet is adjusted, especially related to protein supply, it favors stimulation of protein synthesis. Moreover, active lifestyle maintenance is also associated with increased or maintenance of function and amount of muscle mass.

The main intracellular mechanism involved in these processes is related to a cascade of biochemical signals that modulate the activity of the phosphatidylinositol-3-kinase pathway/protein kinase B/rapamycin target (PI3K/AKT/mTOR pathway) as shown in Fig. 1. In general, insulin and IGF-1, for example, promote the initial stimulation of this pathway. Testosterone and some intermediaries produced by exercise can directly activate AKT [21]. Some nutrients such as amino acids, for example, can directly activate mTOR, the main controller of protein synthesis. mTOR has the function of stimulating the assembly of the ribosomal complex through the 70 kilodaltons (p70s6k) ribosomal protein, incite protein transcription through 4E-BP1 activity, and the new proteins translation [21].

Muscle voluntary contraction and serum creatine kinase levels (a diagnostic marker of skeletal muscle injury) increased equally in both conditions. Regarding hormones and cytokines, no difference was detected in testosterone levels between conditions, but IGF-1, cortisol, total cortisol/testosterone ratio, and IL-6 increased in total sleep deprivation condition. Thus, it was postulated that total sleep deprivation after eccentric exercise-induced muscle damage did not delay the recovery of muscle strength, but modifies inflammatory and hormonal responses [31].

Taken this information together, it is speculated about possible strategies that could minimize and/or even reverse the deleterious effects of sleep debt in skeletal muscle tissue. However, what are these strategies?

3.1 Sleep Debt and Skeletal Muscle: The Role of Physical Exercise and Protein Supplementation

Physical exercise and protein supplementation are non-pharmacological strategies that have gained notoriety in the field of skeletal muscle tissue health in sleep debt conditions [32, 33].

In the context of physical exercise, more specifically to the resistance model, it is the main choice to be adopted when aiming at skeletal muscle health. The mechanical load, hormonal, metabolic changes, and several intracellular events resulting from the practice of resistance exercise contribute to the improvement of strength and increase muscle protein synthesis [34].

Resistance exercise generates acute hormonal responses, especially the increase of IGF-1 levels, which plays an important role in the remodeling of skeletal muscle tissue [35]. The anabolic effects of IGF-1 involve activation of the PI3K/AKT/mTOR pathway and stimulation for proliferation, survival and differentiation of satellite cells [36], which collectively favor protein synthesis, resulting in muscle growth [37]. In addition, the mechanical deformation of muscle fibers (contraction and/or stretching) is already able to stimulate the AKT/mTOR pathway, independently of hormonal changes and immune/inflammatory responses [38].

In parallel, molecular pathways involved with protein degradation and consequent muscular atrophy, such as the ubiquitin-proteasome system, present a reduction of their activity by resistance exercise stimulating. This occurs because of the increased activity of the PI3K/ AKT/ mTOR pathway, which promotes higher phosphorylation of the FOXO, becoming inactive [13, 39].

Against this scenario, some researchers hypothesized [40] these physiological adaptations caused by resistance exercise could minimize or even delete the harmful effects of sleep debt on skeletal muscle (Fig. 1). In an experimental investigation to test this hypothesis, 50 adult male rats were allocated into 5 groups: (1) control group; (2) resistance training group; (3) the SHAM group; (4) 96-hour sleep deprivation group (PSP96); and (5) resistance training group subsequently subjected to 96-hour sleep deprivation (TR/PSP96). The resistance training protocol adopted was of high intensity, with a duration of 8 weeks, performed 5x/week. Resistance training performed prior to sleep deprivation exerted a protective effect on skeletal muscle, minimizing the reduction of IGF-1 and testosterone levels, increasing the expression of proteins involved in protein synthesis (mTOR and p70S6K), and attenuating those involved in degradation pathways [33, 40].

Another potential intervention to minimize sleep deprivation-induced muscle atrophy was amino acid supplementation, more specifically leucine supplementation. Leucine is an essential branched-chain amino acid known to exert anabolic effects through its ability to stimulate protein synthesis and inhibit protein degradation [32]. The mechanisms involved include activation of the mTOR direct signaling pathway and, consequently, phosphorylation of p70S6K and 4E-BP1 proteins, resulting in increased protein synthesis (Fig. 1) [27, 32, 41, 42].

In conditions that lead to muscular atrophy, such as cancer-induced cachexia [43], aging [44], and limb immobilization [27], leucine supplementation has promoted the maintenance of muscle trophism. But what about the sleep debt condition? In this way, De Sá Souza et al. submitted rats to 7 consecutive days of leucine supplementation, whose last 4 days coincided with the protocol of sleep deprivation for 96 hours. The daily dose of leucine supplementation used was 1.35 g/kg of body mass of each animal. At the end of the study, the authors came across an interesting finding. Muscle atrophy caused by sleep deprivation preferentially affected muscles composed of muscle fibers of glycolytic predominance (type II), compared to muscles composed of muscle fibers of oxidative predominance (type I). In relation to leucine supplementation, it was able to attenuate part of the observed muscular atrophy, but only in the type IIb muscle fibers [32].

Although there is no certainty, there is evidence pointing out to humans experiencing the same phenomena supporting these hypotheses [18, 33, 45].

4 Sleep and Skeletal Muscle in the Aging Process and Its Interface with Sarcopenia

The relationship between sleep and skeletal muscle has been explored in the context of adequate sleep and, mainly, in specific conditions of inadequate sleep. Nevertheless, how does this relationship happen in less acute conditions or during health-disease processes?

First, it is necessary to understand that the aging process is a *continuum* and is associated with quantitative and qualitative changes of several body systems. Among these changes, it is possible to mention sleep (see chapter "Sleep and Aging") and skeletal muscle tissue itself. Specifically, on skeletal muscle, some older people (about 10%) may experience an important change until they develop sarcopenia.

Sarcopenia is a disease characterized by the reduction or deterioration of muscle mass and function, commonly related to the aging process [46]. Its pathophysiology is multifactorial and comprises genetic, neuroendocrine, inflammatory factors, nutritional status, and level of physical activity [47, 48].

There exists a scenario in which skeletal muscle is influenced by healthy aging process, added with the changes in sleep pattern across aging [49]. In this sense, the aging process, similar to the condition of sleep debt, is recognized by the imbalance of the anabolism/catabolism relationship. Anabolic hormone pathways deteriorate with advancing age [50, 51] while catabolic pathways are enhanced. Hypercortisolemia is related to muscle catabolism in aging, muscle weakness, and weight loss [52].

In older people, there is a "U" form association between the prevalence of sarcopenia and sleep duration. Elderly individuals with short or long sleep duration have a higher prevalence of sarcopenia compared to those with normal sleep duration [47].

Among the most plausible pathophysiological hypotheses that relate sarcopenia to inadequate sleep, hormonal dysregulation and the pro-inflammatory scenario play an imperative role. The first refers to the increase in cortisol levels in contrast to the decrease in IGF-1 and testosterone levels; creating a catabolic environment, which promotes muscle degradation and thus the loss of muscle mass [53]. The latter concerns the increase of pro-inflammatory cytokines such as C-reactive protein, which appears to be involved in the process of muscle atrophy [54].

In this context, the practice of physical exercise combined with a good diet gains notoriety, by promoting benefits to muscle health, playing an important role in the prevention and/or attenuation of sarcopenia, as well as improving the quality of sleep.

5 Final Words

Adequate sleep plays a key role in maintaining and recovering the physiology of skeletal muscle. Maintaining the integrity of skeletal muscle depends on the balance between protein synthesis and degradation, both processes sensitive to several factors, including sleep, adequate nutrition, and physical exercise. In the same way, the evidence points out that the skeletal muscle healthy seems to positively influence sleep quality.

References

1. Banks S, et al. Chapter 5 - Sleep deprivation. In: Kryger M, Roth T, Dement WC, editors. Principles and practice of sleep medicine. Sixth ed. Philadelphia: Elsevier; 2017. p. 49–55.e4.
2. Dattilo M, et al. Sleep and muscle recovery: endocrinological and molecular basis for a new and promising hypothesis. Med Hypotheses. 2011;77(2):220–2.
3. Frontera WR, Ochala J. Skeletal muscle: a brief review of structure and function. Calcif Tissue Int. 2015;96(3):183–95.
4. Heymsfield SB, et al. Skeletal muscle mass and quality: evolution of modern measurement concepts in the context of sarcopenia. Proc Nutr Soc. 2015;74(4):355–66.

5. Pedersen BK. Muscle as a secretory organ. Compr Physiol. 2013;3(3):1337–62.
6. Siegel JM. Clues to the functions of mammalian sleep. Nature. 2005;437(7063):1264–71.
7. Porkka-Heiskanen T, Zitting KM, Wigren HK. Sleep, its regulation and possible mechanisms of sleep disturbances. Acta Physiol (Oxf). 2013;208(4):311–28.
8. Gronfier C, et al. A quantitative evaluation of the relationships between growth hormone secretion and delta wave electroencephalographic activity during normal sleep and after enrichment in delta waves. Sleep. 1996;19(10):817–24.
9. Holl RW, et al. Thirty-second sampling of plasma growth hormone in man: correlation with sleep stages. J Clin Endocrinol Metab. 1991;72(4):854–61.
10. Auyeung TW, et al. Sleep duration and disturbances were associated with testosterone level, muscle mass, and muscle strength-a cross-sectional study in 1274 older men. J Am Med Dir Assoc. 2015;16(7):630 e1–6.
11. Baumgartner A, et al. Neuroendocrinological investigations during sleep deprivation in depression. I. Early morning levels of thyrotropin, TH, cortisol, prolactin, LH, FSH, estradiol, and testosterone. Biol Psychiatry. 1990;28(7):556–68.
12. Schiaffino S, et al. Mechanisms regulating skeletal muscle growth and atrophy. FEBS J. 2013;280(17):4294–314.
13. Sandri M. Signaling in muscle atrophy and hypertrophy. Physiology (Bethesda). 2008;23:160–70.
14. Bonaldo P, Sandri M. Cellular and molecular mechanisms of muscle atrophy. Dis Model Mech. 2013;6(1):25–39.
15. West DW, Burd NA, Phillips SM. Comment and reply on: interactions of cortisol, testosterone, and resistance training: influence of circadian rhythms. Chronobiol Int. 2010; 27(4): 675–705. Chronobiol Int. 2010;27(9–10):1943–5; author reply 1945–6.
16. Miljkovic N, et al. Aging of skeletal muscle fibers. Ann Rehabil Med. 2015;39(2):155–62.
17. Santos RV, Tufik S, De Mello MT. Exercise, sleep and cytokines: is there a relation? Sleep Med Rev. 2007;11(3):231–9.
18. Dattilo M, et al. Paradoxical sleep deprivation induces muscle atrophy. Muscle Nerve. 2012;45(3):431–3.
19. Kraemer WJ, Ratamess NA. Hormonal responses and adaptations to resistance exercise and training. Sports Med. 2005;35(4):339–61.
20. Monico-Neto M, et al. Resistance exercise: a non-pharmacological strategy to minimize or reverse sleep deprivation-induced muscle atrophy. Med Hypotheses. 2013;80(6):701–5.
21. White JP, et al. Testosterone regulation of Akt/mTORC1/FoxO3a signaling in skeletal muscle. Mol Cell Endocrinol. 2013;365(2):174–86.
22. Tobaldini E, et al. One night on-call: sleep deprivation affects cardiac autonomic control and inflammation in physicians. Eur J Intern Med. 2013;24(7):664–70.
23. Cote KA, et al. Sleep deprivation lowers reactive aggression and testosterone in men. Biol Psychol. 2013;92(2):249–56.
24. Leproult R, Van Cauter E. Effect of 1 week of sleep restriction on testosterone levels in young healthy men. JAMA. 2011;305(21):2173–4.
25. Hardy MP, et al. Stress hormone and male reproductive function. Cell Tissue Res. 2005;322(1):147–53.
26. Martins PJ, et al. Orexin activation precedes increased NPY expression, hyperphagia, and metabolic changes in response to sleep deprivation. Am J Physiol Endocrinol Metab. 2010;298(3):E726–34.
27. Monico-Neto M, et al. REM sleep deprivation impairs muscle regeneration in rats. Growth Factors. 2017;35(1):12–8.
28. Maggio M, et al. Stress hormones, sleep deprivation and cognition in older adults. Maturitas. 2013;76(1):22–44.
29. Chase JD, et al. One night of sleep restriction following heavy exercise impairs 3-km cycling time-trial performance in the morning. Appl Physiol Nutr Metab. 2017;42(9):909–15.
30. Rae DE, et al. One night of partial sleep deprivation impairs recovery from a single exercise training session. Eur J Appl Physiol. 2017;117(4):699–712.

Part VII
Sleep Assessment for Physical Therapy Clinical Practice

Subjective Assessment of Sleep

Cristina Frange, Maria Júlia Figueiró Reis, Eliana Lottenberg Vago, and Fernando Morgadinho Santos Coelho

The intention of sleep assessment is to provide sufficient and accurate data to determine treatment. Accurate sleep assessment is the first step in effective sleep management by the physiotherapist. Information on the nature of sleep disturbance, physiologic, behavioral, and emotional aspects, as previous experiences with sleep, are crucial for the beginning of the treatment and also for managing treatment. Valid and reliable measurements of sleep are needed to identify patients who require intervention and to evaluate the effectiveness of an intervention.

A detailed anamnesis includes an assessment of numerous variables that may interfere with sleep and may play crucial roles in sleep management. Patient characteristics such as age, gender, ethnicity, profession, and marital status should never be missed in the assessment. It is interesting to have height, weight (to calculate body

C. Frange (✉)
Department of Neurology and Neurosurgery, Escola Paulista de Medicina, Universidade Federal de São Paulo, São Paulo, SP, Brazil

Certified in Sleep Physiotherapy by the Brazilian Sleep Society (ABS), and The Brazilian Association of Cardiorespiratory Physiotherapy and Physiotherapy in Intensive Care (ASSOBRAFIR), São Paulo, SP, Brazil

World Physiotherapy Network for Health Promotion in Life and Work, São Paulo, SP, Brazil

M. J. F. Reis
Psychobiology Department, Escola Paulista de Medicina, Universidade Federal de São Paulo, São Paulo, SP, Brazil

E. L. Vago
Neurology and Neurosurgery Department, Escola Paulista de Medicina, Universidade Federal de São Paulo, São Paulo, SP, Brazil

F. M. S. Coelho
Neurology and Neurosurgery Department; Department of Psychobiology, Paulista de Medicina, Universidade Federal de São Paulo, São Paulo, SP, Brazil

C. Frange, F. M. S. Coelho (eds.), *Sleep Medicine and Physical Therapy*, https://doi.org/10.1007/978-3-030-85074-6_35

Table 1 (continued)

Condition	Questionnaire	Characteristics	Purpose + Score + Cut off values
Insomnia	Insomnia Severity Index Bastien et al., 2001 [7]	Evaluates last 1-month measures: severity of sleep-onset, sleep maintenance, early morning awakening problems, satisfaction with current sleep, interference with daily functioning, impairment attributed to the sleep problem, level of distress caused by a sleep problem 7 questions Likert scale of 5 points: 0–4 Recently, it has been described in three sub-domains: nocturnal sleep difficulties, the sum of questions 1 + 2 + 3, the impact of insomnia during the day, the sum of questions 5 + 6 + 7, and dissatisfaction sleep with the sum of questions 1 + 4 + 7	Cognitive-behavioral (b) Insomnia screening (c) Assessment of treatment response Overall score: 0–28 Scores 0–7: no clinically significant insomnia; 8–14: sub-threshold insomnia; 15–21: moderate insomnia; and 22–28: severe insomnia
	Athens Insomnia Scale Soldatos et al., 1999 [8]	Evaluates last 1-month The 8-item questionnaire evaluates sleep onset, night and early-morning waking, sleep time, sleep quality, frequency and duration of complaints, distress caused by the experience of insomnia, and interference with daily functioning Each question could be rated from 0 (no problem) to 3 (very serious problem), leaving two intermediate scores	The severity of insomnia using diagnostic criteria set forth by the International Classification of Diseases (ICD-10) Overall score: 0–24 Cutoff >6 define the presence of insomnia
	Insomnia Symptom Questionnaire Okun et al., 2009 [9]	Weeks, months, or years 13 questions Questions 1–5 are multiple choices on an ordinal scale to assess the presence, frequency, and/or severity of the complaint For example, the "During the past month have you had difficulty falling asleep?" item includes choices ranging from 0 = never to 5 = always (5–7 days per week), and a follow-up contingency question asks about the problem's duration Questions 6–13 assess the extent to which the individual's endorsed sleep complaints affect daytime activities, with response choices ranging from 0 = not at all to 4 = extremely	Designed to identify insomnia

Obstructive sleep apnea	STOP-Bang Chung et al. 2012 [10] http://www.stopbang.ca/osa/screening.php	Easy-to-use 8 yes" or "no" questions + anthropometric measures such as BMI, age, neck circumference, and male sex	Screen for symptoms of obstructive sleep apnea Cutoff ≥3 define having a risk for OSA
	Berlin Netzer et al. 1999 [11] www.sleepapnea.org/wp-content/uploads/2017/02/berlin-questionn	Focuses on 3 categories of apnea signs and symptoms: snoring, daytime sleepiness, and obesity/high blood pressure 11 questions	To identify individuals at high risk for sleep apnea 3 categories related to the risk of having sleep apnea Classification: High risk (≥2 positive answers) or low risk (<2 positive answers)
	NoSAS Score Marti-Soler et al., 2016 [12]	5 items: neck circumference, BMI, snoring, age >55 years, and male sex	Prescreening for sleep-disordered breathing Maximum score = 19 a score of ≥8 indicates an increased probability of sleep-disordered breathing
Narcolepsy	Narcolepsy Severity Scale Dauvilliers et al., 2017 [13]	15 questions to evaluate the frequency and severity of sleepiness, cataplexy, hypnagogic hallucinations, paralysis of sleep, and fragmentation of sleep	Maximum total score = 57 Higher total scores indicate greater severity of narcolepsy at the time of the evaluation
Restless legs syndrome	IRLSSG Restless Legs Syndrome Rating Scale for Severity The International Restless Legs Syndrome Study Group, 2002 [14] http://irlssg.org/RLS-Ratings	Evaluates last week 10 item scale: 5 addressing symptom frequency and intensity +5 addressing the impact of them Likert scale from 0–4, 1 is	Classifies the intensity of the symptoms Overall score: 0–40 points Scores: 0–10 mild; 11–20, moderate; 21–30, severe; and 31–40 very severe
	Johns Hopkins Restless Legs Severity Scale Allen et al., 2001 [15]	Based on the time of day at which symptoms begin to appear 1. Single question	RLS severity

(continued)

Table 1 (continued)

Condition	Questionnaire	Characteristics	Purpose + Score + Cut off values
Pain	Pain and Sleep Questionnaire Three-Item Index (PSQ-3) Ayearst et al., 2012 [16]	Direct measure of the impact of chronic pain on sleep 8 questions: 6 are scored on a 100 mm VAS (ranging from 0 ["never"] to 100 ["always"]) and asks respondents to rate how often they have trouble falling asleep; how often they need pain medication to fall asleep; how often they need sleeping medication to fall asleep; how often they are awakened by pain during the night and in the morning; and how often their partner is awakened. The seventh item is also scored using a VAS; however, it uses different anchor points (0 ["very poor"], 100 ["excellent"]) and asks individuals to rate the overall quality of their sleep. The final item asks individuals to indicate, using a number that can range from 1 to 24, the average number of hours of sleep they get each night	Impact of pain on sleep in chronic pain patients
	Chronic Pain Sleep Inventory (CPSI) https://cpsi-sleep.com [17]	5-item tool measured on a 100 mm VAS assessing: Trouble falling asleep because of pain, needed sleep medication to help you fall asleep, awakened by pain during the night, awakened by pain in the morning, rate overall quality of your sleep	Impact of pain on sleep quality
	Sleep assessment instrument for older adults with pain (SAIOAP) Santana et al., 2021 [18]	Simple and practical tool Sleep dimensions, namely, sleep onset and maintenance, physical discomfort, diurnal repercussions of sleep such as excessive daytime sleepiness, self-perception of health status and medication used for sleep 7 questions: yes and no +4 questions on time to go to bed and wake up, sleep latency, and sleep duration	Score: 1 point for each "yes" answer to produce the total score
Circadian preference	Morningness-Eveningness Questionnaire Horn & Osteberg, 1976 [19] www.cet.org	19 multiple-choice questions, each having 4 or 5 response options	Overall score: 16–86 points Scores: ≤41 indicate "evening types," ≥59 indicate "morning types," between 42 and 58 indicate "intermediate types"
	Munich Chronotype Questionnaire Roenneberg et al., 2015 [20] www.thewep.org/documentations/mctq	Evaluates past 4 weeks 4 subscales: work schedule, workday sleep schedule, free day sleep schedule, self-assessment of chronotype 17 questions	Assess individual phase of entrainment on work and work-free days Scored electronically by the website
Sleep Diary	www.thensf.org/nsf-sleep-diary www.sleepfoundation.org/sleep-diary	A simple and practical tool evaluates how many days desired (suggested to evaluate weekdays and weekends) routine	Detailed information on morning and evening pre-sleep and post-sleep collects data overtime on self-reported sleep

There are several questionnaires for sleep assessment, which are easy, costless, and very manageable at the physiotherapist clinic. Here we present questionnaires that have reliability and validity against objective measures and can be incorporated into physical therapists' (PTs) anamnesis and treatment outcomes evaluation (Table 1). These are subjective measures that assess self-perception of quality and quantity of sleep and can assist in the diagnosis of sleep disorders. Just a reminder that the questionnaires are not designed to provide clinical diagnoses by themselves.

For the evaluation of general sleep, the Pittsburgh Sleep Quality Index (PSQI) [1] is one of the most used in research and clinical practice, assessing sleep quality

---

THE EPWORTH SLEEPINESS SCALE

Name: ______________________________

Today's date: ______________ Your age (years): ______________

Your sex (male = M; female = F): ______________

How likely are you to doze off or fall asleep in the following situations, in contrast to feeling just tired? This refers to your usual way of life in recent times. Even if you have not done some of these things recently try to work out how they would have affected you. Use the following scale to choose the *most appropriate number* for each situation:

0 = would *never* doze
1 = *slight* chance of dozing
2 = *moderate* change of dozing
3 = *high* chance of dozing

Situation	**Chance of dozing**
Sitting and reading	________
Watching TV	________
Sitting, inactive in a public place (e.g. a theater or a meeting)	________
As a passenger in a car for an hour without a break	________
Lying down to rest in the afternoon when circumstances permit	________
Sitting and talking to someone	________
Sitting quietly after a lunch without alcohol	________
In a car, while stopped for a few minutes in the traffic	________

Thank you for your cooperation

Fig. 1 Epworth sleepiness scale. (Reprinted with permission from Johns. Publisher: Oxford University Press [4])

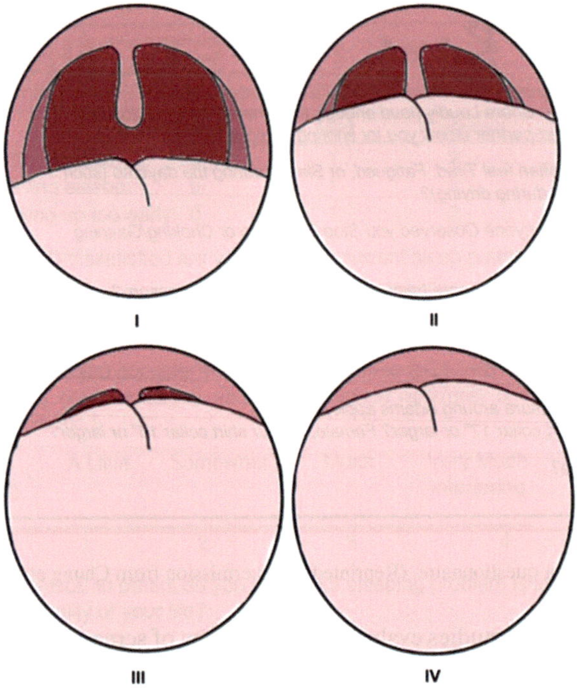

Fig. 4 Modified Mallampati Classification, classes I to IV. Mallampati classes: Class I corresponds to all structures visible (soft palate, uvula, fauces, and pillars); Class II, pillars are no more visible (soft palate, major part of uvula, and fauces visible); Class III, fauces are no more visible (soft palate and base of the uvula visible); finally, class IV, only the hard palate is visible. (Image courtesy from Dr. Maria Júlia Figueiró Reis. Original figure)

designed and validated for the older ones is the Sleep Assessment Instrument for Older Person with Pain (SAIOAP) [18](Fig. 6).

To assess circadian preferences (i.e., whether a person's circadian rhythm or biological clock produces peak alertness in the morning, in the evening, or in between) the Morningness Eveningness Questionnaire (MEQ) [19], which helps to determine individual differences in sleep-wake patterns, and the time-of-day people feel and perform best can be used (Fig. 7). Munich Chronotype Questionnaire (MCTQ) can assess individuals' chronotypes – diurnal preferences that manifest in personal sleep-wake rhythms [20].

The sleep diary is a record of an individual's routine of sleeping and waking times. It can be fulfilled by the proper patient, by a caregiver, or by the parents. The sleep diary records the subjective perception of the sleep period (Fig. 8) and can be recorded for at least 10 days, in order to include weekdays and weekends, or more, depending on the case. Often patients record information such as the time the patient

In the past week:	Score
Overall, how would you rate the RLS discomfort in your legs or arms? **4** Very severe **3** Severe **2** Moderate **1** Mild **0** None	
Overall, how would you rate the need to move around because of your RLS symptoms? **4** Very severe **3** Severe **2** Moderate **1** Mild **0** None	
Overall, how much releif of your RLS arm or leg discomfort did you get from moving around? **4** No relief **3** Mid relief **2** Moderate relief **1** Either complete or almost complete relief **0** No RLS symptoms to be relieved	
How severe was your sleep disturbance from your RLS symptoms? **4** Very severe **3** Severe **2** Moderate **1** Mild **0** None	
How severe was your tiredness or sleepiness during the day due to your RLS symptoms? **4** Very severe **3** Severe **2** Moderate **1** Mild **0** None	
How severe was your RLS as a whole? **4** Very severe **3** Severe **2** Moderate **1** Mild **0** None	
How often did you get RLS symptoms? **4** Very severe (6-7 days in 1 week). **3** often (4-5 days in 1 week). **2** Sometimes (2-3 days in 1 week). **1** Occasionally (1 day in 1 week). **0** None	
When you had RLS symptoms, how severe were they on average? **4** Very severe (8 h or more per 24 h). **3** Severe (3-8 h per 24 h). **2** Moderate (1-3 h per 24 h). **1** Mild (less than 1 h per 24 h). **0** None	
Overall, how severe was the impact of your RLS symptoms, on your ability to carry out your daily affairs, for example, carrying out a satisfactory family, home, social, school, or work life? **4** Very severe **3** Severe **2** Moderate **1** Mild **0** None	
How severe was your modd disturbance from your RLS symptoms-for example angry, depressed, sad, anxious, or irritable? **4** Very severe **3** Severe **2** Moderate **1** Mild **0** None	
Add the scores from above and share the total with your patient. **Mild** 0 to 10 **Moderate** 11 to 20 **Severe** 21 to 30 **Very Severe** 31 to 40	Total Score

Fig. 5 Restless legs syndrome rating scale for severity. (Reprinted with permission from Walters et al. [14])

Sleep Assessment Instrument for Older Person with Pain - SAIOAP

1. Do you take more than 30 minutes to fall asleep due to pain? Yes / No

During the last month, on typical nights:

- **A.** What time do you usually go to bed?
- **B.** How long does it take you to fall asleep?

2. Do to pain, do you wake up earlier than you would like to, and have difficulty getting back to sleep?

During the last month, on typical nights:

- **A.** What time do you get up in the morning?
- **B.** How much did you sleep?

3. Do you wake up in the middle of the night or earlier in the morning due to pain? Yes / No

4. Do you still feel tired when you wake up in the morning? Yes / No

5. Do you have a bad/very bad perception of your sleep? Yes / No

6. Do you feel sleepy during the day? Yes / No

7. Do you take any medication to sleep? Yes / No

Fig. 6 Sleep assessment instrument for older person with pain. (Reprinted with permission from Santana et al. [18])

Morningness-Eveningness Questionnaire

Instructions:

1. Please read each question very carefully before answering.
2. Answer ALL questions
3. Answer questions in numerical oeder.
4. Each question should be answered independently of others. Do NOT go back and cheek your answers.
5. All questions have a selection of answers. For each question place a cross alongside ONE answer only. Some questions have a scale instead of a selection of answers. Place a cross at the appropriate point along the scale.
6. Please answer each question as honestly as possible. Both your answers and the results will be kept, in strict confidence.
7. Please feel free to make any comments in the section provided below each question.

The Questionnaire with scores for each choice

1. Considering only your own "feeling best" rhythm, at what time would you get up if you were entirely free to plan your day?

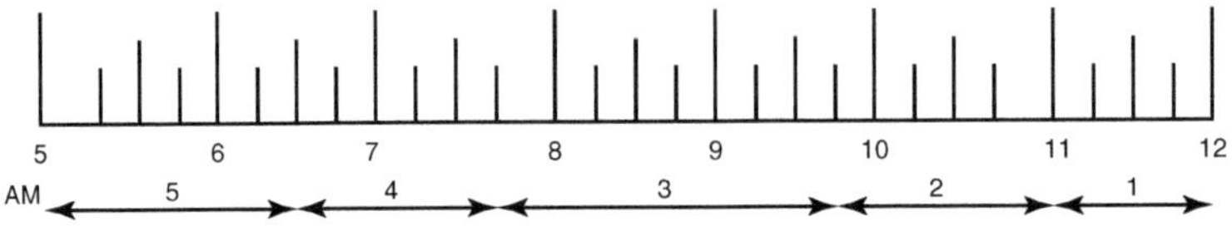

2. Considering only your own "feeling best" rhythm, at what time would you get to bed if you were entirely free to plan your evening?

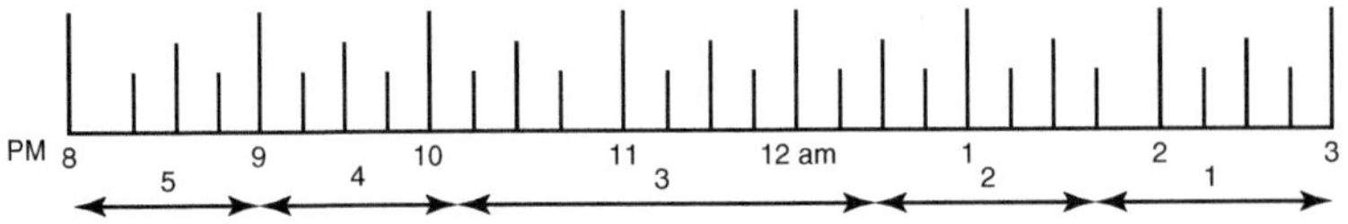

3. If there is a specific time at which you have to get up in the morning, to what extent are you dependent on bring woken up by an alarm clock?

Not at all dependent ☐ 4
Slightly dependent ☐ 3
Fairly dependent ☐ 2
Very dependent ☐ 1

4. Assuming adequate environmental conditions, how easy do you find getting up in the mornings?

Not at all easy ☐ 1
Not very easy ☐ 2
Fairly easy ☐ 3
Very easy ☐ 4

5. How alert do you feel during the first half hour after having woken in the mornings?

Not at all alert ☐ 1
Slightly alert ☐ 2
Fairly alert ☐ 3
Very alert ☐ 4

6. How is your appetite during the first half-hour after having woken in the mornings?

Very poor ☐ 1
Fairly poor ☐ 2
Fairly good ☐ 3
Very good ☐ 4

Fig. 7 Morningness eveningness questionnaire. (Reprinted with permission from Terman et al. [28])

7. During the first half-hour after having woken in the morning, how tired do you feel?

- Very tired ☐ 1
- Fairly tired ☐ 2
- Fairly refreshed ☐ 3
- Very refreshed ☐ 4

8. When you have no commitments the next day, at what time do you go to bed compared to you usual bedtime?

- Seldom or never later ☐ 4
- Less than one hour later ☐ 3
- 1-2 hours later ☐ 2
- More than two hours later ☐ 1

9. You have decided to engage in some physical exercise. A friend suggests that you do this one hour twice a week and the best time for him is between 7:00-8:00 a.m. Bearing in mind nothing else but your own "feeling best" rhythm, how do you think you would perform?

- Would be on good form ☐ 4
- Would be on reasonable form ☐ 3
- Would find it difficult ☐ 2
- Would find it very difficult ☐ 1

10. At what time in the evening do you feel tired and as a result in need of sleep?

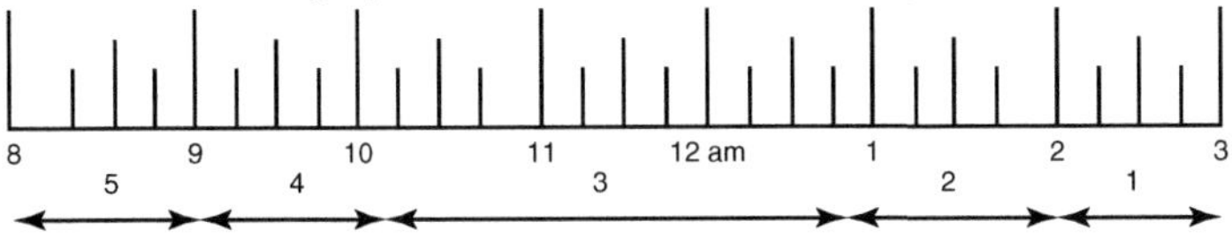

11. You wish to be at your peak performance for a test which you know is going to be mentally exhausting and lasting for two hours. You are entirely free to plan your day and considering only your own "feeling best" rhythm which ONE of the four testing times would you choose?

- 8:00-10:00 a.m. ☐ 6
- 11:00 a.m.-1:00 p.m. ☐ 4
- 3:00-5:00 p.m. ☐ 2
- 7:00-9:00 p.m. ☐ 0

12. If you went to bed at 11 p.m. at what level of tiredness would you be?

- Not at all tired ☐ 0
- A little tired ☐ 2
- Fairly tired ☐ 3
- Very tired ☐ 5

13. For some reason you have gone to bed several hours later than usual, but there is no need to get up at any particular time the next morning. Which ONE of the following events are you most likely to experience?

- Will wake up at usual time and will NOT fall asleep ☐ 4
- Will wake up at usual time and will doze thereafter ☐ 3
- Will wake up at usual time but will fall asleep again ☐ 2
- Will NOT wake up until later than usual ☐ 1

14. One night you have to remain awake between 4-6 a.m. in order to carry out a night watch. You have no commitments the next day, Which ONE of the following alternatives will suit you best?

- Would NOT go to bed until watch was over ☐ 1
- Would take a nap before and sleep after ☐ 2
- Would take a good sleep before and nap after ☐ 3
- Would take ALL sleep before watch ☐ 4

Fig. 7 (continued)

How often and when do I fill out the sleep diary? It is necessary for you to complete your sleep diary every day. If possible, the sleep diary should be completed within one hour of getting out of bed in the morning. The Nighttime Sleep Diary questions can be completed before you go to bed at night.

What should I do if I miss a day? If you forget to fill in the diary or are unable to finish it, leave the diary blank for that day.

What if something unusual affects my sleep or how I feel in the daytime? If your sleep or daytime functioning is affected by some unusual event (such as an illness, or an emergency), you may make brief notes on your diary.

What do the words "bed" and "day" mean in the diary? This diary can be used for people who are awake or asleep at unusual times. In the sleep diary, the word "day" is the time when you choose or are required to be awake. The term "bed" means the place where you usually sleep.

Will answering these questions about my sleep keep me awake? This is not usually a problem. You should not worry about giving exact times, and you should not watch the clock. Just give your best estimate.

Morning Sleep Diary Item Instructions

Use the guide below to clarify what is being asked for each item of the Sleep Diary. Date: Write the date of the morning you are filling out the diary.

1. **What time did you get into bed?** Write the time that you got into bed. This may not be the time you began "trying" to fall asleep.
2. **What time did you try to go to sleep?** Record the time that you began "trying" to fall asleep.
3. **How long did it take you to fall asleep?** Beginning at the time you wrote in question 2, how long did it take you to fall asleep?
4. **How many times did you wake up, not counting your final awakening? How** many times did you wake up between the time you first fell asleep and your final awakening?
5. **In total, how long did these awakenings last?** What was the total time you were awake between the time you first fell asleep and your final awakening? For example, if you woke 3 times for 20 minutes, 35 minutes, and 15 minutes, add them all up (20 + 35 + 15 = 70 min or 1 hr. and 10 min).

6a. What time was your final awakening? Record the last time you woke up in the morning.

6b. After your final awakening, how long did you spend in bed trying to sleep? After the last time, you woke up

(Item #6a), how many minutes did you spend in bed trying to sleep? For example, if you woke up at 8 am but continued to try and sleep until 9 am, record 1 hour.

6c. Did you wake up earlier than you planned? If you woke up or were awakened earlier than you planned, check yes. If you woke up at your planned time, check no.

6d. If yes, how much earlier? If you answered "yes" to question 6c, write the number of minutes you woke up earlier than you had planned on waking up. For example, if you woke up 15 minutes before the alarm went off, record 15 minutes here.

7. **What time did you get out of bed for the day?** What time did you get out of bed with no further attempt at sleeping? This may be different from your final awakening time (e.g., you may have woken up at 6:35 a.m. but did not get out of bed to start your day until 7:20 a.m.)
8. **In total, how long did you sleep?** This should just be your best estimate, based on when you went to bed and woke up, how long it took you to fall asleep, and how long you were awake. You do not need to calculate this by adding and subtracting; just give your best estimate.
9. **How would you rate the quality of your sleep?** "Sleep Quality" is your sense of whether your sleep was good or poor.
10. **How restful or refreshed did you feel when you woke up for the day?** This refers to how you felt after you were done sleeping for the night, during the first few minutes that you were awake.

Nighttime Sleep Diary Item Instructions

Please complete the following items before you go to bed.

Date: Write the date of the evening you are filling out the diary.

11a. **How many times did you nap or doze?** A nap is a time you decided to sleep during the day, whether in bed or not in bed. "Dozing" is a time you may have nodded off for a few minutes, without meaning to, such as while watching TV. Count all the times you napped or dozed at any time from when you first got out of bed in the morning until you got into bed again at night.

11b. **In total, how long did you nap or doze?** Estimate the total amount of time you spent napping or dozing, in hours and minutes. For instance, if you napped twice, once for 30 minutes and once for 60 minutes, and dozed for 10 minutes, you would answer "1 hour 40 minutes." If you did not nap or doze, write "N/A" (not applicable).

12a. **How many drinks containing alcohol did you have?** Enter the number of alcoholic drinks you had where 1 drink is defined as one 12 oz. beer (can), 5 oz. wine, or 1.5 oz. liquor (one shot).

12b. **What time was your last drink?** If you had an alcoholic drink yesterday, enter the time of day in hours and minutes of your last drink. If you did not have a drink, write "N/A" (not applicable).

13a. **How many caffeinated drinks (coffee, tea, soda, energy drinks) did you have?** Enter the number of caffeinated drinks (coffee, tea, soda, energy drinks) you had where for coffee and tea, one drink = 6–8 oz.; while for caffeinated soda one drink = 12 oz.

13b. **What time was your last drink?** If you had a caffeinated drink, enter the time of day in hours and minutes of your last drink. If you did not have a caffeinated drink, write "N/A" (not applicable).

14. **Did you take any over-the-counter or prescription medication(s) to help you sleep?** If so, list medication(s), dose, and time taken: List the medication name,

how much and when you took EACH different medication you took tonight to help you sleep. Include medication available over the counter, prescription medications, and herbals (e.g., "Sleepwell 50 mg 11 pm"). If every night is the same, write "same" after the first day.

15. Comments: If you have anything that you would like to say that is relevant to your sleep, feel free to write it here.

References

1. Buysse DJ, et al. The Pittsburgh Sleep Quality Index: a new instrument for psychiatric practice and research. Psychiatry Res. 1989;28(2):193–213.
2. Jenkins CD, et al. A scale for the estimation of sleep problems in clinical research. J Clin Epidemiol. 1988;41(4):313–21.
3. Health R Sleep scale from the medical outcomes study. 1986 [cited 2020 Jan 11]. Available from: http://www.rand.org/health/surveys_tools/mos/mos_sleep_survey.pdf
4. Johns MW. A new method for measuring daytime sleepiness: the Epworth sleepiness scale. Sleep. 1991;14(6):540–5.
5. Hoddes E, Dement W, Zarcone V. The development and use of the Stanford sleepiness scale. Psychophysiology. 1972;9:150.
6. Akerstedt T, Gillberg M. Subjective and objective sleepiness in the active individual. Int J Neurosci. 1990;52(1–2):29–37.
7. Bastien CH, Vallieres A, Morin CM. Validation of the Insomnia Severity Index as an outcome measure for insomnia research. Sleep Med. 2001;2(4):297–307.
8. Soldatos CR, Dikeos DG, Paparrigopoulos TJ. Athens Insomnia Scale: validation of an instrument based on ICD-10 criteria. J Psychosom Res. 2000;48(6):555–60.
9. Okun ML, et al. Psychometric evaluation of the Insomnia Symptom Questionnaire: a self-report measure to identify chronic insomnia. J Clin Sleep Med. 2009;5(1):41–51.
10. Chung F, et al. STOP questionnaire: a tool to screen patients for obstructive sleep apnea. Anesthesiology. 2008;108(5):812–21.
11. Netzer NC, et al. Using the Berlin Questionnaire to identify patients at risk for the sleep apnea syndrome. Ann Intern Med. 1999;131(7):485–91.
12. Marti-Soler H, et al. The NoSAS score for screening of sleep-disordered breathing: a derivation and validation study. Lancet Respir Med. 2016;4(9):742–8.
13. Dauvilliers Y, et al. Measurement of narcolepsy symptoms: the narcolepsy severity scale. Neurology. 2017;88(14):1358–65.
14. Walters AS, et al. Validation of the International Restless Legs Syndrome Study Group rating scale for restless legs syndrome. Sleep Med. 2003;4(2):121–32.
15. Allen RP, Earley CJ. Validation of the Johns Hopkins restless legs severity scale. Sleep Med. 2001;2(3):239–42.
16. Ayearst L, Harsanyi Z, Michalko KJ. The Pain and Sleep Questionnaire three-item index (PSQ-3): a reliable and valid measure of the impact of pain on sleep in chronic nonmalignant pain of various etiologies. Pain Res Manag. 2012;17(4):281–90.
17. Kosinski M, et al. Psychometric testing and validation of the Chronic Pain Sleep Inventory. Clin Ther. 2007;29 Suppl:2562–77.
18. de Andrade Santana MV, R.H.F, de Figueiredo Bersani AL, Frange C, Coelho FMS, Custódio O, Santos FC. Development and validation of the sleep assessment instrument for older adults with pain (SAIOAP). Neuro-Psychiatry Archives. 2021. in press.
19. Horne JA, Ostberg O. A self-assessment questionnaire to determine morningness-eveningness in human circadian rhythms. Int J Chronobiol. 1976;4(2):97–110.

20. Roenneberg T, et al. Human activity and rest in situ. Methods Enzymol. 2015;552:257–83.
21. Samsoon GL, Young JR. Difficult tracheal intubation: a retrospective study. Anaesthesia. 1987;42(5):487–90.
22. Amra B, et al. The prediction of obstructive sleep apnea severity based on anthropometric and Mallampati indices. J Res Med Sci. 2019;24:66.
23. Lavigne GJ, et al. Critical issues in dental and medical management of obstructive sleep apnea. J Dent Res. 2020;99(1):26–35.
24. Bittencourt LRA, Martinho Haddad F, Fabbro CD, Cintra FD, Rios L. General approach in patient with obstructive sleep apnea syndrome. Rev Bras Hipertens. 2009;16(3):158–63.
25. Dauvilliers Y, et al. Narcolepsy severity scale: a reliable tool assessing symptom severity and consequences. Sleep. 2020;43(6).
26. Pimentel Filho LH, et al. Validation of the Brazilian Portuguese version of the narcolepsy severity scale. Sleep Med. 2020;76:134–9.
27. Ouyang H, et al. Chinese version of narcolepsy severity scale: a validation study. BMC Neurol. 2019;19(1):334.
28. Terman M, Williams J, White TM. Assessment instruments. In: Partonen P-PT, editor. Seasonal affective disorder. Oxford: Oxford University Press; 2010. p. 255–64.
29. Natale V, et al. The consensus sleep diary: quantitative criteria for primary insomnia diagnosis. Psychosom Med. 2015;77(4):413–8.
30. Carney CE, et al. The consensus sleep diary: standardizing prospective sleep self-monitoring. Sleep. 2012;35(2):287–302.

1 Polysomnography

Diagnostic overnight polysomnography (PSG) examination, also known as a sleep study, is the main exam for assessment and diagnosis of sleep disorders and must be prescribed by a physician. PSG monitors the sleep stages and cycles to identify if or when our sleep patterns are disrupted and why. Sleep staging and marking of the associated events can be performed by a single trained PSG technician based on the criteria recommended by the Standard Manual for Staging Sleep and Associated Events at the American Academy of Sleep Medicine [1]. Physical therapists (PTs) can act as PSG technicians (as any other health professional) and learn how to "read" and interpret the exam, after attending some courses and being approved in the examination of the Board of Registered Polysomnographic Technologists.

The PSG records multiple physiological variables that are monitored simultaneously: electroencephalogram (EEG), electrooculogram (EOG), electrocardiogram (ECG), airflow, surface electromyogram (EMG, submental, temporal, masseter, and tibialis anterior muscles), respiratory effort of the thorax and abdomen (using inductance plethysmography belts), snoring, body position, saturation of peripheral oxygen (SpO_2), and heart rate (Fig. 1). Sleep staging is based on EEG, EOG, and submental (chin) EMG criteria. To detect stage R in particular, EOG and EMG submental recordings are mandatory for detecting saccadic eye movements and muscle atonia [2]. The nomenclature of EEG electrodes follows the International 10–20 system [3].

In a sleep recording study, that is PSG, it is possible to visualize brain waveforms derived from EEG by multiple time windows, known as epochs. An *epoch* can have a duration of 10, 15, 30, 60, 90, 120, or 240 seconds. A 30-second window is used to stage sleep, whereas a 10-second window is used for clinical EEG monitoring. Nowadays sleep is staged in sequential 30-second *epochs*, but digital PSG allows for use of different time windows based on the examiner's purpose, as for scoring of respiratory events, when 60 to 120-second epochs are frequently used. Many variables appear in a PSG examination, including sleep architecture (sleep structure, sleep pattern), and they depend on the duration of sleep and exam (Table 1). In addition, heart rate, saturation index, mean, minimum and maximum saturation (oximetry evolution), snoring, movement of limbs (legs and arms) during sleep and respiratory data, such as obstructive, central and mixed apneas and hypopneas, respiratory effort related arousal, the duration of each of these events in specific sleep stages, and the decubitus in which these events happened can also be described (Fig. 2).

Many monitoring PSG types can be prescribed by the physician, specifically when there is suspicion of associated diseases, such as (i) PSG with neurological assembly, which includes an increased number of "channels" or electrodes added to the EEG compared to the basal PSG. It is requested by the physician in cases of suspected epilepsy or other neurological conditions; (ii) PSG for bruxism, focusing on the evaluation of chewing movements or jaw contraction, which may include video recordings; (iii) PSG for positive air pressure (PAP) titration in patients with sleep-related breathing disorders, to define the adequate treatment pressure for each patient and mask type. It is possible for technicians, during titration, to make adjustments in the level of air pressure necessary to completely eliminate respiratory events. Adjusting

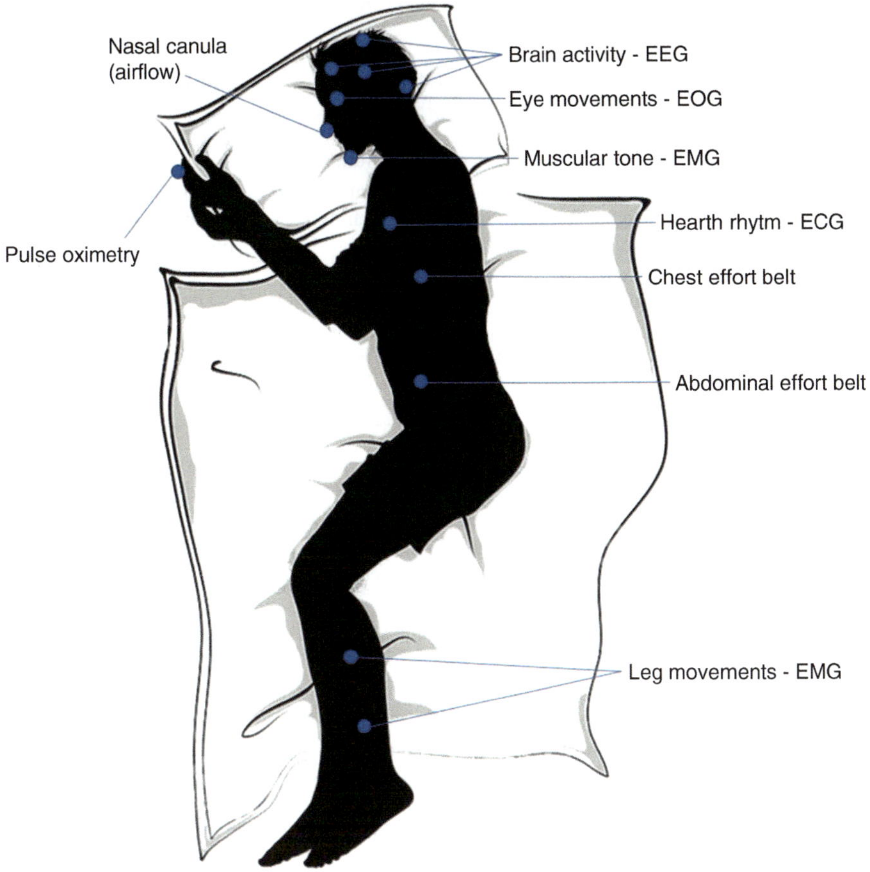

Fig. 1 Schematic representation of basic electrodes for sleep monitoring – polysomnography examination
Brain activity is measured bilaterally, at frontal, central, occipital, mastoid, central midline (vertex), and frontopolar midline (above and between the eyes). Eye movements are recorded using electrodes poisoned near the eyes, below and above, and at both sides. Chin activity is monitored via one electrode poisoned above the inferior edge of the mandible and two electrodes positioned below the inferior edge of the mandible, right and left. EEG electroencephalography, EOG electrooculography, EMG electromyography, ECG electrocardiography. (Image courtesy Dr. Cristina Frange. Original figure.)

the pressure of the PAP device is a simple procedure, but requires great knowledge from the technician and patient's collaboration, as the degree of airway "closure" can vary throughout the night, depending on the stages of sleep or the sleeping position; (iv) PSG for ventilation therapy adjustment, including types of PAP devices such as Bilevel or Servo Ventilator, which treat more complex respiratory or neuromuscular diseases, and are also adjusted during a PSG night examination; (v) PSG for confirmation of the efficacy of Mandibular Advancement Device (MAD) after subjective titration or, more recently, for its objective titration [4]. MAD promotes changes in the position of the mandible by bringing it forward and increasing the space for air to

Table 1 American Academy of Sleep Medicine recommended reporting parameters of polysomnographic examination

Parameter		Definition	Values for normal adults
Lights out time (h:min)		Time of the start of the recording	–
Lights on time (h:min)		Time of the ending of the recording	–
Time in bed or total recording time (TRT, min)		Total time spent in bed, from lights out to lights on, which includes sleep and wakefulness	Varies accordingly to age, chronotype, and circadian preferences
Total sleep time (TST, min)		Total time of sleep recorded over the PSG, time spent in stages N1, N2, N3, or R (Most PSGs arc performed in the hope that at least 6–7 hours of TST will be recorded, but useful data can be acquired in many patients even with 2–3 hours of TST)	
Sleep efficiency (SE, %)		Total sleep time divided by The total time in bed multiplied by 100% (SE in sleep laboratories are highly variable, and this value is usually not given all that much weight in clinical practice unless the SE is very low or very high)	>85%
Sleep latency or sleep onset latency (SL, min)		The amount of time it takes to go from being fully awake to sleeping	<30 min
Stage R latency (REMSL, min)		The elapsed time between sleep onset and the onset of the first REM sleep period	70–120 min
Wake after sleep onset (WASO, min)		Total time of scored wakefulness that occurred after the initial epoch of sleep, linked to the fragmentation of sleep	<30 min
Arousal index (#/hr)		Total number of arousals divided by TST	<10–25 (large variation by age)
Stage wake (W, min)		All minutes of stage wake during TRT	
Sleep stages	N1 (%)	Total time in each sleep stage divided by TST and multiplied by 100% Also shown in minutes	2–5% of TST
	N2 (%)		45–55% of TST
	N3 (%)		20% of TST
	R (%)		20–25% of TST
Periodic limb movement index (PLMi)		PLMi is calculated by dividing the total number of PLMs by sleep time in hours	Normal: PLMi ≤5 Mild: >5 PLMi <25 Moderate: >25 PLMi <50 Severe: PMLi ≥50
Apnea hypopnea index (AHI)		Represents the number of apnea and hypopnea events per hour of sleep	Normal: AHI < 5 Mild: 5 ≤ AHI < 15 Moderate: ≥15 AHI <30 Severe: AHI ≥30
Respiratory disturbance index (RDI)		Apnea hypopnea index + hypopnea + RERA: Respiratory effort related arousal	

Adapted with permission from Carskadon and Dement [12]
H hour, *Min* minutes

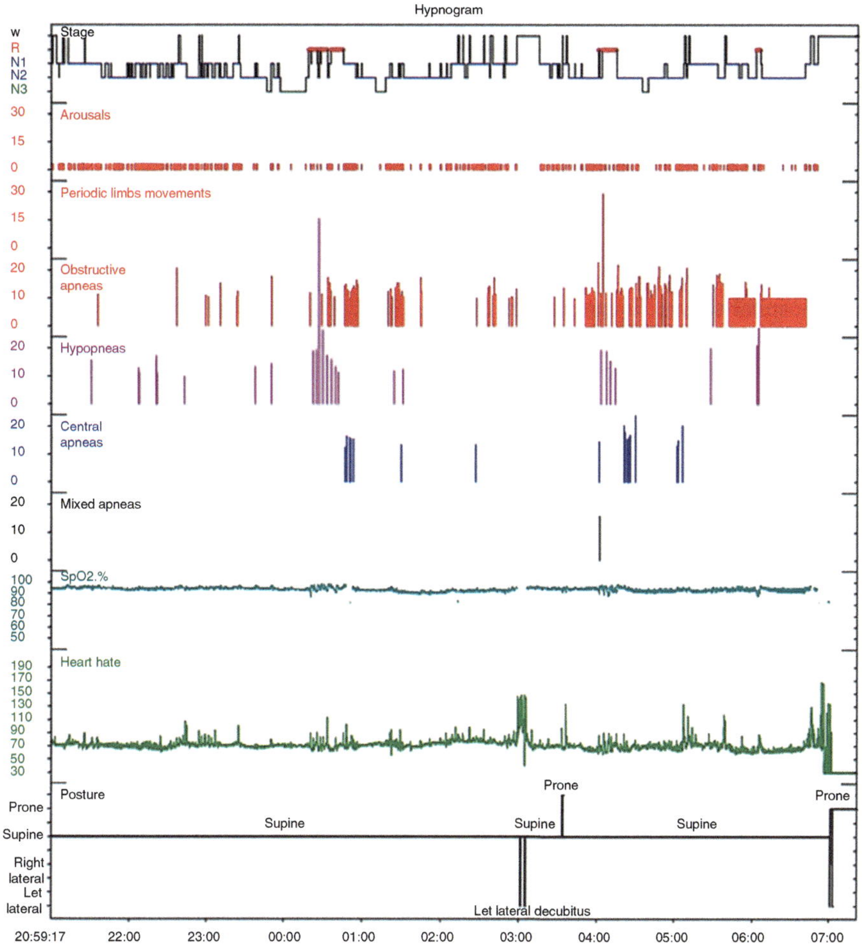

Fig. 2 Result sheet from an overnight polysomnography examination in the laboratory, from 20:59 until 7 hours in the morning (time at the bottom). Hypnogram showing each sleep stage according to time of the night, R stage (red line), N1 (black line), N2 (blue line) and N3, green line; arousal (in red); periodic limb movements (this patient had none); obstructive sleep apnea (in red lines, seconds); hypopneas (in pink lines, seconds); central apneas (blue lines, seconds); mixed apnea (black line, seconds); oxygen saturation (in, %); heart rate (in green, bpm); and time spent in each posture (supine, prone, left or right lateral decubitus). Note that this patient slept in the supine position for the most part of the night, and during the R sleep stage, when obstructive sleep apneas and hypopneas occurred, he had a desaturation of oxygen at both moments, and increased heart rate. W wake, R REM sleep stage, N1 NREM N1 sleep stage, N2 NREM N2 sleep stage, N3 NREM N3 sleep stage. (Image courtesy Dr. Cristina Frange)

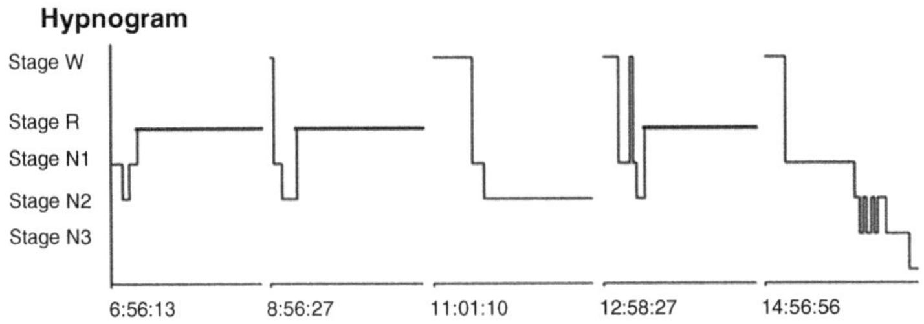

Summary

	Nap 1	Nap 2	Nap 3	Nap 4	Nap 5
Lights off	6:56:13	8:56:27	11:01:10	12:58:27	14:56:56
Sleep onset	6:56:13	8:56:57	11:06:10	13:00:27	14:59:26
Lights on	7:16:13	9:16:27	11:22:10	13:18:27	15:16:56
Time in bed	20'00"	20'00"	21'00"	20'00"	20'00"
Total sleep time	20'00"	19'30"	16'00"	17'30"	17'30"
Sleep latency	00'00"	00'30"	05'00"	02'00"	02'30"
REM sleep latency	03'30"	03'00"	/	03'30"	/

Mean sleep latency (5 episodes) : 02'00"
Mean REM sleep latency (3 episodes) : 03'20"

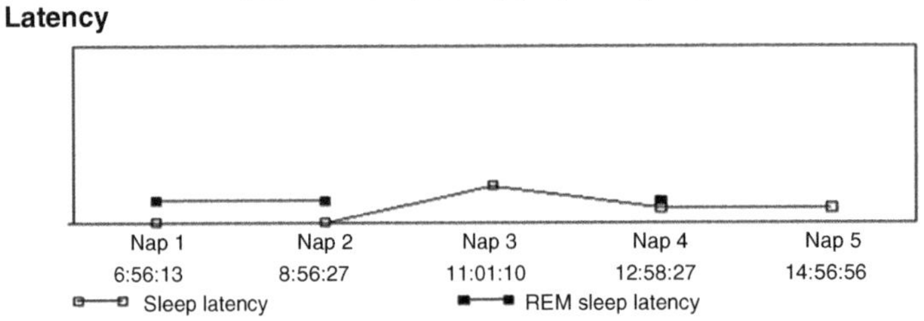

Fig. 4 Example of abnormal findings on the Multiple Sleep Latency Test. (Image courtesy from Dr. Fernando Morgadinho Santos Coelho. Original figure)

the mean sleep latency is ≤8 minutes (more precisely, 2 minutes), also suggesting hypersomnolence and reinforcing Narcolepsy diagnosis.

4 Maintenance of Wakefulness Test

The Maintenance of Wakefulness Test (MWT) assesses the individual's ability to stay awake for a period of time in a calm environment and without stimulation, also during the day. It measures wakefulness, showing whether an individual is able to stay awake for a defined period of time, usually beginning 90–180 minutes after the patient's usual wake-up time. Polysomnography and sleep logs may be useful before the test protocol, in selected cases [8]. Sleep latency is assessed by how long individuals take to fall asleep during the test. Four records are made with a duration of 40 minutes each, in which the patient is advised to try not to sleep, followed by intervals of 1h20min, in which one cannot sleep either (Fig. 5). The test is performed with the patient sited in bed with head supported and in dim light. MWT is

Example A – normal MW1

Nap	Initial sleep latency (minutes)	Unequivocal sleep latency (minutes)	SOREM?
1	40.0	40.0	No
2	40.0	40.0	No
3	34.0	34.0	No
4	40.0	40.0	No
Summary	Mean ISL: 38.5 min	Unequiv Mean ISL: 38.5 min	SOREMs: 0

Example B – abnormal MWT – indicative of hypersomnia

Nap	Initial sleep latency (minutes)	Unequivocal sleep latency (minutes)	SOREM?
1	20.0	20.0	No
2	24.0	24.0	No
3	12.0	15.0	No
4	30.0	30.0	No
Summary	Mean ISL: 21.5 min	Unequiv Mean ISL: 22.25 min	SOREMs: 0

Fig. 5 Example of normal and abnormal findings on the Maintenance of Wakefulness Test These are findings from a patient who is hypersomnolent on the MWT despite regular use of CPAP for OSA. A wake-promoting agent or psychostimulant may be indicated in this patient. MWT Maintenance of Wakefulness Test, ISL initial sleep latency, SOREM Sleep onset REM period. (Reprinted with permission from Boeve [13])

an indicator of how well individuals may be able to function and remain alert during quiet periods of inactivity [9].

The main difference between MWT and MSLT is that the former is intended to measure the ability to stay awake, while the latter quantifies the ability to fall asleep, although both express results based on the mean values of sleep latencies. MSLT is used as part of the diagnostic criteria of central disorders of hypersomnolence, especially narcolepsy and idiopathic hypersomnia [10]. On the other hand, MWT can be used to estimate safety in work environments in which somnolence would represent a risk and evaluate response to treatment in patients with excessive daytime sleepiness [8]. Nevertheless, because somnolence is a multifactorial clinical parameter, MWT results are difficult to interpret and predictive value for assessing accident risk is not clear [11].

5 Actigraphy

Due to its use in clinical practice for PTs, actigraphic devices will be explained in the next chapter.

References

1. Berry RB, et al. AASM scoring manual updates for 2017 (version 2.4). J Clin Sleep Med. 2017;13(5):665–6.
2. Berry RB, Brooks R, Gamaldo CE, et al., for the American Academy of Sleep Medicine. The AASM manual for the scoring of sleep and associated events: rules, terminology and technical specifications. Version 2.0. Darien: American Academy of Sleep Medicine; 2012.
3. Klem GH, et al. The ten-twenty electrode system of the International Federation. The International Federation of Clinical Neurophysiology. Electroencephalogr Clin Neurophysiol Suppl. 1999;52:3–6.
4. Dieltjens M, et al. Remotely controlled mandibular positioning of oral appliance therapy during polysomnography and drug-induced sleep endoscopy compared with conventional subjective titration in patients with obstructive sleep apnea: protocol for a randomized crossover trial. Trials. 2019;20(1):615.
5. Zancanella E, et al. Home sleep apnea testing: an accuracy study. Sleep Breath. 2021.
6. Pinheiro GDL, et al. Validation of an overnight wireless high-resolution oximeter plus cloud-based algorithm for the diagnosis of obstructive sleep apnea. Clinics (Sao Paulo). 2020;75:e2414.
7. Carskadon MA, et al. Guidelines for the multiple sleep latency test (MSLT): a standard measure of sleepiness. Sleep. 1986;9(4):519–24.
8. Littner MR, et al. Practice parameters for clinical use of the multiple sleep latency test and the maintenance of wakefulness test. Sleep. 2005;28(1):113–21.
9. Mitler MM, Gujavarty KS, Browman CP. Maintenance of wakefulness test: a polysomnographic technique for evaluation treatment efficacy in patients with excessive somnolence. Electroencephalogr Clin Neurophysiol. 1982;53(6):658–61.
10. (AASM), A.A.o.S.M. International classification of sleep disorders (ICSD-3). 3rd ed. Darien: American Academy of Sleep Medicine; 2014.
11. Malhotra RK. Evaluating the sleepy and sleepless patient. Continuum (Minneap Minn). 2020;26(4):871–89.
12. Carskadon MA, Dement WC. Monitoring and staging human sleep. In: Kryger MH, Roth T, Dement WC, editors. Principles and practice of sleep medicine. 5th ed. St. Louis: Elsevier Saunders; 2011.
13. Boeve FB. Chapter 27 - Sleep issues in dementia. In: Miller BL, editor. The behavioral neurology of dementia. University of California, San Francisco: Cambridge University Press. p. 446–69; 2016.

Actigraphy

Mario A. Leocadio-Miguel and John Fontenele-Araújo

It seems a new idea to predict a person's sleep health status based on the information of a simple wrist-worn device, like an ordinary wristwatch but equipped with multiple sensors, almost infinite memory, and state-of-the-art artificial intelligence (Fig. 1). However, this idea is far from being new. The desire to study someone's sleep in ordinary life, outside the domains and restrictions of a sleep laboratory, arose in the mid-1970s and that is the origin of actigraphy, the graphic representation of locomotor activity as a function of time. Actigraphy is being developed by the joint efforts of reasonably distinct science fields, including chronobiology, sports, and locomotor sciences, and, of course, sleep science. In the last decades, actigraphy has benefited from impressive technological advances in terms of sensors, battery, and memory constraints, allowing researchers and clinicians to explore this tool in sleep health research and sleep medicine. This chapter is dedicated to cover the basic science behind actigraphy, its main methods, its application in sleep medicine, as well as to present actigraphy as an already applied and promising tool to support physical therapy and rehabilitation practices.

M. A. Leocadio-Miguel (✉)
Department of Physiology and Behavior, Postgraduate Course on Psychobiology, Federal University of Rio Grande do Norte, Natal, Rio Grande do Norte, Brazil; Brazilian Sleep Society, Natal, Rio Grande do Norte, Brazil

J. Fontenele-Araújo
Department of Physiology and Behavior, Postgraduate Course on Psychobiology, Federal University of Rio Grande do Norte, Natal, Rio Grande do Norte, Brazil

C. Frange, F. M. S. Coelho (eds.), *Sleep Medicine and Physical Therapy*, https://doi.org/10.1007/978-3-030-85074-6_37

proposal by Gonçalves et al., we can even access, through non-parametric analysis of the rest-activity rhythm, indicators of the circadian and homeostatic components that control the sleep-wake cycle, measuring the stability of the rhythm over the days (interdaily stability) and the degree of fragmentation throughout the day (intradaily variation), respectively [5].

2 Actigraphy in the Assessment of Sleep

In parallel with the advances in the determination of the parameters of the rest-activity rhythm by actigraphy, the analysis of sleep through actimetry has undergone a succession of significant advances. Through the polysomnographic examination (PSG), it is possible to objectively determine sleep variables, such as sleep duration, markers of the sleep onset, sleep offset, sleep latency, number of nocturnal awakenings, time awake after sleep has started (WASO), sleep efficiency and total time in bed, besides, of course, the determination of the alternating phases during a sleep episode, culminating in the construction of the hypnogram [6]. To accomplish this goal, PSG requires the processing of multiple signals, both electrical (e.g., EEG) and mechanical (e.g., breathing), which provide enough information to help the analysis carried out by a trained and certified professional. However, the PSG is free of problems, especially since it is commonly performed outside the patient's home (in the sleep laboratory); it generates relative discomfort due to the number of elements connected to the patient during data collection, the high cost, and the need for trained and certified professionals. It is in this scenario that the original proposal of actigraphy is inserted, offering itself as a low-cost alternative, less cumbersome than PSG, with the ability to collect multiple days and nights in the individual's real sleep scenario, being essential for both long-term monitoring of patients and the screening of large groups of people [7].

However, can we measure and extract sleep variables using actigraphy? This is a question that has guided the efforts of different research groups. Partially based on the excellent performance of specialists in the visual analysis of the PSG traces, which demonstrates the capacity of our nervous system to recognize visual patterns, Kripke and collaborators described, still in 1978, that the actigraphy would be able to estimate, with agreement close to 90% with polysomnography, total sleep time, waking time after the sleep episode started, sleep onset, and, to a lesser degree, sleep latency [8]. However, despite enough performance, the analysis of the actigraphy data moved toward the automation of the processes, looking for cost reduction, velocity, and, fundamentally, an increase in the reproducibility capacity. In this sense, it was developed, in 1982, the first algorithm for automatic analysis of actigraphy, already with excellent results. This simple algorithm was based on the assessment, on a minute basis, of the degree of locomotor activity, and the determination of sleep or wakefulness for each minute was dependent on the measurement of the minutes around that given point, using a linear combination [9]. Multiple algorithms have been developed in the last decades, specially designed to validate actigraphy against PSG for distinct populations, from young adults (91% agreement with PSG) to postmenopausal women (85% agreement with PSG) [10].

Even with all the described advantages of actigraphy over polysomnography, the need for multiple channels of PSG signals makes clear the complexity, or rather, the difficulty of estimating the characteristics of human sleep. Therefore, considering the relative simplicity of actigraphy, it is expected that there are limitations to its performance. It has been achieved a consensus that actigraphy has high accuracy and high sensitivity, that is, it is perfect for the correct identification of the presence of sleep. However, despite the efforts of different research groups and their algorithms, actigraphy has low specificity, that is, there is a difficulty in identifying epochs of wakefulness during sleep [11]. This represents the difficulty in differentiating rest with relative immobility and a real episode of sleep. Therefore, there is a tendency for an overestimation of total sleep time and an underestimation of wake time after the start of the sleep episode (WASO), in addition to a clear difficulty in identifying the sleep onset, especially in the presence of increased sleep latency, as commonly observed in insomnia patients. Outside the sleep laboratory, there is still a difficulty in specifying the exact interval in which the individual is in bed, something essential for calculating sleep latency and sleep efficiency (ratio between total sleep time and time total in bed). For this purpose, different algorithms use additional information, such as an input from the patient himself, through an event button, indicating going to and leaving the bed, as well as additional signal channels, such as the light exposure channel [12]. A final limitation, so far not overcome, is the inability to estimate sleep stages through actigraphy, despite the efforts of different research groups [13]. By far, from the technical point of view, we should highlight the effort of Ancoli-Israel and collaborators, acting as a board of specialists from the Society of Behavioral Sleep Medicine (SBSM) of the United States of America, that developed the most comprehensive guide to actigraphy monitoring, for both the clinical and the research applications [7].

3 Actigraphy in the Monitoring of Sleep Disorders

Considering the advantages and disadvantages of actigraphy, especially in the view of the gold standard of polysomnography, how useful is actigraphy to help us in screening, diagnosing, and monitoring the treatment of sleep disorders? Actigraphy can be considered a consolidated tool in the sleep field. Actigraphy can provide consistent objective sleep data, as recently stated by the American Academy of Sleep Medicine task force [14].

Sadeh and collaborators were the precursors in demonstrating, back in 1989, the validation and clinical potential of actigraphy for sleep disorders, though making clear the methodological challenge of its application. Despite the success in the minute-by-minute comparison with polysomnography in healthy populations, in which the degree of agreement for identifying sleep and wakefulness was 90.2% for normal adults, 89.9% for children, clinical populations represent a real challenge:

78.2% of the agreement for patients with insomnia and 85.7% for patients with sleep apnea [15].

However, is actigraphy useful or recommended to assist researchers and clinicians to correctly identify, design a treatment, or perform follow-up evaluations to treat every sort of sleep disturbance? Here we summarize the use of actigraphy based on the established recommendations found in the literature.

Considering the characteristics of the actigraphic examination, this tool is absolutely recommended in the scenario of a rather specific class of sleep disorders known as sleep disorders linked to circadian rhythmicity. They primarily result from the phenomena of desynchronization or friction between the endogenous expression of an individual's biological rhythmicity and external synchronizing agents, such as the environmental light-dark cycle, or even by the imposition of an incompatible sleep phase with high quality, restful sleep, as in night shift situations [16]. We can include here the challenges of working schedules that involve alternating shifts and night work, resulting in the imposition of an unnatural time allocation on workers' sleep, resulting in superficial, non-restorative, fragmented sleep, incompatible with health [17]. Moreover, usually, night workers exhibit short sleep duration, presence of naps, and great variability in sleep episodes [18]. Importantly, not all subjects submitted to shift work develop a sleep disorder. However, for those with shift work disorder, the treatment aims to improve sleep quality and adjust the circadian rhythms. Actigraphy is recommended to assess the allocation of the sleep phase and to quantify the irregularity of the sleep-wake cycle. One possibility is also the determination of the light phase, as actigraphy devices also register the light exposition. Therefore, it is possible to assess whether the worker is sleeping in a lighted environment or not and, thereby, impairing the quality of his sleep. With the actigraphic data, both activity and light, it is possible to instruct the patients on good practices of sleep hygiene.

In this group of diseases, we can also include the advanced and delayed syndromes of the sleep-wake cycle, in which patients have extreme times of sleep onset and offset, conditions often overlapping or confused with insomnia (Fig. 3). Finally, it is important to highlight the presence of a non-24-hour sleep-wake disorder (Fig. 4), or free-running sleep cycle, resulting from the inability to synchronize with external synchronizers. In this condition, common in individuals with total blindness or lesions of the central nervous system, sleeping and waking times are irregular, commonly happening with a cumulative delay day after day [19]. Actigraphy plays a central role in its diagnosis and monitoring here, mainly because the gold standard for diagnosis and monitoring of sleep disorders, polysomnography, is not useful in these cases (Fig. 5). Therefore, through actigraphy it is possible to monitor multiple days, multiple episodes of sleep, and, at the same time, assess their synchronization situation, allowing the determination of the most common therapeutic approaches of treating these disorders, such as melatonin therapy or light therapy for example [20].

Affecting a significant proportion of the world's population, reaching values above 30% in prevalence, as the case of Sao Paulo, Brazil [21], insomnia is an

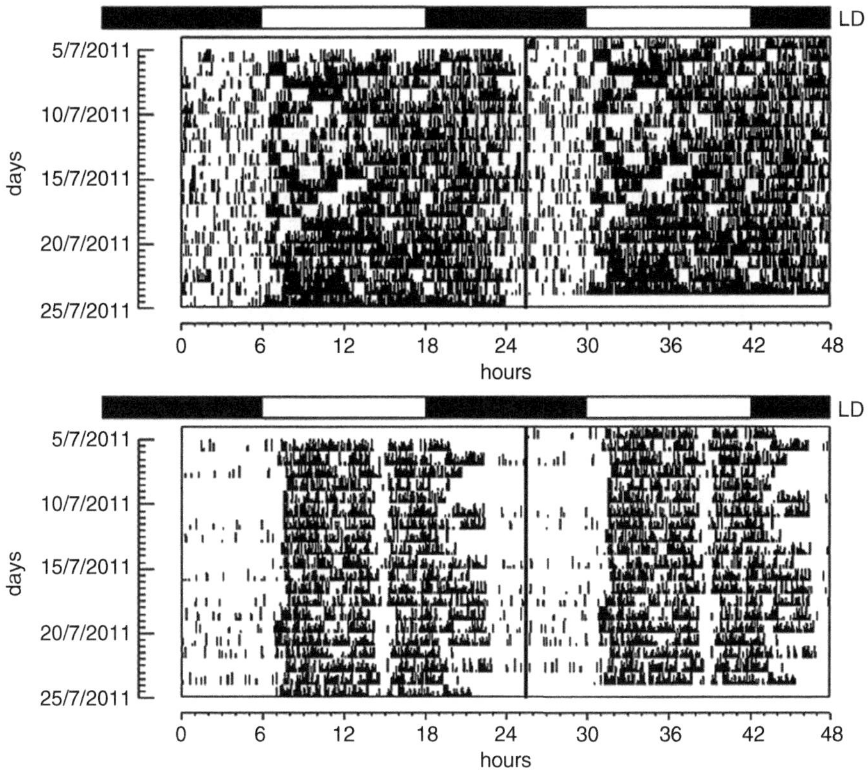

Fig. 3 Sleep-wake phase disorders. Upper actogram depicting a patient with delayed sleep phase disorder, highlighting late offset and onset of activity. Bottom actogram representative of a patient with advanced sleep phase disorder, highlighting daily long nap episodes. Created with El Temps software, using data from the authors (LNRB-UFRN). (Image courtesy from Dr. Mario A. Leocadio-Miguel and John Fontenele-Araújo. Original figure)

example of a condition that can benefit from actigraphy, especially since it provides continuous monitoring of the patient for multiple days in the natural, real scenario of occurrence of sleep, without the difficulties and artifacts arising from the laboratory polysomnographic examination [22]. Typically, patients with insomnia tend to overestimate their sleep latency, as well as to underestimate total sleep time, when compared to objective data from polysomnography, especially in sleep diary reports. Also, considering the high variability between nights, the collection of actigraphy data must be carried out as long as possible, with a duration of 1 week as a minimum recommendation [23].

Despite the controversy in the literature about the actual validation of actimetry for patients with insomnia, the adoption of this methodology is recommended for this type of sleep disorder. Williams and colleagues recently compared objective data of home polysomnography and actigraphy in insomnia patients, demonstrating that actigraphy can be considered a valid objective measure for measuring sleep monitoring sleep fragmentation and the presence of outbreaks of locomotor activity during sleep, which follows the potential multiple awakenings throughout the night in these patients [30]. Not by chance, monitoring the effectiveness of therapeutic measures, as in the case of the adoption of ventilatory support during sleep, is a possible use for actigraphy in patients with obstructive sleep apnea. Moreover, it is known that the addition of the actigraphic measure to cardiopulmonary sensors or apnea detectors is beneficial because it allows the study of sleep measures associated with ventilatory interruptions. After all, it provides a better analysis of the total sleep time and sleep efficiency [31].

Actigraphy also presents itself as an interesting tool in the pictures of periodic limb movement disorder (PLMD). The typical assessment of this condition involves the analysis of the surface electroneuromyography (EMG) of the anterior tibial muscle performed during polysomnography. However, considering periodic movement as an essential phenomenon of this disorder, actigraphy could be applied successfully. Importantly, there is a positive correlation between the amplitude of EMG of the anterior tibial muscle and the actigraphy, precisely regarding the number of movements per hour of sleep. Still, considering the high variability between nights in patients with PLMS, actigraphy is even more important, which includes its potential for monitoring the treatment of this condition [32].

Actigraphy is also fundamental in the assessment of total sleep time as a first step before the multiple sleep latency test (MSLT) in patients suspected of disorders of hypersomnolence, such as narcolepsy [33]. Importantly, actigraphy is an underestimated tool in clinics able to discriminate narcolepsy type 1 from primary insomnia [34]. Finally, actigraphy is essential in the assessment of daytime sleep, naps, and could reflect daytime somnolence in those suffering from hypersomnolence.

4 Actigraphy in the Context of Rehabilitation

Considering the fundamental role of actigraphy as a tool for measuring the amount of locomotor activity as a function of time, are we allowed to use actigraphy in the diagnosis and the follow-up of patients with secondary sleep disorders? The most direct answer is yes, particularly in conditions that compromise, either acutely or chronically, the motor function, although the particularities of the distinct motor phenotypes of the different disorders affect the generalization and efficiency of sleep detection algorithms [35].

One of the most well-known associations is between pain and sleep. It is a bidirectional relationship where poor sleep and increased pain positively feedback one another [36]. A clear example of this relationship is the recent report of postmenopausal women suffering from insomnia and chronic pain. Actigraphy was essential to disclose that sleep duration is a predictor of pain intensity in the following morning and that pain intensity at bedtime predicts both time in bed and sleep duration [37].

The use of accelerometry to monitor motor patterns, the amount of physical activity, and even the metabolic equivalent associated with energy expenditure is already established in the literature, including for patients with motor limitations [38]. Most studies in this area, however, use the actigraph in the hip region, which limits the ability to estimate total sleep time, sleep efficiency, and WASO, but could be overcome when the actigraph device is worn on the wrist [39]. However, actigraphy can provide measures of locomotor activity, an essential feature because multiple clinical conditions have a clear association with impairments in biological rhythms, especially regarding the sleep-wake cycle, highlighting the potential of this methodology beyond sleep medicine. An especially useful example for the rehabilitation field is the use of the total activity score, derived from the sum of locomotor activity over the 24 hours, that has successfully been used to monitor the evolution of patients with motor disorders, as in the case of stroke [40]. In a recent effort, Fleming and colleagues studied the relationship between the evolution of functional independence in patients with injuries in the central nervous system and the degree of sleep fragmentation measured through actigraphy. The authors demonstrated that the degree and speed of recovery in these patients can be predicted by sleep fragmentation [41]. The non-parametric analysis of actigraphy is also a powerful tool in the context of rehabilitation, and it has been shown that in patients with spinal cord injury, both the measurement of intraday variability (a proxy of sleep fragmentation) and the relative amplitude between the phases of maximum and minimal locomotor activity (wakefulness and sleep, respectively) are associated with poor sleep quality. Besides, the variable called interdaily stability (a proxy of synchronization of the sleep-wake cycle) is a predictor of pain in these patients [42].

5 Final Words

Multidisciplinary since its beginning, the limits of the usefulness of actigraphy are yet to be determined. However, it must be crystal clear that actigraphy is not meant to be a mere substitute for polysomnography, despite the relatively high agreement in some sleep variables. Rather, it must be considered as a broad-spectrum tool that may also be used as a supplement in sleep health. Actigraphy is mandatory in the assessment of sleep disorders related to circadian rhythmicity. Moreover, it is also highly recommended for differential diagnosis, especially for young patients with insomnia complaints and delayed syndrome of the sleep-wake cycle. Another interesting role of actigraphy is in sleep misperception (Fig. 6), in which the actogram can be adopted to clarify, directly to the patient, the pattern of the sleep-wake cycle. This approach is also useful for sleep education and as a follow-up tool in interventions. Finally, as a graphical representation of the motor output, actigraphy is being progressively more applied in the scenario of rehabilitation, ideally in patients recovering from neurological diseases or other pathologies compromising the movement expression and locomotion, usually displaying concurrent alterations of the sleep-wake cycle.

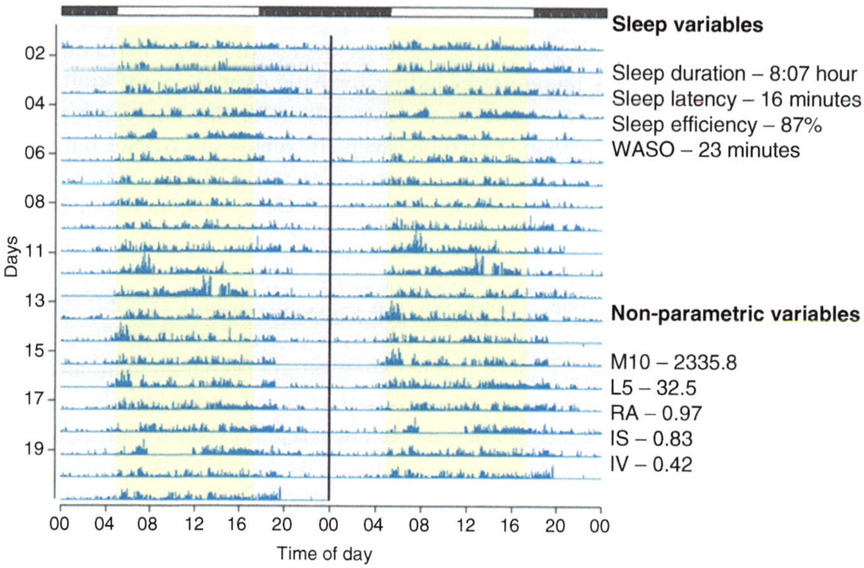

Fig. 6 Actogram of 21 days of actigraphy assessment of a patient with complaints of short sleep, but with an absence of diurnal sleepiness. Actigraphy revealed a regular 24-hour rest-activity rhythm, high levels of M10 (activity phase), and low level of activity during sleep (rest phase), with an estimated sleep duration of 7:30 hours, suggesting a sleep-wake cycle within a normal range. A patient diagnosed with sleep misperception. Actigraphy examination was essential as an explanation tool for the patient. Graphics created with ActStudio Software, using data from the authors (LNRB-UFRN). (Image courtesy from Dr. Mario A. Leocadio-Miguel and John Fontenele-Araújo. Original figure)

References

1. Foster FG, Kupfer D, Weiss G, Lipponen V, McPartland R, Delgado J. Mobility recording and cycle research in neuropsychiatry. J Interdiscipl Cycle Res. 1972;3:61–72.
2. Nelson W, Tong YL, Lee JK, Halberg F. Methods for cosinor-rhythmometry. Chronobiologia. 1979;6:305–23.
3. Refinetti R, Cornlissen G, Halberg F. Procedures for numerical analysis of circadian rhythms. Biol Rhythm Res. 2007;38:275–325.
4. van Someren EJ, Hagebeuk EE, Lijzenga C, Scheltens P, de Rooij SE, Jonker C, Pot AM, Mirmiran M, Swaab DF. Circadian rest-activity rhythm disturbances in Alzheimer's disease. Biol Psychiatry. 1996;40:259–70.
5. Gonçalves BSB, Adamowicz T, Louzada FM, Moreno CR, Araujo JF. A fresh look at the use of nonparametric analysis in actimetry. Sleep Med Rev. 2015;20:84–91.
6. Berry RB, Brooks R, Gamaldo C, Harding SM, Lloyd RM, Quan SF, Troester MT, Vaughn BV. AASM scoring manual updates for 2017 (version 2.4). J Clin Sleep Med. 2017;13:665–6.
7. Ancoli-Israel S, Martin JL, Blackwell T, Buenaver L, Liu L, Meltzer LJ, Sadeh A, Spira AP, Taylor DJ. The SBSM guide to actigraphy monitoring: clinical and research applications. Behav Sleep Med. 2015;13(Suppl 1):S4–S38.
8. Kripke DF, Mullaney DJ, Atkinson M, Wolf S. Circadian rhythm disorders in manic-depressives. Biol Psychiatry. 1978;13:335–51.

9. Webster JB, Kripke DF, Messin S, Mullaney DJ, Wyborney G. An activity-based sleep monitor system for ambulatory use. Sleep. 1982;5:389–99.
10. Jean-Louis G, Kripke DF, Cole RJ, Assmus JD, Langer RD. Sleep detection with an accelerometer actigraph: comparisons with polysomnography. Physiol Behav. 2001;72:21–8.
11. Boe AJ, McGee Koch LL, O'Brien MK, Shawen N, Rogers JA, Lieber RL, Reid KJ, Zee PC, Jayaraman A. Automating sleep stage classification using wireless, wearable sensors. NPJ Digit Med. 2019;2:131.
12. Fekedulegn D, Andrew ME, Shi M, Violanti JM, Knox S, Innes KE. Actigraphy-based assessment of sleep parameters. Ann Work Expo Health. 2020;64:350–67.
13. Winnebeck EC, Fischer D, Leise T, Roenneberg T. Dynamics and Ultradian structure of human sleep in real life. Curr Biol. 2018;28:49–59.e5.
14. Smith MT, McCrae CS, Cheung J, Martin JL, Harrod CG, Heald JL, Carden KA. Use of actigraphy for the evaluation of sleep disorders and circadian rhythm sleep-wake disorders: an American Academy of Sleep Medicine systematic review, meta-analysis, and GRADE assessment. J Clin Sleep Med. 2018;14:1209–30.
15. Sadeh A, Alster J, Urbach D, Lavie P. Actigraphically based automatic bedtime sleep-wake scoring: validity and clinical applications. J Ambulatory Monitoring. 1989;2:209–16.
16. Sack RL, Auckley D, Auger RR, Carskadon MA, Wright KP, Vitiello MV, Zhdanova IV. Circadian rhythm sleep disorders: part I, basic principles, shift work and jet lag disorders. Sleep. 2007;30:1460–83.
17. Moreno CR de C, Louzada FM. What happens to the body when one works at night? Cad Saude Publica. 2004;20:1739–45.
18. Reid KJ, Weng J, Ramos AR, Zee PC, Daviglus M, Mossavar-Rahmani Y, Sotres-Alvarez D, Gallo LC, Chirinos DA, Patel SR. Impact of shift work schedules on actigraphy-based measures of sleep in Hispanic workers: results from the Hispanic Community Health Study/Study of Latinos ancillary Sueño study. Sleep. 2018; https://doi.org/10.1093/sleep/zsy131.
19. Skene DJ, Arendt J. Circadian rhythm sleep disorders in the blind and their treatment with melatonin. Sleep Med. 2007;8:651–5.
20. Mitolo M, Tonon C, La Morgia C, Testa C, Carelli V, Lodi R. Effects of light treatment on sleep, cognition, mood, and behavior in Alzheimer's disease: a systematic review. Dement Geriatr Cogn Disord. 2018;46:371–84.
21. Castro LS, Poyares D, Leger D, Bittencourt L, Tufik S. Objective prevalence of insomnia in the São Paulo, Brazil epidemiologic sleep study. Ann Neurol. 2013;74:537–46.
22. Lichstein KL, Stone KC, Donaldson J, Nau SD, Soeffing JP, Murray D, Lester KW, Aguillard RN. Actigraphy validation with insomnia. Sleep. 2006;29:232–9.
23. Natale V, Plazzi G, Martoni M. Actigraphy in the assessment of insomnia: a quantitative approach. Sleep. 2009;32:767–71.
24. Williams JM, Taylor DJ, Slavish DC, Gardner CE, Zimmerman MR, Patel K, Reichenberger DA, Francetich JM, Dietch JR, Estevez R. Validity of actigraphy in young adults with insomnia. Behav Sleep Med. 2020;18:91–106.
25. Auger RR, Burgess HJ, Emens JS, Deriy LV, Thomas SM, Sharkey KM. Clinical practice guideline for the treatment of intrinsic circadian rhythm sleep-wake disorders: advanced sleep-wake phase disorder (ASWPD), delayed sleep-wake phase disorder (DSWPD), non-24-hour sleep-wake rhythm disorder (N24SWD), and irregular sleep-wake rhythm disorder (ISWRD). An update for 2015: an American Academy of Sleep Medicine clinical practice guideline. J Clin Sleep Med. 2015;11:1199–236.
26. Harvey AG, Tang NKY. (Mis)perception of sleep in insomnia: a puzzle and a resolution. Psychol Bull. 2012;138:77–101.
27. Te Lindert BHW, Blanken TF, van der Meijden WP, Dekker K, Wassing R, van der Werf YD, Ramautar JR, Van Someren EJW. Actigraphic multi-night home-recorded sleep estimates reveal three types of sleep misperception in Insomnia Disorder and good sleepers. J Sleep Res. 2020;29:e12937.

Index

C. Frange, F. M. S. Coelho (eds.), *Sleep Medicine and Physical Therapy*,
https://doi.org/10.1007/978-3-030-85074-6

R

S